Canadian Perspectives
on Advanced Practice Nursing

Canadian Perspectives
on Advanced Practice Nursing

Edited by

Eric Staples, Susan L. Ray, and Ruth A. Hannon

Canadian Scholars' Press
Toronto

Canadian Perspectives on Advanced Practice Nursing
Edited by Eric Staples, Susan L. Ray, and Ruth A. Hannon

First published in 2016 by
Canadian Scholars' Press Inc.
425 Adelaide Street West, Suite 200
Toronto, Ontario
M5V 3C1
www.cspi.org

Library and Archives Canada Cataloguing in Publication

Canadian perspectives on advanced practice nursing
/ edited by Eric Staples, Susan L. Ray, and Ruth A. Hannon.

Includes bibliographical references and index.
Issued in print and electronic formats.
ISBN 978-1-55130-909-5 (paperback).—ISBN 978-1-55130-910-1 (pdf).—
ISBN 978-1-55130-911-8 (ebook)

    1. Nursing—Canada—Textbooks. 2. Nursing—Study and teaching (Graduate)—Canada.
I. Ray, Susan L. (Susan Lynn), 1950–, editor II. Staples, Eric, editor III. Hannon, Ruth A., editor

RT41.C36 2016   610.730971   C2016-903457-7   C2016-903458-5

Text design by Susan MacGregor/Digital Zone
Cover design by Gord Robertson
Cover image by Serg Myshkovsky

16 17 18 19 20   5 4 3 2 1

Printed and bound in Canada by Webcom.

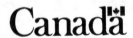

MIX
Paper from
responsible sources
FSC® C004071

This book is dedicated to the memory of a close friend and colleague, Dr. Susan L. Ray, who unfortunately left us before seeing the dream of a Canadian APN textbook become a reality.

Table of Contents

Foreword

Canadian nurses, the Canadian Nurses Association (CNA), provincial nursing organizations, and others have been advancing the importance of advanced practice nurses (APNs) for decades. The evolution has been slow and efforts have been made by too many to list. Today's reality of clinical nurse specialists (CNSs), nurse practitioners (NPs), and multiple specialties speak to the success of the commitment and efforts of both Canadian nursing organizations generally, and the Canadian nursing community at large.

This book is another historical step in these efforts. *Canadian Perspectives on Advanced Practice Nursing* is the first Canadian book on APN and will benefit registered nurses (RNs) in APN roles, university APN programs, policy- and decision-makers, professional nursing organizations, and leaders in health care. Furthermore, as communities consider building stronger health care services, this book will be a great resource for them. This text should also be considered in the context of the different roles that need to be played by clinicians, leaders, researchers, and educators, as well as associations and advocacy groups, nationally and internationally, to move from idea to reality. While realizing that it can take decades to bring an idea to fruition, we also need to acknowledge that while we have made tremendous strides, our work in the arena of APNs is not yet done.

As the 27th president of the International Council of Nurses (ICN), and only the second Canadian to hold this extremely important position, I am privileged to see both the global reality and the needs on the ground from this position. Much of the global agenda for the next couple of decades will continue to focus on primary health care, universal health coverage, non-communicable diseases, emerging and existing infectious diseases, and maternal child health. Outside of health care, we will continue to focus on poverty, economic stability, education, housing, and more. Health and social determinants factors are all essential elements to build healthy people, healthy communities, healthy nations, and healthy global communities.

APNs are the solution to many global health care challenges and agendas. APNs, as you will see from the various chapters in this book, provide a broad base of care from mental to community health, and acute care and beyond. In spite of the extensive contribution that APNs can make to health, there isn't sufficient appreciation of and investment in these important roles.

Over the last few decades, ICN has recognized the need to have a global nursing voice and shared agreement among the nursing community to articulate the elements associated with the APN role. The ICN has established a formal network of advanced practice nurses, which can be found at the following URL: www.icn-apnetwork.org.

The International Council of Nurses (ICN) defines the role of an APN as follows:

> A nurse practitioner/advanced practice nurse is a registered nurse who has acquired the expert knowledge base, complex decision-making skills and clinical competencies for expanded practice, the characteristics of which are shaped by the context and/or country in which s/he is credentialed to practice. A Master's degree is recommended for entry level. (2008)

The roles of APNs have been in existence globally (and under discussion in many countries) for several decades. While developed countries such as Canada and others have made progress in introducing these roles through legislation, regulation, and education, in many countries the roles of APNs have not been formalized. Overall, the roles of APNs have not yet been developed to the level that the nursing community thinks will best serve global health and the citizens of the world.

Furthermore, in my international engagement, I see great need for APNs. I also see interest and some progress in introducing the role. The evidence to date has clearly demonstrated the safety, value, and impact of the APN role, but closing the "knowledge" and "policy" gap is not so easy.

In Canada, we need to recognize and celebrate that a book like this is relevant and possible because of what we have accomplished through having legislation, regulations, licensing, and educational programs to prepare individuals that have a clear scope and authority to practice the roles that the public requires.

This book, as well as getting to this stage of APNs in Canada, should be a policy primer. I would suggest that both future APNs and policy-makers will benefit from becoming familiar with the role of the CNA and various provincial governments and nursing associations in making this dream a reality. We also need to acknowledge the tremendous contribution of Canadian research that provided the evidence for the APN role and its impact.

Canadian Perspectives on Advanced Practice Nursing should be on the desk of every health funding and system decision-maker, as the book demonstrates the richness of the work that has been and can be carried out by APNs across the country. Furthermore, this book is testimony to how to manage costs, and social and clinical challenges. Canada has been falling behind some of the Organisation for Economic Co-operation and Development (OECD) countries on some health indicators; a broad introduction of NPs, coupled with some policy decisions, can turn the tide around and put us on top of the list of the healthiest, most socially responsible, and economically vibrant societies.

Canadians, along with the global community, are watching with great interest the continued role and positions that APNs play in the Canadian health care tapestry. I am often asked about how we were able to achieve what we have now, and what can be learned from the Canadian experience. This book will be a great addition to the research, policy papers, and other Canadian documents to tell the story.

Finally, I would be remiss if I did not mention the role of Dr. Susan L. Ray, who passed away far too early in her very productive life. Susan and Dr. Eric Staples recognized the importance of having a Canadian text dedicated to the APN agenda and took on the challenge of producing this important book. With Susan's early passing while the book was in its development phase, Eric continued to embrace the project and charged full steam ahead. Later in the process, Ruth Hannon, NP–PHC and Teaching Professor at McMaster University, was brought on board to support this vision. Nursing is a community with a shared vision and acts on what needs to be done. Susan, Eric, Ruth, and all the other contributors are great examples that demonstrate the spirit of Canada.

Judith Shamian
President, International Council of Nurses (ICN)

Contributors

Michelle Acorn, DNP, NP–PHC/Adult, MN/ACNP, ENC(C), GNC(C)
APN Professional Practice Leader
Lakeridge Health, Whitby, ON
Lecturer and Primary Health Care/Global Health NP Program Coordinator
Lawrence S. Bloomberg Faculty of Nursing
University of Toronto, Toronto, ON

Cynthia Baker, RN, PhD
Executive Director
Canadian Association of Schools of Nursing (CASN), Ottawa, ON
Professor Emerita
Queen's University, Kingston, ON

Marilyn Ballantyne, RN(EC), PhD
Chief Nurse Executive & Clinician Investigator
Holland Bloorview Kids Rehabilitation Hospital, Toronto, ON
Adjunct Professor, Lawrence S. Bloomberg Faculty of Nursing
University of Toronto, Toronto, ON

Marcia Carr, RN, BN, MS, GNC(C), NCA
CNS–Medicine Clinical Service Network
Fraser Health Authority, Delta, BC

Kristina Chapman, RN, MN, NP
NP–Pediatrics, Hematology/Oncology
IWK Health Centre, Halifax, NS

Dana Edge, RN, PhD
Associate Professor, School of Nursing
Queen's University, Kingston, ON

Cheryl Forchuk, RN, PhD
Distinguished Professor and Associate Director of Nursing Research
Arthur Labatt Family School of Nursing
Scientist and Assistant Director, Lawson Health Research Institute

Professor, Department of Psychiatry
Schulich Medicine & Dentistry
Western University, London, ON
Associate Clinical Professor, School of Nursing
McMaster University, Hamilton, ON

Doris Grinspun, RN, MSN, PhD, LLD(hon), O.ONT
Chief Executive Officer
Registered Nurses' Association of Ontario (RNAO), Toronto, ON

Ruth A. Hannon, NP–PHC, MHA, MSFNP-BC, DNP(c)
Teaching Professor, School of Nursing
McMaster University, Hamilton, ON

Roberta Heale, RN(EC), PHCNP, DNP, PhD(c)
Associate Professor, School of Nursing
Laurentian University, Sudbury, ON

Kathleen F. Hunter, PhD, RN, NP–GNC(C), NCA
Associate Professor & Coordinator—MN Entry to Practice as an NP Program
Faculty of Nursing
Assistant Adjunct Professor, Division of Geriatric Medicine
University of Alberta, Edmonton, AB
Nurse Practitioner-Specialized Geriatric Services
Glenrose Hospital, Edmonton, AB

Laura Johnson, RN, MN, NP, DNP
Professor, BScN Program
Faculty of Health & Human Services
Vancouver Island University, Victoria, BC

Jane MacDonald, RN, MN, NP
Winnipeg Regional Health Authority
Winnipeg, MB

Mary-Lou Martin, RN, MScN, MEd
CNS–Mental Health, Forensic Program
St. Joseph's Healthcare, Hamilton, ON
Associate Clinical Professor, School of Nursing
McMaster University, Hamilton, ON

Mary McAllister, RN, PhD
Associate Chief, Nursing Practice
The Hospital for Sick Children, Toronto, ON

Patricia A. McQuinn, RN, MScN, CHPCC(C)
Clinical Nurse Specialist–Palliative Care
Extra-Mural Program
Horizon Regional Health Authority, Moncton, NB

Gloria McInnis-Perry, RN, PhD
Associate Professor, School of Nursing
University of Prince Edward Island, Charlottetown, PE

Lynn Miller, DNP, NP
Policy Consultant–Policy, Practice, and Legislative Services
College of Registered Nurses of Nova Scotia (CRNNS), Halifax, NS

Josephine Muxlow, RN, MS
Clinical Nurse Specialist–Adult Mental Health
Professional Practice Directorate
First Nations & Inuit Health Branch, Atlantic Region, Halifax, NS
Adjunct Professor, School of Nursing
Dalhousie University, Halifax, NS

Carole Orchard, RN, EdD
Professor, Arthur Labatt Family School of Nursing
Coordinator, Interprofessional Health Education and Research Office
Western University, London, ON

Tammy O'Rourke, RN, PhD, NP
Assistant Professor, School of Nursing
University of Alberta, Edmonton, AB

Monica Parry, NP–Adult, MEd, MSc, PhD, CCN(C)
Assistant Professor and Director, Nurse Practitioner Programs
Lawrence S. Bloomberg Faculty of Nursing
University of Toronto, Toronto, ON

Joanna Pierazzo, RN, PhD
Assistant Professor and BScN Curriculum Chair, School of Nursing
McMaster University, Hamilton, ON

Jennifer Price, RN, BNSc, MScN, ACNP, CCN(C), PhD
APN–Women's Cardiovascular Health Initiative
Women's College Hospital, Toronto, ON

Susan L. Ray, RN, CNS/APN, PhD (deceased)
Associate Professor/Associate Scientist, Arthur Labatt Family School of Nursing
Western University, London, ON

Josette Roussel, RN, MSc, M. Ed. l, inf. aut., M. Sc., M. Ed.
Senior Nurse Advisor
Policy, Advocacy and Strategy
Canadian Nurses Association, Ottawa, ON

Esther Sangster-Gormley, PhD, RN, ARNP (Florida, US)
Associate Professor and Nurse Practitioner Program Coordinator, School of Nursing
University of Victoria, Victoria, BC

Judith Shamian, RN, PhD, D.Sc, (Hon), LLD (Hon), FAAN
President–International Council of Nurses (ICN), Geneva, Switzerland

Eric Staples, RN, BAA(N), MSc, ACNP (cert.), DNP
Independent Nursing Practice Consultant, Ancaster, ON

Amanda Symington, RN(EC), BSc, BScN, MHSc
Nurse Practitioner–Pediatrics, Neonatal Intensive Care Unit
McMaster Children's Hospital, Hamilton, ON
Assistant Clinical Professor, School of Nursing
McMaster University, Hamilton, ON

Bernadine Wallis, RN, BN, MEd
Instructor
College of Nursing
University of Manitoba, Winnipeg, MB

Margaret (Marnee) Wilson, MSc(N), CDE, NP–Adult
NP–Adult and Professional Practice Leader for NPs & NP Cardiovascular Surgery
St. Michael's Hospital, Toronto, ON
Adjunct Lecturer, Lawrence Bloomberg Faculty of Nursing
University of Toronto, Toronto, ON

Rosemary Wilson, RN(EC), PhD
Assistant Professor
School of Nursing & Department of Anesthesiology and Perioperative Medicine
Queen's University, Kingston, ON

Preface

This textbook came about in response to a question asked by a Western University advanced practice nursing (APN) student. Dr. Susan L. Ray was professor of an elective course, *Issues in Advanced Nursing Practice*, and Dr. Eric Staples had been invited as a guest speaker on the role of nurse practitioners (NPs) in Canada. At the end of the class, a student enquired about the lack of an advanced nursing textbook in Canada.

This question lit the spark that ultimately led to this publication, as faculty (particularly Susan and Eric) realized that there was a reliance upon American APN textbooks that did not represent the context of APN education and practice in Canada.

There is a wealth of knowledge about APN in Canada and it has been said, for example, that NPs have been the most researched and scrutinized nursing group within the umbrella of APN. Yet, with all of the published reports, journal articles, and research data related to APN, there had never been a published textbook on APN from a uniquely Canadian perspective.

This textbook is intended for graduate nursing students, practicing APNs in all roles, educators, policy-makers, and leaders in nursing. Canada is a vast country; there are many similarities but also many differences across jurisdictions related to APN education, titling, title protection, integration, legislation, and regulation. The contributors to this textbook are from across the country and come from backgrounds in academia, practice, health policy, and professional nursing organizations, both provincially and nationally. They were chosen to represent and showcase the essential components of APN from distinctly Canadian perspectives. One of the main goals, unique to this textbook, was to provide practical application for faculty and students, in the form of case studies and critical thinking questions, of the essentials for APN roles and practice competencies relevant to any APN context across the country.

Please note that not every topic that may be related to APN could be covered in this first edition. There is a dearth of strong evidence relating to many areas of advanced practice, such as the use of informatics technology or outcomes measurement that includes the cost benefit of APNs. These oversights are due to significant variations in these measures across APN specialties, jurisdictions, workplace settings, role characteristics, and experience, but they point to a need for integration of technology into existing APN curricula. Topics related to vulnerable populations (including Aboriginal and immigrant health), ethical principles and decision-making, and professional negligence are not just relevant to APN. These considerations are well discussed by the nursing profession as a whole, and are taken into account in practice, as well as by the health care disciplines we collaborate with interprofessionally.

Some content and concepts pertaining to APN roles and topics may, at times, appear to be repetitive. Efforts were made to reduce repetition but some material was left as it provided context, informed, reinforced, or substantiated discussions across the chapters, and lent consistency in how the textbook progresses through Sections I to IV. Where there is repetition, the reader is reminded to go back to the original chapter where the topic can be read in greater detail.

Finally, some may feel that the textbook is Ontario-centric but the reality is that Ontario has the largest number of APNs in the country. The province has been an APN leader, contributing to the majority of publications related to APN. The challenge is for other provinces to "grow your own APNs" who will document the introduction, integration, and evaluation of APNs from each provincial and territorial context.

Best wishes to APNs, APN students, and educators who utilize this textbook as a Canadian resource in your professional library.

Eric Staples
Ruth A. Hannon

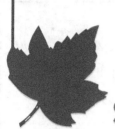

SECTION I

Historical and Developmental Overview of Advanced Practice Nursing in Canada

This section provides an overview of the evolutionary timeline of advanced practice nursing (APN) in a Canadian context, from early beginnings in outpost settings to the present day. Highlights of this section include the strides that have been made to develop and integrate the clinical nurse specialist (CNS) and nurse practitioner (NP) roles. Educational, regulatory, legal, and credentialing influences that have acted as facilitators and barriers to these two integral APN roles are discussed. The Canadian APN framework and other advanced practice frameworks utilized or developed in Canada are highlighted to illuminate the evolution of APN in this country.

Chapter 1

A Historical Overview of Advanced Practice Nursing in Canada

Eric Staples and Susan L. Ray

Eric Staples is an Independent Nursing Practice Consultant who previously worked as an APN. He has served as an Assistant Professor at Dalhousie University in Halifax, Nova Scotia, where he was involved in implementing the Advanced Nursing Practice stream in 1998; at McMaster University, where he worked as NP coordinator in the Ontario Primary Health Care Nurse Practitioner Program; and at the University of Regina. He has served on a number of Canadian Association of Schools of Nursing (CASN) committees related to NP education, preceptorship, prescribing, and the development of the position statement on doctoral education in Canada.

Susan L. Ray was an Associate Professor as well as an Associate Scientist at the Arthur Labatt Family School of Nursing at Western University in London, Ontario. Having completed the Tertiary Care NP certificate, she was a CNS–Mental Health in London, Ontario. Susan was a visionary for this textbook, but passed away after a short battle with cancer during the initial stages of development. Susan was a prolific researcher in many areas, including the impact of psychological trauma on contemporary peacekeepers, military personnel, veterans, and military families; PTSD and homeless veterans; male survivors of sexual abuse and incest; the immigrant/refugee population; and survivors of natural disasters. In 2014, Susan was co-editor of the Canadian edition of Varcarolis's *Canadian Psychiatric Mental Health Nursing*.

KEY TERMS

acute care nurse practitioner (ACNP)
advanced practice nursing (APN)
clinical nurse specialist (CNS)
nurse practitioner (NP)
primary health care nurse practitioner (PHCNP)

OBJECTIVES

1. Appraise the origins of advanced practice nursing (APN) in Canada.
2. Explore the development of the clinical nurse specialist (CNS) role.
3. Explore the development of nurse practitioner (NP) roles.

Introduction

In order to fully understand and appreciate APN in Canada, it is necessary to investigate the historical evolution of the roles that today define a level of nursing practice that utilizes extended and expanded clinical competencies, as well as experience and knowledge that include (but are not limited to) the assessment, diagnosis, planning, implementation, and evaluation of patient care. **Advanced practice nursing (APN)**, as defined by the Canadian Nurses Association (CNA), is

> an umbrella term describing an advanced level of clinical nursing practice that maximizes the use of graduate educational preparation, in-depth knowledge and expertise in meeting the health needs of individuals, families, groups, communities and populations. It involves analyzing and synthesizing knowledge; understanding, interpreting and applying nursing theory and research; and developing and advancing nursing knowledge and the profession as a whole. (2008, p. 10)

This chapter highlights the development of APN roles in Canada from early beginnings to the present day, and examines the CNS and NP roles in the context of the socio-political, educational, regulatory, legislative, and economic environments that have shaped them.

Early Beginnings of Advanced Practice Nursing

Nurses in expanded roles have safely accepted responsibilities traditionally taken by family and general practitioners in rural and remote areas of Canada for over 100 years (Hodgkin, 1977). The demand for nurses to work in these underserviced areas was a result of the chronic shortage of physicians in remote areas of Canada. They were known as outpost nurses and were introduced by religious organizations to improve primary health care services for underserviced populations (Kaasalainen et al., 2010; Kulig et al., 2003). The first formally trained nurses to work in Canada arrived from England as part of the Grenfell Mission in 1894 (Higgins, 2008; Kulig et al., 2003). Wilfred Grenfell, a British medical missionary, led the Grenfell Mission with the intent to provide the earliest medical services in Labrador and northern Newfoundland (Higgins, 2008). Before the Mission, essentially no health care resources or formally trained nurses existed in these remote rural areas. Demand for nurses to work in underserviced areas of Canada continued to grow following the Grenfell Mission, as nurses in expanded roles accepted responsibilities traditionally held by family and general practitioners (Hodgkin, 1977). These early beginnings of advanced practice nursing (APN) have been noted but largely remain unrecognized within the Canadian health care system (McTavish, 1979).

Evolution of the Clinical Nurse Specialist Role

In 1943, Reiter first introduced the term *nurse clinician* to describe nurses with advanced knowledge and clinical skills capable of providing a high level of patient care (Davies & Eng, 1995; Hamric, Spross, & Hanson, 2009; Montemuro, 1987). After World War II, the term *specialist* was one of the first used to describe what the clinical nurse specialist (CNS) is today.

In the aftermath of two world wars, the federal government encouraged the building of hospitals and by 1960 the majority of nurses (59%) worked in hospitals, compared with 25% in 1930 (Haines, 1993). Guided by this change in environment, current CNS practice grew to span the continuum of care from pediatric to adult, including long-term and acute care settings such as in-patient units, critical care units, and hospital-based clinics (Bryant-Lukosius et al., 2010; Mayo et al., 2010). CNSs now provide an advanced level of nursing practice through the integration of in-depth knowledge and skills as a clinician, educator, researcher, consultant, and leader (CNA, 2009a) in a variety of clinical specialties that include oncology (Ream et al., 2009), cardiology (Avery & Schnell-Hoehn, 2010), acute and critical care (Jenkins & Lindsey, 2010; Wetzel & Kalman, 2010), gerontology (Smith-Higuchi, Hagen, Brown & Zeiber, 2006), and mental health (Mayo et al., 2010). Three substantive areas of CNS practice, identified by Lewandowski and Adamle (2009), include the management and care of complex and vulnerable populations, the education and support of interdisciplinary staff, and the facilitation of change and innovation within health care systems.

In the 1960s, a shortage of skilled nurses and the increasing complexity in health care and technology became the driving force for the introduction of the CNS role into the Canadian health care system. The changes to modern health care following World Wars I and II generated a need for more advanced and specialized nurses with the knowledge and skills to support nursing practice at the bedside of patients (CNA, 2003; Kaasalainen et al., 2010).

By the 1970s, decentralization of political and administrative authority, consumer participation, a shift in emphasis to community-based care, and increased emphasis on health care outcomes combined with physician shortages, a trend toward specialization by physicians, and baccalaureate-level preparation for nurses had created an impetus to critically examine the scope of nursing practice (MacDonald, Herbert, & Thibeault, 2006). The University of Toronto introduced a master's degree program in nursing in 1970, and although it was not specifically designed to educate or produce CNSs the program focused on clinical specialization.

There has been a consensus in the literature that the minimum level of education required for CNS practice should be a master's degree (CNA, 2009a, 2009b; DiCenso et al., 2010b). This level of educational preparation has been found to influence the extent to which CNSs practice at an advanced level and how they implement their roles. For example, CNSs holding a master's degree can influence patient and population health, nursing practice, and health systems because they are more likely to implement a range of

role activities that are consistent with the national framework for advanced nursing practice. These activities include: caring for the most complex patients; working with specific
populations; working with staff, patients, and families to develop a plan of care; and policy
and program development. In contrast, clinical practice that is focused on the direct care of
individuals is the major concern of baccalaureate-prepared CNSs (Schreiber et al., 2005a).

By 1986, most practicing CNSs were prepared at a master's level (Montemuro, 1987).
Beaudoin, Besner, and Gaudreault (1978) argued that the CNS role was more in keeping
with nursing values than the **nurse practitioner** (NP) role, which they described as an
extension of medicine because of the medical role functions it incorporated. Stevens (1976)
agreed and added that the CNS role contributed vastly in attempts to not only professional-
ize nursing, but to substantiate its existence as an independent profession. However, there
are currently no mandatory credentials, educational requirements, nor title protection for
CNSs in Canada (Profetto-McGrath, Negrin, Hugo, & Smith, 2010).

The CNA released its first position statement on the CNS role in 1986, describing it as

> an expert practitioner who provides direct care to clients and serves as a role
> model and consultant to other practicing nurses. The nurse participates in
> research to improve the quality of nursing care and communicates and uses
> research findings. The practice of the clinical nurse specialist is based on
> in-depth knowledge of nursing and the behavioural and biological sciences.
> … A CNS is a registered nurse who holds a master's degree in nursing and has
> expertise in a clinical nursing specialty. (p. 1)

Following this report, Ontario and British Columbia released two provincial statements on
the CNS role. Both statements identified the major components of the CNS role as clinical
practice, education, research, consultation, and leadership/change agent. Over time, the
CNA has put forth many definitions of the CNS role (1978, 1986) but these components
of the CNS role remained constant throughout two subsequent iterations of CNA position
statements (CNA, 2003, 2009a).

In 1989, one of the most significant developments in advancing the CNS role across Canada
was the formation of a national interest group, initially called the Canadian Clinical Nurse
Specialist Interest Group (CCNSIG). Leaders within this group worked closely with CNSs
from other provinces to help develop their own provincial organizations, as well as organize
conferences to advance their professional practice. In 1991, CCNSIG became an associate group
of CNA. CCNSIG was renamed in 1998 to the Canadian Association of Advanced Practice
Nurses (CAAPN) for the purpose of including other types of APNs (Kaasalainen et al., 2010).

Unlike that of the NP, the CNS role has continued to formally exist over the last 40 years;
however, hospital budget cutbacks in the 1980s and 1990s led to the elimination of many of

these positions (DiCenso & Bryant-Lukosius, 2010). The development and implementation of the CNS role was often challenged by issues related to role ambiguity, lack of involvement or recognition in the organizational structure, and lack of administrative support (Davies & Eng, 1995; Montemuro, 1987).

In early 2000, interest in the CNS role returned, with the intent to bring clinical leadership back into health care environments. Emphasis on helping staff nurses apply evidence to practice was necessary, as this leadership was lacking due to reductions in executive and educator positions for nurses (Kaasalainen et al., 2010). Currently, the most significant challenges facing the CNS role in Canada include a lack of common vision and understanding of the CNS role, limited access to CNS-specific graduate education programs, and the continued lack of title protection or credentialing (DiCenso et al., 2010a).

Based on the Canadian Institute for Health Information (CIHI), there were about 2,227 CNSs in Canada in 2008, and the largest numbers of CNSs are found in British Columbia, Quebec, and Ontario (2010). However, the true number of CNSs is unknown because current CNS estimates are based on self-report and many of these individuals lack graduate education or specialty-based experience.

CNSs have played an important part in the delivery of advanced nursing services in Canada (Kaasalainen et al., 2010). In several Canadian studies, CNSs described how they promote evidence-based practice (Pepler et al., 2006), influence clinical and administrative decision-making (Profetto-McGrath, Smith, Hugo, Taylor, & El-Hajj, 2007), and integrate research, education, and leadership expertise to improve patient care at three levels: individual patients and nurses/health care providers, the clinical unit, and the organization (Schreiber et al., 2005a, 2005b).

However, their full integration into the health care system will require high-quality research evidence. To date, very little research has been conducted on CNSs in Canada (Bryant-Lukosius et al., 2010). Over the next decade, research will play a critical role in forecasting the evolution, needs-based deployment, and impact of the CNS role in Canada.

In recognition of the valuable contributions of the CNS role in Canada, the CNA (2014) published the *Pan-Canadian Core Competencies for the Clinical Nurse Specialist* framework, which defines core competencies for CNS practice. The purpose of the framework is to clarify the CNS role, demonstrate its contribution to health care, and facilitate role utilization. This framework provides the most up-to-date definition of the CNS role:

> The CNS is a registered nurse who holds a graduate degree in nursing and has a high level of expertise in a clinical specialty. Areas of specialization may focus on expertise related to a specific population, a practice setting, a disease or subspecialty, a type of care or a type of health problem. The CNS improves client, population and health system outcomes by integrating knowledge, skills

and expertise in clinical care, leadership, consultation, education and collaboration. . . . The CNS role can change in response to the dynamic needs of clients, nursing staff and practice settings, the changing strategic directions of the organization, and the economic and policy priorities of health care funders and ministries of health. Despite role variability, all CNS work is aimed at ensuring safety, quality of care, and positive health outcomes. (CNA, 2014, p. 1)

The framework may be of great value for CNSs, nurse researchers, regulators, and leaders in further defining, integrating, and evaluating the role's scope and influence across diverse practice settings in response to population health needs, and a changing practice and health care landscape.

Evolution of the Nurse Practitioner Role in Primary Health Care

The earliest **primary health care nurse practitioners (PHCNPs)** began practicing in northern Canada over 100 years ago as outpost nurses (Kaasalainen et al., 2010; Kulig et al., 2003).

In 1967, the first nursing education programs in Canada that began training midwives and outpost nurses were started at Dalhousie University in Halifax, Nova Scotia. By 1971, other NP programs had been developed at McMaster University in Hamilton, Ontario, and McGill University in Montreal, Quebec, that focused on preparing "family practice nurses" to work in urban settings. The University of British Columbia, as well as Memorial University in St. John's, Newfoundland, followed soon after with similar programs (Chambers & West, 1978). Six more universities—Alberta, Manitoba, Western Ontario, Toronto, McGill, and Sherbrooke—followed by 1972. The Kergin Report (1970) was highly influential in the development of curriculum for the new programs, which focused on preparing clinically trained nurses (CTNs) to practice in isolated settings (Hazlett, 1975).

In 1972, the Boudreau Report, commissioned by the Department of National Health and Welfare, was released by the Committee on Nurse Practitioners. The report strongly recommended that the implementation of the NP role be of the highest priority in meeting primary health care needs of Canadians. Based on this report, pilot and demonstration projects were initiated across Canada. The evaluation of these projects was favourable: 93% of NPs found employment, more time was reported being spent with patients, and NPs reported role satisfaction (Scherer, Fortin, Spitzer, & Kergin, 1977; Spitzer et al., 1973; Spitzer & Kergin, 1975). Chenoy, Spitzer, and Anderson (1973) found that patients supported nurses being involved in primary health care promotion activities, but in some situations still preferred a physician.

Research also supported the role of NPs in pediatric settings (McFarlane & Norman, 1972), outpatient clinics (King, Spaulding, & Wright, 1974; Ramsay, McKenzie, & Fish,

1982), and emergency settings (Vayda, Gent, & Paisley, 1973). However, in northern Newfoundland and Ontario, outpost nurses were still responsible for providing primary health care to communities in clinics that focused on preventative health and treating episodic illnesses (Dunn & Higgins, 1986). The evaluation of one pilot project of four NPs in rural Saskatchewan showed mixed results, with the conclusion that role implementation was dependent on specific community needs (Cardenas, 1975).

Two distinct streams of educational programs developed across the country; those continuing to prepare the outpost nurses that provided health services in remote areas of northern Canada, and those that focused on developing nurses with primary health care skills to work in family practices and community nursing settings (The Canadian Nurse, 1978). The length and educational level of these programs varied: outpost programs were typically two years in length at the post-diploma level, while NP programs were eight months in length at the post-baccalaureate level. Debate about educational requirements for NP practice was an issue during the early 1970s. There were several recommendations for baccalaureate education for NPs (Buzzell, 1976) and graduate education for CNSs (Boone & Kikuchi, 1977). A nation-wide consensus in the 1970s determined that additional education beyond a baccalaureate or diploma level was required to prepare nurses for NP roles (Donald et al., 2010). Collaborative practice became an essential expectation of the PHCNP role, and was integral to defining role functions. Arguments for increased standardization of NP education, however, continued to be debated up until the past decade, when graduate education for all APN roles was deemed necessary (Canadian Nurse Practitioner Initiative [CNPI], 2006a; Schreiber et al., 2005a, 2005b).

Family physicians were not initially interested in NP practice (Kilpatrick et al., 2010), but by 1973 the CNA and the Canadian Medical Association (CMA) released a joint statement on the role of the NP that signalled medical support and cooperation in revisiting the need for the NP role (Canadian Medical Association Journal, 1973). Several provincial nursing groups, as well as NPs, were prolific during this time and worked to legitimize expanded nursing roles (Cardenas, 1975). The Lalonde Report (1974) was instrumental in linking the concepts of primary health care and the influence of the determinants of health on societal health and well-being, with the impact of expanded RN roles in health promotion and disease prevention.

Despite these efforts, by the 1980s NP education program implementation ceased due to a perceived oversupply of physicians; weak support from medicine, nursing, and policy-makers; little public awareness; lack of funding; and a failure to develop regulation, legislation, and remuneration processes (CIHI, 2006). Although this initial attempt to implement NP roles failed, interest in an expanded role for RNs continued across Canada. NPs continued to work in several provinces (including Ontario and Saskatchewan) in urban community health centres, northern nursing stations, and First Nations communities. When a perceived undersupply of physicians and a shift to primary health care led to a renewal of the health care system in the 1990s, the role of the NP was again revisited.

Provincial nursing groups, including former graduates of ceased NP education programs, continued to lobby government for NPs legitimization. In the early 1990s, these groups were instrumental in creating new initiatives with the Ontario Ministry of Health and Long-Term Care (MOHLTC) as part of the government's primary health care reform strategy. This eventually resulted in the re-establishment of NP university education programs in 1995, and the Expanded Nursing Services for Patients Act was passed in 1998. This legislation gave NPs registered in the new, extended class with the College of Nurses of Ontario (CNO) the authority to practice within a broader scope by adding three controlled acts: communicating a diagnosis; prescribing a limited range of drugs; and ordering certain diagnostic tests, X-rays, and ultrasounds (NPAO, n.d.).

During the latter part of the 1990s into the early 2000s, federal and provincial government reports called for primary health care reform, and identified the unique role of nurses in improving timely access to health care delivery services (Kirby, 2002; Romanow, 2002). Reform efforts were fuelled by unprecedented federal and provincial investments in primary health care infrastructure and interdisciplinary health care teams, leading to a countrywide emphasis on enhancing health promotion and improving equitable health care access and quality (Hutchison, 2008). This context prompted the revival of governments' interest in the PHCNP role and initiated the second wave of PHCNP role implementation, supported by legislation, regulation, remuneration mechanisms, and funded education programs. Foundational to implementing the role was the abundant research that strongly demonstrated PHCNPs as effective, safe practitioners who positively influenced patient care, as well as provider and health system outcomes (Dierick-van Daele et al., 2010).

Many provinces introduced university-based education programs and legislation to support the renewal of PHCNPs, and improve access to primary care amidst the growing concerns about shortages of doctors and burgeoning interests in developing team-based approaches to health care delivery. In Ontario, the MOHLTC, in conjunction with the Council of Ontario University Programs in Nursing (COUPN), announced in 1994 a new NP initiative as part of a broader effort to improve access to primary care. This was supported by a newly funded, ten-university consortium education program in 1995 (CIHI, 2006; DiCenso et al., 2010b; NPAO, n.d.).

Other provinces and territories followed suit, with some developing programs at the post-diploma or post-baccalaureate level and others at the master's level (CNPI, 2006c). As of 2008, a master's degree from an approved graduate-level PHCNP program became the recommended educational standard, both in Canada and internationally (CNA, 2008; International Council of Nurses [ICN], 2008). By the end of 2014, all PHCNP programs across Canada were at the graduate and/or post-graduate level, with the newest NP program being a Collaborative Nurse Practitioner Program (CNPP) between the Schools of Nursing of the University of Regina and Saskatchewan Polytechnic, formerly the Saskatchewan Institute of Applied Science and Technology (SIAST) (Saskatchewan Collaborative Programs in Nursing, 2015).

Nursing leaders, realizing that a national, integrated approach was required for continued sustainability of the role, proposed the development of a Canadian APN framework. The CNPI, funded federally by Health Canada and sponsored by CNA, was instrumental in developing literature related directly to practice, education, legislation, implementation, and social marketing of the NP role across Canada (CNA, 2008). Accomplishments of this group included: the development, and later revision, of the *Canadian Nurse Practitioner Core Competency Framework* (CNA, 2010), which identified the core competencies required for all NPs in practice, regardless of individual clinical specialization; the Canadian Nurse Practitioner Examination (CNPE) (CNPI, 2006b); the Implementation and Evaluation Toolkit for Nurse Practitioners in Canada (CNPI, 2006a); and frameworks for practice, education, legislation, and regulation (CNPI, 2006c).

Prior to the CNPI, each provincial/territorial regulatory body had their own examination for licensing/credentialing of PHCNPs. In 2005, the CNA announced, in collaboration with all nursing regulatory bodies (with the exception of Quebec), the first national examination: the Canadian Nurse Practitioner Examination (CNPE). This also marked a change, led by the CNA, from care-based licensure/credentialing to a population-based focus that was called Family/All Ages.

Today, although there is not a national definition for the PHCNP role, it is understood that they provide primary health care services to individuals, groups, and families across their lifespan, and work in a variety of community-based settings (DiCenso, Paech, & IBM Corporation, 2003; DiCenso et al., 2007). The focus of their practice is health promotion, illness prevention, the diagnosis and treatment of episodic conditions and injuries, and monitoring and managing stable chronic conditions (DiCenso et al., 2003; Sidani, Irvine, & DiCenso, 2000; Way, Jones, Baskerville, & Busing, 2001). PHCNPs utilize an evidence-informed holistic approach that emphasizes health promotion and community partnership development, and practice complementarily with physicians rather than as a replacement.

Patient satisfaction with the PHCNP continues to be high. Heightened awareness of the NP role has made the Canadian public more comfortable with NPs, and most are willing to see an NP instead of their physician for health care needs (Harris/Decima, 2009). PHCNPs, now commonly referred as Family/All Ages NPs, are the fastest-growing advanced practice nursing role in Canada.

Evolution of the Nurse Practitioner Role in Acute/Tertiary Care

At the same time that PHCNP programs were being phased out in the 1980s, there was increasing interest in an advanced nursing practice role in acute/tertiary care settings. Government cutbacks in medical school funding had led to decreased numbers of medical residency positions. Compounded by an exodus of medical graduates to the United States, Canadian physicians were experiencing increased workloads in acute care settings. Health care administrators, medical directors, and nurses described a lack of continuity in patient care, leading to a growing concern regarding the rising acuity in acute/tertiary patients and the increasing complexity of care delivery. Additionally, in neonatal intensive care units (NICU) a concern for maintaining a high standard of new-born care in the face of these economic and workforce issues generated the development of a post-graduate diploma NP program at McMaster University in Hamilton, Ontario, in 1986 (Paes et al., 1989).

The role title that evolved from this program was that of the neonatal nurse practitioner (NNP). The introduction of the NNP in Ontario was based on a comprehensive assessment (DiCenso, 1998) that began with a needs assessment (Paes et al., 1989). Surveys were con-ducted to delineate the role (Hunsberger et al., 1992), evaluate the graduate-level education program that was developed (Mitchell et al., 1995), create a randomized controlled trial to evaluate the effectiveness of the role (Mitchell-DiCenso et al., 1996), and assess team satisfaction within the role (Mitchell-DiCenso, Pinelli, & Southwell, 1996). Around this time, the term *clinical nurse specialist* (CNS) was also attached to the NP title: CNS/NP. This was a deliberate action aimed to legitimize the non-clinical advanced practice role domains that included education, research, and leadership (DiCenso, 1998; Hunsberger et al., 1992).

The term **acute care nurse practitioner (ACNP)** was first coined in the United States to describe NPs working in critical care areas (Kleinpell, 1997). In Canada, the term was adopted in the mid-1990s for NPs working in specialty disciplines within acute care settings (Simpson, 1997). ACNPs, also known as *specialty* or *specialist NPs*, provide advanced nursing care for patients who are acutely, critically, or chronically ill with complex conditions (CNA, 2008).

The ACNP program at the University of Toronto began in 1993 and was the first NP program to offer post-graduate level education outside of neonatology (Simpson, 1997). Some provinces continue to offer generalist graduate ACNP programs, for example, in an adult-focused specialty discipline (CNA, 2008), where the knowledge and skills specific to the desired clinical specialty are obtained through both graduate education and preceptored clinical learning placements.

Neonatology, however, remains the most specialized acute care program in the English speaking provinces (Rutherford & Rutherford Consulting Group Inc., 2005). In Quebec, the ACNP was the first NP role formally introduced into the health care system and remains the most specialized acute care program (OIIQ, 2009). ACNPs in Quebec are authorized to practice only in the clinical specialty areas—such as neonatology, nephrology, cardiology, and primary care—in which they are prepared (Allard & Durand, 2006; OIIQ & CMQ, 2006) and specialty preparation and certification are required for using the title "specialized" (Bussières & Parent, 2004).

ACNP programs and roles were also developed and introduced in London, Ontario, at the University of Western Ontario and at the University of Calgary, Alberta. These programs focused on specialty areas within hospitals in response to the shortage of medical residents and lack of continuity of care for seriously ill patients (Pringle, 2007).

In contrast to the PHCNP programs, all ACNP educational programs were developed at the graduate or post-graduate level throughout Canada (Alcock, 1996; Faculté des sciences infirmières, Université de Montréal, 2008; Roschkov et al., 2007). The first wave of graduates from these programs specialized in neonatal ICU, cardiology/cardiovascular, oncology, gerontology, and nephrology. Kilpatrick et al. (2010) found that internal politics influenced the selection of these particular specialty areas over primary health care, specifically one specialist in the university teaching hospitals who was responsible for lobbying in support of educating ACNPs focused on these areas.

Canadian and international literature agrees on the components of the ACNP role (Almost & Laschinger, 2002; Royal College of Nursing, 2008; Sidani & Irvine, 1999). ACNP and CNS roles share core competencies with other types of advanced practice nursing roles, including direct patient care, research, education, consultation, and leadership activities (CNA, 2009b; Schreiber et al., 2005a). Studies have also demonstrated the effective and safe practice of ACNPs in a variety of clinical settings—emergency rooms, in-patient settings, NICU, outpatient clinics—based on a range of patient and health care system identified outcomes (e.g., patient health status, quality of care, patient or provider satisfaction, health system costs, length of stay). ACNPs contribute to the delivery of complex, patient-centred care and are capable of utilizing both pharmacological and non-pharmacological approaches (D'Amour et al., 2007). Additionally, ACNPs promote patient self-care abilities, improve symptom management, and increase patients' abilities to perform activities of daily living (Sidani, 2008; Sidani et al., 2006a). RNs, physicians, administrators, and ACNPs have all reported that the ACNP role has led to improvements in the continuity of care for acutely ill patients (van Soeren & Micevski, 2001).

Although ACNPs engage predominantly in direct patient care activities, diagnostic activities, care planning, and coordination (Sidani et al., 2000), balancing these patient-focused clinical activities are non-clinical activities that are generally performed with, or for the benefit of, nursing or other organization staff. In Quebec, it is recommended that 70% of ACNP practice constitutes direct clinical activities and 30% non-clinical activities such as leadership, education, and research (OIIQ & CMQ, 2006). Clearly identifying ACNP non-clinical activities are important because these activities distinguish this particular role's strong, combined clinical and leadership focus. It is this unique combination that enables ACNPs to contribute so effectively to the improvements of patient care quality, as well as health care provider and system outcomes (Irvine et al., 2000).

Many ACNPs, however, have difficulty integrating all of the domains of their advanced practice nursing role, given their patient care responsibilities (D'Amour et al., 2007). The struggle to balance direct clinical and non-clinical functions has created high, even unrealistic expectations of the ACNP role, and confusion with the similar role functions of the CNS. Griffiths (2006) highlighted the importance of clearly articulating and defining each role's purpose and scope of practice, since the overlap of role function may be significant between CNSs and ACNPs in the same medical discipline, given that they both have graduate-level education and share many care coordination functions (Sidani et al., 2006a, 2006b).

There is also a discrepancy between the expectations of administrators and the expectations of physicians in regards to the amount of time ACNPs spend on direct patient care activities. Physicians believe that the ACNPs' time should be devoted predominantly to direct clinical practice, whereas administrators have recognized the importance of protecting the time ACNPs spend engaging in leadership, education, and research aligned with their role because these activities supports nursing practice within the organization (Kilpatrick et al., 2010). This situation stems from neonatology, when CNS and NP roles were purposefully combined in order to distinguish and legitimize non-clinical nursing activities (DiCenso, 1998; Hunsberger et al., 1992).

The exploration of nursing administrators' roles and perspectives when introducing an ACNP role within the health care team by Reay, Golden-Biddle, and Germann (2006) found that nursing administrators faced three major challenges: task reallocation, management of altered working relationships, and management of the team in an evolving situation. Successful implementation of ACNPs into health care teams was reliant on administrators' abilities to clearly communicate ACNP role expectations (van Soeren & Micevski, 2001), provide a clear vision of the ACNP role to both ACNPs and team members, and support ACNP roles across the organization (Reay et al., 2006).

The development of detailed role descriptions (Cummings, Fraser, & Tarlier, 2003), with input from ACNPs (Nhan & Zuidema, 2007) and open dialogue between administrators and team members, promotes a greater understanding of the ACNP role (Wall, 2006) and helps to define clear expectations of the ACNP role (Rosenthal & Guerrasio, 2009). These strategies have increased job satisfaction and assisted the facilitation of ACNP integration into the health care team (Cummings, Fraser, & Tarlier, 2003).

Notoriously, physicians have had the final say on whether or not they will accept the implementation of an ACNP in their practice (D'Amour et al., 2007), directly affecting the ability of ACNPs to work to their full scope of practice (McNamara, Giguère, St-Louis, & Boileau, 2009). Disagreement related to the scope of ACNP practice has created interprofessional barriers that impede the development of the role in Quebec (Desrosiers, 2009; D'Amour et al., 2007; D'Amour, Tremblay, & Prouix, 2009; McNamara et al., 2009; OIIQ, 2009). Professional territoriality has been highlighted in acute care setting literature. Some medical residents have expressed concern about losing control of patient care decisions and competing with ACNPs for opportunities to perform medical skills (D'Amour et al., 2007; Fédération des médecins résidents du Québec, 2003a, 2003b, 2003c, 2004).

Findings regarding nurses' views of ACNP roles, however, are mixed. D'Amour et al. (2007) reported that in Quebec, RNs expressed concern over a perceived increase in hierarchy within the nursing profession following the introduction of ACNP roles. Others studies (Harwood, Wilson, Heidenheim, & Lindsay, 2004; Mitchell-DiCenso et al., 1996b) found that nurses had a positive view of the ACNP role because ACNPs were a ready source of patient information, attended to team member concerns about patients in a timely manner, improved communication among team members, and provided consistency in patient care because they were always visible (unlike medical residents, who are clinically rotated). The results vary, in part due to the length of time nurses had been exposed to ACNPs prior to the study being conducted, since further studies demonstrated that nurses did not feel that their roles were threatened by the introduction and integration of ACNPs (Irvine et al., 2000).

Until 2008, ACNPs were referred to (in keeping with the CNPE population-based focus) as NP–Adult and NP–Pediatrics (CNA, 2010). At that time, these roles were not licensed/credentialed and, therefore, were not included in the regulatory data. However, the number of ACNPs increased between 2003 and 2007 in all provincial jurisdictions by 5% (CIHI, 2008). Roots and MacDonald (2008) conducted an exploratory study of NPs and stakeholders to identify the factors influencing NP role implementation in British Columbia and reported a mismatch between NP education and available positions. For example, some NPs educated in primary health care were working in acute care, or with specialized populations. Schreiber et al. (2003, 2005a) found that APNs in British Columbia needed to engage in both formal and informal education opportunities to further role development. However, access to clinical specialty education in Canada is limited. This is notable because specialty education is significant in developing role confidence, job satisfaction (Bryant-Lukosius et al., 2007), self-confidence, and the ability to solve complex problems (Richmond & Becker, 2005). Researchers (CNA, 2006; D'Amour et al., 2007; DiCenso et al., 2010a; OIIQ, 2009) question the long-term survival of ACNP roles without stable funding, affecting salaries that clearly recognize their scope of practice and the level of responsibility involved once they have been successfully incorporated into the health care delivery organization.

The status of ACNP roles continues to evolve across the nation and ongoing leadership and research continue to be vital to the enhancement and the integration of these roles into the Canadian health care system.

Conclusion

Nurses have practiced in several expanded roles across Canada for over a century. The role that began with outpost nurses and war-time "nurse clinicians" and "specialists" has undergone an intense evolution and emerged as the CNS, PHCNP, NP, ACNP, and other streams of advanced practice nursing that are visible today.

The recent definition of the CNS role (CNA, 2014) provides direction for role clarity and ongoing role integration across practice settings within a changing health care environment. There continues to be only one definition for all NP roles in Canada, which focuses on the required educational preparation and experience required to autonomously practice within a regulated scope. Through the integration of in-depth knowledge and skills, each of the APN roles provides an advanced level of nursing practice that are diverse and span all aspects of clinical practice.

Although neonatal nurse practitioners (NNP) were the first to be termed acute care NP (ACNP) in Canada, today ACNPs are found in all areas of practice and predominantly engage in direct patient care activities, diagnostic activities, care planning, and care coordination. However, the continued sustainability of CNS and NP roles, once they have been successfully incorporated into a health care system without stable funding and salaries that recognize both their scope of practice and level of responsibility, is in question. Ongoing leadership and continued research are required to enhance development and integration of all APN roles into the Canadian health care system.

Critical Thinking Questions

1. What are the differences between the roles of clinical nurse specialist (CNS) and nurse practitioner (NP)?
2. What has been the impact of the clinical nurse specialist (CNS) role in the delivery of health care services?
3. Can you trace the introduction of either the CNS or NP roles within your organization?
4. What have been the facilitators of and barriers to implementing NP roles in Canada?

References

Alcock, D.S. (1996). The clinical nurse specialist, clinical nurse specialist/nurse practitioner and other titled nurse in Ontario. *Canadian Journal of Nursing Administration, 9*(1), 23–44.

Allard, M., & Durand, S. (2006). L'infirmière praticienne spécialisée: un nouveau rôle de pratique infirmière avancée au Québec. *Perspective Infirmière: Revue Officielle de l'Ordre des Infirmières et Infirmiers du Québec, 3*(5), 10–16.

Almost, J., & Laschinger, H.K. (2002). Workplace empowerment, collaborative work relationships and job strain in nurse practitioners. *Journal of the American Academy of Nurse Practitioners, 14*(9), 408–420.

Avery, L.J., & Schnell-Hoehn, K.N. (2010). Clinical nurse specialist practice in evidence-informed multidisciplinary cardiac care. *Clinical Nurse Specialist, 24*(2), 76–79.

Beaudoin, M.L., Besner, G., & Gaudreault, G. (1978). Praticienne? Clinicienne? *Infirmière Canadienne, 20*(12), 23–25.

Boone, M., & Kikuchi, J. (1977). The clinical nurse specialist. In B. LaSor & R. Elliott (Eds.), *Issues in Canadian nursing* (pp. 101–125). Scarborough, ON: Prentice-Hall.

Boudreau, T.J. (1972). *Report of the committee on nurse practitioners.* Ottawa, ON: Department of National Health and Welfare.

Bryant-Lukosius, D., Carter, N., Kilpatrick, K., Martin-Misener, R., Donald, F., Kaasalainen, S., ... DiCenso, A. (2010). The clinical nurse specialist role in Canada. *Nursing Leadership, 23*(Special Issue December), 140–166.

Bryant-Lukosius, D., Green, E., Fitch, M., Macartney, G., Robb-Blenderman, L., McFarlane, S., ... Milne, H. (2007). A survey of oncology advanced practice nurses in Ontario: Profile and predictors of job satisfaction. *Nursing Leadership, 20*(2), 50–68.

Bussières, J., & Parent, M. (2004). Histoire de la spécialisation en santé au Québec – 1re partie. *Pharmactuel, 37*(1), 39–50.

Buzzell, E.M. (1976). Baccalaureate preparation for the nurse practitioner: When will we ever learn? *Nursing Papers, 8*(3), 2–9.

Canadian Institute for Health Information (CIHI). (2006). *The regulation and supply of nurse practitioners in Canada: 2006 update.* Ottawa, ON: CIHI. Retrieved from https://secure.cihi.ca/free_products/The_Nurse_Practitioner_Workforce_in_Canada_2006_Update_final.pdf

CIHI. (2008). *Regulated nurses: Trends, 2003 to 2007: Registered nurses, licensed practical nurses, registered psychiatric nurses.* Ottawa, ON: CIHI. Retrieved from https://secure.cihi.ca/free_products/nursing_report_2003_to_2007_e.pdf

CIHI. (2010). *Regulated nurses: Canadian trends, 2005 to 2009.* Ottawa, ON: CIHI. Retrieved from https://secure.cihi.ca/free_products/nursing_report_2005-2009_en.pdf

Canadian Medical Association Journal. (1973). Canadian medical, nurses associations agreed on expanded role for nurses. *Canadian Medical Association Journal, 108*(10), 1306–1307.

Canadian Nurses Association (CNA). (1978). *Position statement: Clinical nurse specialist.* Ottawa, ON: CNA.

CNA. (1986). *Position statement: Clinical nurse specialist.* Ottawa, ON: CNA.

CNA. (2003). *Position statement: Clinical nurse specialist.* Ottawa, ON: CNA.

CNA. (2006). *Report of 2005 dialogue on advanced nursing practice.* Ottawa, ON: CNA.

CNA. (2008). *Advanced nursing practice: A national framework.* Ottawa, ON: CNA. Retrieved from http://www.cna-aiic.ca/~/media/cna/page-content/pdf-en/anp_national_framework_e.pdf

CNA. (2009a). *Position statement: Clinical nurse specialist.* Ottawa, ON: CNA. Retrieved from https://www.cna-aiic.ca/~/media/cna/page-content/pdf-en/clinical-nurse-specialist_position-statement.pdf?la=en

CNA. (2009b). *Position statement: The nurse practitioner.* Ottawa, ON: CNA. Retrieved from http://cna-aiic.ca/~/media/cna/page-content/pdf-fr/ps_nurse_practitioner_e.pdf

CNA. (2010). *Canadian nurse practitioner core competency framework.* Ottawa, ON: CNA. Retrieved from https://www.cna-aiic.ca/~/media/cna/files/en/competency_framework_2010_e.pdf

CNA. (2014). *Pan-Canadian core competencies for the clinical nurse specialist.* Ottawa, ON: CNA. Retrieved from http://cna-aiic.ca/en/news-room/news-releases/2014/canadian-nurses-association-launches-core-competencies-for-clinical-nurse-specialists

Canadian Nurses Association (CNA) and the Canadian Medical Association (CMA). (1973). *The joint committee on the expanded role of the nurses: Statement of policy.* Ottawa, ON: CNA/CMA.

Canadian Nurse Practitioner Initiative (CNPI). (2006a). *Implementation and evaluation toolkit for nurse practitioners in Canada.* Ottawa, ON: CNA. Retrieved from https://nurseone.ca/~/media/nurseone/files/en/toolkit_implementation_evaluation_np_e.pdf

CNPI. (2006b). *Nurse practitioners: The time is now: A solution to improving access and reducing wait times in Canada.* Ottawa, ON: CNA. Retrieved from http://www.npnow.ca/docs/tech-report/section1/01_Integrated_Report.pdf

CNPI. (2006c). *Nurse practitioners: The time is now: Technical reports.* Ottawa, ON: CNA.

Cardenas, B.D. (1975). The independent nurse practitioner. Alive and well and living in rural Saskatchewan. *Nursing Clinics of North America, 10*(4), 711–719.

Chambers, L.W., & West, A.E. (1978). The St. John's randomized trial of the family practice nurse: Health outcomes of patients. *International Journal of Epidemiology, 7*(2), 153–161.

Chenoy, N.C., Spitzer, W.O., & Anderson, G.D. (1973). Nurse practitioners in primary care. II. Prior attitudes of a rural population. *Canadian Medical Association Journal, 108*(8), 998–1003.

Cummings, G.G., Fraser K., & Tarlier, D.S. (2003). Implementing advanced nurse practitioner roles in acute care: An evaluation of organizational change. *Journal of Nursing Administration, 33*(3), 139–145.

D'Amour, D., Morin, D., Dubois, C., Lavoie-Tremblay, M., Dallaire, C., & Cyr, G. (2007). *Évaluation de l'implantation du programme d'intéressement au titre d'infirmière praticienne.* Montreal, QC: Ministère de la Santé et des services sociaux du Québec.

D'Amour, D., Tremblay, D., & Proulx., M. (2009). Déploiement de nouveaux rôles infirmiers au Québec et pouvoir médical. *Recherches sociographiques, 50*(2), 301–320.

Davies, B., & Eng, B. (1995). Implementation of the CNS role in Vancouver, British Columbia, Canada. *Clinical Nurse Specialist, 9*(1), 23–30.

Desrosiers, G. (2009). Toutes les infirmières sont importantes, mais alors, pourquoi encore parler des infirmières praticiennes spécialisées? *Le Journal, 6*(3), 2.

DiCenso, A. (1998). The neonatal nurse practitioner. *Current Opinion in Pediatrics,10*(2), 151–155.

DiCenso, A., Auffrey, L., Bryant-Lukosius, D., Donald, F., Martin-Misener, R., Matthews, S., & Opsteen, J. (2007). Primary health care nurse practitioners in Canada. *Contemporary Nurse, 26*(1), 104–115. doi: 10.5172/conu.2007.26.1.104

DiCenso, A., & Bryant-Lukosius, D. (2010). The long and winding road: Integration of nurse practitioners and clinical nurse specialists into the Canadian health-care system. *Canadian Journal of Nursing Research, 42*(2), 3–8.

DiCenso, A., Bryant-Lukosius, D., Bourgeault, I., Martin-Misener, R., Donald, F., Abelson, J., ... Harbman, P. (2010a). *Clinical nurse specialists and nurse practitioners in Canada: A decision support synthesis.* Ottawa, ON: Canadian Health Services Research Foundation.

DiCenso, A., Martin-Misener, R., Bryant-Lukosius, D., Bourgeault, I., Kilpatrick, K., Donald, F.,... Charbonneau-Smith, R. (2010b). Advanced practice nursing in Canada: Overview of a decision support synthesis. *Nursing Leadership, 23*(Special Issue, December), 15–34.

DiCenso, A., Paech, G., & IBM Corporation. (2003). *Report on the integration of primary health care nurse practitioners into the province of Ontario.* Toronto, ON: MOHLTC.

Dierick-van Daele, A., Steuten, L., Metsemakers, J., Derckx, E., Spreeuwenberg, C., & Vrijhoef, H. (2010). Economic evaluation of nurse practitioners versus GPs in treating common conditions. *British Journal of General Practice, 60*(570), e28–e35.

Donald, F., Martin-Misener, R., Bryant-Lukosius, D., Kilpatrick, K., Kaasalainen, S., Carter, N., … DiCenso, A. (2010). The primary healthcare nurse practitioner role in Canada. *Nursing Leadership, 23*(Special Issue, December), 88–113.

Dunn, E.V., & Higgins, C.A. (1986). Health problems encountered by three levels of providers in a remote setting. *American Journal of Public Health, 76*(2), 154–159.

Faculté des sciences infirmières, Université de Montréal. (2008). *Une maîtrise, quatre options.* Montréal, QC: Université de Montréal.

Fédération des médecins résidents du Québec. (2003a). *Avis consultatif de la FMRQ déposé dans le cadre des activités du comité conjoint consultatif paritaire OIIQ-CMQ concernant l'infirmière praticienne en cardiologie – Volet chirurgie cardiaque.* Montréal, QC: Fédération des médecins résidents du Québec.

Fédération des médecins résidents du Québec. (2003b). *Avis consultatif de la FMRQ déposé dans le cadre des activités du comité conjoint consultatif paritaire OIIQ-CMQ concernant l'infirmière praticienne en néonatologie.* Montréal, QC: Fédération des médecins résidents du Québec.

Fédération des médecins résidents du Québec. (2003c). *Avis consultatif de la FMRQ déposé dans le cadre des activités du comité conjoint consultatif paritaire OIIQ-CMQ concernant l'infirmière praticienne en néphrologie.* Montréal, QC: Fédération des médecins résidents du Québec.

Fédération des médecins résidents du Québec. (2004). *Avis consultatif de la FMRQ déposé dans le cadre des activités du comité conjoint consultatif paritaire OIIQ-CMQ concernant la création du rôle de l'infirmière praticienne spécialisée en cardiologie – Volet cardiologie médicale au Québec.* Montréal, QC: Fédération des médecins résidents du Québec.

Griffiths, H. (2006). Advanced nursing practice: Enter the nurse practitioner. *Nursing BC, 38*(2), 12–16.

Haines, J. (1993). *The nurse practitioner: A discussion paper.* Ottawa, ON: CNA.

Hamric, A.B., Spross, J. A., & Hanson, C. (2009). *Advanced nursing practice: An integrative approach* (4th ed.). Philadelphia, PA: W.B. Saunders.

Harris/Decima. (2009, August 13). *Canadians very comfortable with expanded role for nurse practitioners.* Ottawa, ON: Harris/Decima. Retrieved from http://sdnpc.ca/images/stories/Canadians_very_comfortable_with_expanded_role_for_nurse_practitioners.doc

Harwood, L., Wilson, B., Heidenheim, A.P., & Lindsay, R.M. (2004). The advanced practice nurse-nephrologist care model: Effect on patient outcomes and hemodialysis unit team satisfaction. *Hemodialysis International, 8*(3), 273–282.

Hazlett, C.B. (1975). Task analysis of the clinically trained nurse (C.T.N.). *Nursing Clinics of North America, 10*(4), 699–709.

Higgins, J. (2008). *Grenfell Mission: Newfoundland and Labrador heritage.* St. John's, NL: Memorial University of Newfoundland.

Hodgkin, K. (1977). The family practice nurse. *Canadian Medical Association Journal 116*(8), 829–830.

Hunsberger, M., Mitchell, A., Blatz, S., Paes, B., Pinelli, J., Southwell, D., ... Soluk, R. (1992). Definition of an advanced nursing practice role in the NICU: The clinical nurse specialist/ neonatal practitioner. *Clinical Nurse Specialist, 6*(2), 91–96.

Hutchison, B. (2008). A long time coming: Primary healthcare renewal in Canada. *Healthcare Papers, 8*(2), 10–24.

International Council of Nurses (ICN). (2008). *The scope of practice, standards and competencies of the advanced practice nurse.* Geneva, CH: ICN.

Irvine, D., Sidani, S., Porter, H., O'Brien-Pallas, L., Simpson, B., McGillis Hall, L., ... Nagel, L. (2000). Organizational factors influencing nurse practitioners' role implementation in acute care settings. *Canadian Journal of Nursing Leadership, 13*(3), 28–35.

Jenkins, S.D., & Lindsey, P.L. (2010). Clinical nurse specialists as leaders in rapid response. *Clinical Nurse Specialist, 24*(1), 24–30.

Kaasalainen, S., Martin-Misener, R., Kilpatrick, K., Harbman, P., Bryant-Lukosius, D., Donald, F., & DiCenso, A. (2010). A historical overview of the development of advanced practice nursing roles in Canada. *Nursing Leadership, 23*(Special Issue, December), 35–60.

Kilpatrick, K., Harbman, P., Carter, N., Martin-Misener, R., Bryant-Lukosius, D., Donald, F., ... DiCenso, A. (2010). The acute care nurse practitioner role in Canada. *Nursing Leadership, 23*(Special, Issue December), 114–139.

King, B., Spaulding, W.B., & Wright, A.D. (1974). Problem-oriented diabetic day care. *The Canadian Nurse, 70*(10), 19–22.

Kirby, M. (2002). *The health of Canadians – The federal role: Final report.* Ottawa, ON: Parliament of Canada. Retrieved from http://www.parl.gc.ca/content/sen/committee/372/soci/rep/repoct02vol6-e.htm

Kleinpell, R.M. (1997). Acute-care nurse practitioners: Roles and practice profiles. *American Association of Clinical-Care Nurses (AACN) Clinical Issues, 8*(1), 156–162.

Kulig, J., Thomlinson, E., Curran, F., Nahachewsky, D., Macleod, M., Stewart N., & Pitblado, R. (2003). *Nursing practice in rural and remote Canada: An analysis of policy documents.* Prince George, BC: University of Northern British Columbia. Retrieved from http://ruralnursing.unbc.ca/reports/jkulig/FinalReportweb.php

Lalonde, M. (1974). *A new perspective on health of Canadians: A working document.* Ottawa, ON: Government of Canada. Retrieved from http://www.phac-aspc.gc.ca/ph-sp/pdf/perspect-eng.pdf

Lewandowski, W., & Adamle, K. (2009). Substantive areas of clinical nurse specialist practice: A comprehensive review of the literature. *Clinical Nurse Specialist, 23*(2), 73–90.

MacDonald, J., Herbert, R., & Thibeault, C. (2006). Advanced practice nursing: Unification through a common identity. *Journal of Professional Nursing, 22*(3), 172–179.

Mayo, A.M., Omery, A., Agocs-Scott, L.M., Khaghani, F., Meckes, P.G., Moti, N., ... Cuenca, E. (2010). Clinical nurse specialist practice patterns. *Clinical Nurse Specialist, 24*(2), 60–68.

McFarlane, A.H., & Norman, G.R. (1972). A medical care information system: Evaluation of changing patterns of primary care. *Medical Care, 10*(6), 481–487.

McNamara, S., Giguère, V., St-Louis, L., & Boileau, J. (2009). Development and implementation of the specialized nurse practitioner role: Use of the PEPPA framework to achieve success. *Nursing and Health Sciences, 11*(3), 318–325.

McTavish, M. (1979). The Nurse Practitioner: An idea whose time has come. *Canadian Nurse* 75(8), 41–44.

Mitchell, A., Watts, J., Whyte, R., Blatz, S., Norman, G., Southwell, D., ... Pinelli, J. (1995). Evaluation of an educational program to prepare neonatal nurse practitioners. *Journal of Nursing Education, 34*(6), 286–289.

Mitchell-DiCenso, A., Guyatt, G., Marrin, M., Goeree, R., Willan, A., Southwell, D., ... Baumann, A. (1996). A controlled trial of nurse practitioners in neonatal intensive care. *Pediatrics, 98*(6), 1143–1148.

Mitchell-DiCenso, A., Pinelli, J., & Southwell, D. (1996). Introduction and evaluation of an advanced nursing practice role in neonatal intensive care. In K. Kelly (Ed). *Outcomes of effective management practice* (pp. 171–186). Thousand Oaks, CA: Sage.

Montemuro, M.A. (1987). The evolution of the clinical nurse specialist: Response to the challenge of professional nursing practice. *Clinical Nurse Specialist 1*(3), 106–110.

Nhan, J., & Zuidema, S. (2007). Nurse practitioners in the northern Alberta renal program. *Canadian Association of Nephrology Nurses and Technologists Journal, 17*(2), 48–50.

Nurse Practitioners' Association of Ontario (NPAO). (n.d.). *Nurse practitioner history in Ontario.* Toronto, ON: NPAO. Retrieved from http://npao.org/nurse-practitioners/history/

Ordre des infirmières et infirmiers du Québec (OIIQ). (2009). *Les infirmières praticiennes spécialisées: Un rôle à propulser, une intégration à accélérer. Bilan et perspectives de pérennité.* Montréal, QC: OIIQ.

Ordre des infirmières et infirmiers du Québec (OIIQ), & Collège des médecins du Québec (CMQ). (2006). *Lignes directrices sur les modalités de la pratique de l'infirmière praticienne spécialisée.* Montréal, QC: OIIQ/CMQ.

Paes, B., Mitchell, A., Hunsberger, M., Blatz, S., Watts, J., Dent, P., ... Southwell, D. (1989). Medical staffing in Ontario neonatal intensive care units. *The Canadian Medical Association Journal, 140*(11), 1321–1326.

Pepler, C.J., Edgar, L., Frisch, S., Rennick, J., Swidzinski, M., White, C., ... Gross, J. (2006). Strategies to increase research-based practice: Interplay with unit culture. *Clinical Nurse Specialist, 20*(1), 23–31.

Pringle, D. (2007). Nurse practitioner role: Nursing needs it. *Canadian Journal of Nursing Leadership, 20*(2), 1–5.

Profetto-McGrath, J., Negrin, K.A., Hugo, K., & Smith, K.B. (2010). Clinical nurse specialists' approaches in selecting and using evidence to improve practice. *Worldviews on Evidence-Based Nursing, 7*(1), 36–50.

Profetto-McGrath, J., Smith, K.B., Hugo, K., Taylor, M., & El-Hajj, H. (2007). Clinical nurse specialists' use of evidence in practice: A pilot study. *Worldviews on Evidence-Based Nursing, 4*(2), 86–96.

Ramsay, J.A., McKenzie, J.K., & Fish, D.G. (1982). Physicians and nurse practitioners: Do they provide equivalent health care? *American Journal of Public Health, 72*(1), 55–57.

Ream, E., Wilson-Barnett, J., Faithfull, S., Fincham, L., Khoo, V., & Richardson, A. (2009). Working patterns and perceived contributions of prostate cancer clinical nurse specialists: A mixed method investigation. *International Journal of Nursing Studies, 46*, 1345–1354.

Reay, T., Golden-Biddle, K., & Germann, K. (2006). Legitimizing a new role: Small wins and micro processes of change. *Academy of Management Journal, 49*(5), 977–998.

Richmond, T.S., & Becker, D. (2005). Creating an advanced practice nurse-friendly culture: A marathon, not a sprint. *American Association of Critical-Care Nurses Clinical Issues,16*(1), 58–66.

Romanow, R.J. (2002). *Building on values: The future of health care in Canada – Final report.* Ottawa, ON: Commission on the Future of Health Care in Canada.

Roots, A., & MacDonald, M. (2008, September 17–20). 3 *years down the road: Exploring the implementation of the NP role in British Columbia, Canada.* Poster presentation at the 5th International Council of Nursing, International Nurse Practitioner/Advanced Practice Nursing (INP/APN) Conference, Toronto, ON.

Roschkov, S., Rebeyka, D., Comeau, A., Mah, J., Scherr, K., Smigorowsky, M., & Stoop, J. (2007). Cardiovascular nurse practitioner practice: Results of a Canada-wide survey. *Canadian Journal of Cardiovascular Nursing, 17*(3), 27–31.

Rosenthal, L., & Guerrasio, J. (2009). Acute care nurse practitioner as hospitalist: Role description. *American Association of Critical-Care Nurses Advanced Clinical Care, 20*(2), 133–136.

Royal College of Nursing (RCN). (2008). *Advanced nurse practitioners: An RCN guide to the advanced nurse practitioner role, competencies and programme accreditation.* London, UK: Royal College of Nursing.

Rutherford, G., & Rutherford Consulting Group Inc. (2005). Appendix B: *Education component: Literature review report.* Ottawa, ON: CNA/CNPI. Retrieved from http://www.npnow.ca/docs/tech-report/section5/03_Education_AppendixB.pdf

Saskatchewan Collaborative Programs in Nursing (2015). *Nurse practitioners – Improving health care in communities.* Regina, SK: Saskatchewan Polytechnic and University of Regina. Retrieved from http://www.sasknursingdegree.ca/cnpp/

Scherer, K., Fortin, F., Spitzer, W.O., & Kergin, D.J. (1977). Nurse practitioners in primary care. VII. A cohort study of 99 nurses and 79 associated physicians. *CMA Journal, 116*(8), 856–862.

Schreiber, R., Davidson, H., MacDonald, M., Crickmore, J., Moss, L., Pinelli, J., ... Hammond, C. (2003). *Advanced nursing practice: Opportunities and challenges in British Columbia.* Ottawa, ON: Canadian Health Services Research Foundation. Retrieved from http://www.fcass-cfhi.ca/Migrated/PDF/ResearchReports/OGC/schreiber_report.pdf

Schreiber, R., MacDonald, M., Pauly, B., Davidson, H., Crickmore, J., Moss, L., ... Regan. S. (2005a). Singing from the same songbook: The future of advanced nursing practice in British Columbia. *Canadian Journal of Nursing Leadership, 18*(2), 1–14.

Schreiber, R., MacDonald, M., Pauly, B., Davidson, H., Crickmore, J., Moss, L., ... Hammond, C. (2005b). Singing in different keys: Enactment of advanced nursing practice in British Columbia. *Canadian Journal of Nursing Leadership, 6,* 1–17.

Sidani, S. (2008). Effects of patient-centered care on patient outcomes: An evaluation. *Research and Theory for Nursing Practice: An international journal, 22*(1), 24–37.

Sidani, S., Doran, D., Porter, H., LeFort, S., O'Brien-Pallas, L., Zahn, C., & Sarkissian, S. (2006a). Outcomes of nurse practitioners in acute care: An exploration. *Internet Journal of Advanced Nursing Practice, 8*(1). Retrieved from https://ispub.com/IJANP/8/1/12232

Sidani, S., Doran, D., Porter, H., LeFort, S., O'Brien-Pallas, L., Zahn, C., ... Sarkissian, S. (2006b). Processes of care: Comparison between nurse practitioners and physician residents in acute care. *Canadian Journal of Nursing Leadership, 19*(1), 69–85.

Sidani, S., & Irvine, D. (1999). A conceptual framework for evaluating the nurse practitioner role in acute care settings. *Journal of Advanced Nursing, 30*(1), 58–66.

Sidani, S., Irvine, D., & DiCenso, A. (2000). Implementation of the primary care nurse practitioner role in Ontario. *Canadian Journal of Nursing Leadership, 13*(3), 13–19.

Sidani, S., Irvine, D., Porter, H., O'Brien-Pallas, L., Simpson, B., McGillis Hall, L., … Redelmeir, D. (2000b). Practice patterns of acute care nurse practitioners. *Canadian Journal of Nursing Leadership, 13*(3), 6–12.

Simpson, B. (1997). An educational partnership to develop acute care nurse practitioners. *Canadian Journal of Nursing Administration, 10*(1), 69–84.

Smith-Higuchi, K.A., Hagen, B., Brown, S., & Zeiber, M.P. (2006). A new role for advanced practice nurses in Canada: bridging the gap in health services for rural older adults. *Journal of Gerontological Nursing, 32*(7), 49–55.

Spitzer, W.O., & Kergin, D.J. (1975). Nurse practitioners in primary care I: The McMaster University educational program. *Health Care Dimensions,* Spring, 95–103.

Spitzer, W.O., Kergin, D.J., Yoshida, M.A., Russell, W.A., Hackett, B.C., & Goldsmith, C.H. (1973). Nurse practitioners in primary care III. The southern Ontario randomized trial. *Canadian Medical Association Journal, 108*(8), 1005.

Stevens, B.J. (1976). Accountability of the clinical specialist: The administrator's viewpoint. *Journal of Nursing Administration, 6*(2), 30–32.

The Canadian Nurse. (1978). Nurse practitioners—The national picture. *The Canadian Nurse, 74*(4), 13.

van Soeren, M.H., & Micevski, V. (2001). Success indicators and barriers to acute nurse practitioner role implementation in four Ontario hospitals. *American Association of Critical-Care Nurses (AACN) Clinical Issues, 12*(3), 424–37.

Vayda, E., Gent, M., & Paisley, L. (1973). An emergency department triage model based on presenting complaints. *Canadian Journal of Public Health, 64*(3), 246–253.

Wall, S. (2006). Living with grey: Role understandings between clinical nurse educators and advanced practice nurses. *Canadian Journal of Nursing Leadership, 19*(4), 57–71.

Way, D., Jones, L., Baskerville, B., & Busing, N. (2001). Primary health care services provided by nurse practitioners and family physicians in shared practice. *Canadian Medical Association Journal, 165*(9), 1210–1214.

Wetzel, C., & Kalman, M. (2010). Critical care clinical nurse specialist. Is this role for you? *Dimensions of Critical Care Nursing, 29*(1), 29–32.

Chapter 2

The Integration of Advanced Practice Nursing Roles in Canada

Michelle Acorn

Michelle Acorn is an NP–Adult and PHC. She is the Lead NP at Lakeridge Health in Whitby, Ontario, which was the first hospital in Canada to implement an NP-led model of care as most responsible provider (MRP). Michelle is also a Lecturer and Primary Health Care/Global Health NP Program Coordinator at the University of Toronto's Lawrence S. Bloomberg Faculty of Nursing.

KEY TERMS

advanced practice nursing (APN)
clinical nurse specialist (CNS)
Doctor of Nursing Practice (DNP)
integration
most responsible provider/practitioner (MRP)
nurse practitioner (NP)
NP-led clinic (NPLC)

OBJECTIVES

1. Appraise the integration of advanced practice nursing (APN) in Canada.
2. Explore the integration of nurse practitioner (NP) roles in Canada.
3. Highlight the integration of clinical nurse specialist (CNS) roles in Canada.

Introduction

This chapter will highlight the integration of **advanced practice nursing** (APN) roles, both **clinical nurse specialists** (CNS) and **nurse practitioners** (NP), in Canada. A historical and innovative practice lens will demonstrate the successes and challenges for both clinical and non-clinical advanced practice role dimensions, which leverage NP sustainability.

Advanced Practice Nursing Integration Influences

The process of integrating advanced practice nurses (APNs) into the Canadian health care system has been occurring for over 40 years. Integration is defined as "the act or process of integrating as equals into society or as an organization of individuals of different groups. Furthermore, integration is the combining or coordinating of separate parts or elements into a unified whole" (Merriam-Webster, 2014). Integration of APNs in Canada will be discussed in relation to primary health care, as well as tertiary and long-term care settings.

The CNS provides an important clinical leadership role for the nursing profession and broader health care system. Key challenges to full integration include fluctuating role prominence, lack of common vision for the CNS role, need for credentialing, and limited CNS-specific graduate education (Bryant-Lukosius et al., 2010).

The acute care nurse practitioner (ACNP) role in Canada evolved in the late 1980s to offset increasing physician workloads and address the lack of continuity in complex care within acute and critical care settings (see Chapter 1). Failure to utilize all APN role components, scope of practice limitations, variability in team acceptance, and funding challenges, however, remain barriers to integration. Clear role communication, tailored messages to stakeholders, supportive leadership, and stable funding are needed to facilitate the role of APNs (Kilpatrick et al., 2010).

In Canada, the primary health care nurse practitioner (PHCNP) role is the fastest-growing APN role. They deliver NP care across all provinces and territories, providing care to families across their lifespans. The introduction of the APN role has led to countrywide health care reform by improving accessibility and quality primary care (Donald et al., 2010b).

A review of the Canadian literature regarding full integration of APNs was found to focus on the CNS, PHCNP, and ACNP roles. Regarding APN role development and systemic planning, enabling factors occurred at the federal, provincial, and territorial levels. A pan-Canadian approach, delivering high-quality education and supportive legislative and regulatory mechanisms, were key requirements for successful APN integration. Implementation strategies for APN roles included recruitment and retention, funding, public awareness, leadership, and intraprofessional relationships between CNSs and NPs. To support the success of implementation, organizational considerations included fostering role clarity, setting support, utilizing all APN role components, and continuing professional development (DiCenso et al., 2010).

Remaining barriers to full integration of APNs can be identified by title confusion and unclear roles. A lack of awareness, ambiguous expectations, scope of practice confusion, and title protection variances exist for both the CNS and NP roles. It is recommended that a focus on consistent role titling that fosters role clarity, along with improved communication strategies that highlight the roles of the CNS and NP, is needed to enhance integration. Attention to team dynamics and interprofessional education is also suggested (Donald et al., 2010a). CNSs are currently seeking title protection similar to that of their NP colleagues. Supportive organizational leadership strategies for both CNS and NP role integration include systematic planning based on needs, stakeholder engagement, utilizing Canadian APN role toolkits, utilizing all role dimensions, and communicating role awareness (Carter et al., 2010).

In 2011, the Canadian Nurses Association (CNA) suggested that a pan-Canadian collaborative integration plan was required for the integration of NPs in Canada. Theoretically, this comprehensive plan could be utilized further to include the CNS role. The strategic areas outlined in the plan include legislation and regulation, education, human resources in the health sector, and communication. Each of these components has key actions to both lead and support APN integration.

Canadian Advanced Practice Nursing Framework

The literature highlights the provincial and national practice of describing and recognizing the APN domains of practice. For clinical and non-clinical practice impacts, it supports common understanding and language across the CNS and NP landscape. To support patients' needs and organizational leadership, the value-added capacities can be optimized to yield the most talented APNs (van Soeren, Hurlock-Chorostecki, & Reeves, 2011). The Canadian APN framework (CNA, 2008), in terms of theoretical underpinnings, was utilized in the majority of NP studies identifying these clinical issues (Acorn, 2015a; Hurlock-Chorostecki, van Soeren, & Goodwin, 2008; van Soeren & Micevski, 2001; van Soeren & Hurlock-Chorostecki, 2009; van Soeren et al., 2011).

Canadian Integration Landscape for Nurse Practitioners

In 2010, 11 Canadian jurisdictions submitted profile data that identified 2,554 NPs, representing 0.9% of all RNs in Canada. Over 97% were employed in nursing, an increase of 85% since 2007; 77.5% worked full-time, 14% part-time, and 5.6% worked on a casual basis. Of these, 72% of NPs had a single employer, while 23% had multiple employers. The data also revealed that men represented 5.1% (128) and women 94.9% (2,358) of NPs. Almost 17% of those were 55 years of age or older (CNA, 2012). A provincial breakdown of the data found that Newfoundland and Labrador employed 65 NPs, Nova Scotia 106, New Brunswick 69, and Quebec 64. Ontario was positioned the strongest with 1,482, followed by Alberta with 262, British Columbia with 129, and Saskatchewan with 122. The Northwest Territories and Nunavut employed a combined 56 NPs (CNA, 2012). Overall, the data showed that the ratio of NPs employed in nursing to the Canadian population was one for every 13,727 persons.

The NP employment profile depicted primary areas of responsibility in direct patient care (93.8%), administration (2.7%), education (3.2%), and research (0.3%) (CNA, 2012).

The number of NPs in Ontario doubled from 1,344 in 2007 to 2,777 in 2011 (Canadian Institute for Health Information [CIHI], 2013). This reflects increased provincial investment in NPs; however, they still account for only 1% of all registered nurses (RNs) in Ontario, with more than half of NPs working in community practice (Acorn 2015a, 2015b; CIHI, 2014; College of Nurses of Ontario [CNO], 2011).

When looking at the educational preparation of NPs in Canada, 47.6% possessed a graduate degree, followed by 42.8% with a baccalaureate degree, and 8.8% with a post-baccalaureate diploma. (Only 0.8% of NPs were educated at the doctoral level.) Almost all (96% or 2,352) NPs were educated in Canada, while the other 4.2% were educated internationally (CNO, 2011).

A paradigm shift regarding the divide traditionally associated with practice settings is narrowing with the alignment of the NP specialties within geographical practice settings (Acorn, 2015b; Hurlock-Chorestecki, van Soeren, & Goodwin, 2008). The notion that primary health care nurse practitioners (PHCNP) can only practice in the community, and NP–Adult or NP–Pediatrics are only authorized to practice in tertiary care settings, is diluting. NP knowledge as generalists or specialists can be portable, transferrable, and responsive to care needs across diverse settings. Professional self-regulation that focuses on NPs matching competence and confidence for care delivery accountabilities is the expectation (Acorn, 2015b, 2015c).

Integration of Nurse Practitioners in Primary Health Care

NP education prepares graduates to provide safe, high-quality, cost-effective, coordinated, and comprehensive care grounded in evidence-based practice (NP Roundtable, 2008). In 2000, a landmark randomized control trial (RCT) in Ontario established that NPs were both effective and safe (Acorn, 2015a, 2015b; Irvine et al., 2000). This trial, involving almost 1,600 families, established that NPs were able to thoroughly manage office-based patient care and request consultation from physician colleagues when required (Sackett, Spitzer, Gent, & Roberts, 1974). The NPs were the first contact for patients and delivered consistent care. Today these actions have paved the way for NPs acting as a **most responsible provider/ practitioner (MRP)** (Acorn, 2015a, 2015b).

One large-sample (over 1,500 patients) Danish RCT studied 12 experienced, senior NPs substituting for general practitioners. Patients reported a high appreciation for the quality of care against the quality of comparable services. No differences between NPs and general practitioners were found in health status, medical resource consumption, or guideline compliance. The study group invited more patient follow-up and conducted longer consultations as a consequence (Acorn, 2015a, 2015b; Dierick-van Daele et al., 2008).

Primary health care outcomes for patients treated by NPs versus physicians in ambulatory care revealed more comparable patient outcomes. Mundinger et al. (2000) conducted a RCT with almost 3,400 patients and found no significant differences in satisfaction, patient heath service utilization, health status, or physiologic test results. In patients with hypertension, the diastolic value was statistically significantly lower for the NPs' patients (p = .04). During the period of study, the NPs, essentially acting as the MRP, had the same authority, responsibility, productivity, administrative requirements, and patient populations as their physician counterparts (Acorn, 2015a, 2015b).

Integrating Nurse Practitioner (NP)-Led Clinics

Within Canada, Ontario is the first province to adopt broader utilization of the NP in PHC by developing and integrating 26 **NP-led clinics (NPLC)**. With NPs now championing interprofessional teams, this model of care delivery (where they function as the MRP) shifts clinical leadership and leverages governance. NPs delivering care in collaborative teams are improving access for more than 43,000 people (Ministry of Health and Long-Term Care [MOHLTC], 2014). PHCNPs or NP–PHCs make up the majority of NPs employed in community practices, however NP–Adult and NP–Pediatrics are also utilized in family health teams (FHT) and community health centres (CHC) (Acorn, 2015a, 2015b).

Similarly, the provincial government in Manitoba has made several investments in the province's health care system by launching five QuickCare clinics and two mobile clinics led by NPs. In an effort to provide a more sustainable health system, other new primary care clinics include access centres and working on My Health Teams. These groups provide health services across patients' lifespans in emergency departments, personal care homes, and remote nursing stations (Government of Manitoba, 2015).

Advanced Practice Nurses and Hospital Integration Practices

Ontario is leading hospital research contributions and informing deeper understanding of NPs as key players in patient-centred practices. A mixed methods study involving nine Ontario hospitals highlighted the contributions that NPs make through improved interprofessional practices (van Soeren et al., 2011). Key findings demonstrated that interprofessional teams valued clinical time and desired more. Useful NP attributes were evidenced in patient-focused care, safety, trust, and approachability. Greater accessibility, engagement between nurses and teams, general knowledge, and bridging care gaps were also valued NP roles (van Soeren et al., 2011). Additionally, assessment and diagnosis of health conditions, treatment, and prescribing medication encompass maximizing the scope of NP practice. These activities, aligned with enablement and empowerment, were necessary for effective integrations of NPs in hospital care. The considerable way in which NPs contributed to consistency in care and knowledge of patients, as well as the capacity to act as liaisons, hold central coordinating roles, and integrate with interprofessional teams were also key findings (Acorn, 2015a, 2015b; van Soeren et al., 2011).

A systematic literature review synthesized fourteen studies (predominately from the United Kingdom) for APN roles within hospital settings, including both NPs and CNSs. Relationships, communication, role definition, and role expectations were found to be the most important facilitators for NP role success (Jones, 2005). Variables such as previous employment, blending credibility with legitimacy in the hospital, political astuteness, established hospital networks or relationships, confidence, and specialty experience were also seen as supportive for the success, integration, and sustainability of the NP role (Acorn, 2015a).

Another pilot study in four Ontario academic hospitals, which included various specialty NP practices, indicated that successful NP role implementation was related to the level of role development (van Soeren & Micevski, 2001). Identified barriers included a lack of mentorship, lack of role knowledge, and perceived lack of support from administrators and physicians. However, the overall themes affecting patient care were shown to be improved NP communication, attention to patient care issues, and understanding the purpose and value of the APN role (Acorn, 2015a; van Soeren & Micevski, 2001).

Academic versus Community Hospital Integration

A propensity to study NPs in academic hospital settings was revealed in the literature, in contrast to the under-represented evaluation of community hospital NP role integration. NPs in Ontario community hospitals were found to spend more time in direct clinical practice than in academic teaching hospitals. Conversely, NPs in Ontario academic hospitals were found to spend more time on research than community hospital–based NPs (van Soeren et al., 2011). Hurlock-Chorestecki et al. (2008) highlighted ACNP practice patterns in Ontario hospitals and found the majority of NPs practicing in academic hospitals spend 75% of their time in direct patient care. Less than 20% of NPs worked in community hospitals (Acorn, 2015c).

Interprofessional Hospital Integration

One study on the integration of specialty NPs, conducted in Ontario, found that 75% of NP practice time was spent within the clinical domain, 8% in leadership, and 7% in research activities. NPs who spent the most time in clinical practice worked in community hospitals, and patient care delivered by NPs was found to be timely and responsive. Pediatric hospital NPs were discovered to have spent the greatest amount of practice in collaboration and consultation, while academic hospital NPs spent more time in research. Among the NP practices highly regarded by the medical team were strong communication, evidence-based care, and timely decision-making (Acorn, 2015b, 2015c; van Soeren & Hurlock-Chorostecki, 2009).

Hurlock-Chorostecki et al. (2013) researched hospital-based NP roles and the impact of interprofessional practice through a scoping review. They mapped eight literature reviews, including relevant Canadian studies, to four countries. Six themes emerged: NP role understanding, role status, workforce description, role integration, role outcomes, and role perceptions (Acorn, 2015a, 2015b).

Quality NP outcomes related to timely care, patient follow-up, improved discharge planning and safe discharges, as well as cost appreciation and improved staff knowledge are all realized by contributions from Canadian NPs. Such efforts also include role enactment, boundary work, and perceptions of team effectiveness, as well as the embedded value-add of NP role integration concepts (Kilpatrick et al., 2012b). Frameworks identified the reciprocal relationship between structure, process, and outcomes to linkages in NP role enactment. In an accountability and evidence-informed era of approach, indicators were intertwined (Acorn, 2015a).

Integration of Nurse Practitioners in Hospitals

In Canada, NPs in just three provinces have in-patient admitting and discharge authorities. Alberta was the first province authorized in 2007, Ontario followed in 2011 (first with discharging and then admission in 2012), and finally British Columbia in 2012 (Registered Nurses' Association of Ontario [RNAO], 2012). Ontario is showcasing NP hospital admission and MRP management, capitalizing on synergizing APN and medical expertise to optimize access to hospital care. Though not legally defined, the MRP refers to the provider who has primary responsibility and accountability for the care of a patient within the hospital (Ontario Hospital Association [OHA], 2012). The definition of the MRP encompasses primary responsibility and consistent care assumed by the NP during admission, treatment, diagnostics, diagnosis, prescribing, and discharge (Acorn, 2015a, 2015b). Many other countries do not have such restrictive hospital legislation and leave the decision to individual hospitals (Acorn 2015a, 2015b; RNAO, 2012).

The NP role is legally recognized as Registered Nurses in the Extended Class (RN(EC)), according to the Ontario Public Hospital Act (PHA). Two types of access to NP hospital practice may exist. The first model is well established for NPs employed at hospitals, who are authorized to diagnose and treat both in-patients and outpatients. These NPs do not require formal credentialing and privileging, but organizational support and endorsement are crucial for success and sustainability. The second track is for NPs not officially employed by the hospital but to whom the hospital board has granted privileges to diagnose and treat patients as professional staff NPs—similar to physicians, dentists, and midwives (OHA, 2012;

RNAO, 2012). These NPs may be employed in external primary- or tertiary-care organizations such as NP-led clinics, CHCs, FHTs, or LTC organizations (Acorn, 2015b, 2015c).

Ultimately, hospital professional staff bylaws, credentialing, and privileging will require amendments to be inclusive of NPs (OHA, 2012; RNAO, 2012). Hospital bylaws that integrate NPs into the privileged/professional staff mixes provide NPs with privileges ranging from courtesy to associate. These NPs move to active privileges after one year of practice and annual reappointment evaluation assurances (Acorn, 2015b, 2015c; OHA, 2012; RNAO, 2012).

Accountability and reporting structures for NPs currently align with the medical advisory council of privileged staff. The Excellent Health Care for All Act has leveraged the role of the chief nurse executive (CNE) to oversee NP and CNS nursing quality of care in hospitals (MOHLTC, 2010; OHA, 2012; RNAO, 2012). The CNE holds a strategic role to leverage senior executive nursing leadership, and support infrastructures for nursing success and sustainability. The CNE role ensures NP appointments and performance reviews are relevant for patient needs and appropriate for the NP role (OHA, 2012; RNAO, 2012). Professional liability coverage should be ensured for all privileged staff. NP employees may have additional coverage through organizational hospital insurance if practicing within scope, additional coverage if unionized, and may choose to carry personal professional liability coverage (Acorn, 2015a, 2015b; OHA, 2012; RNAO, 2012).

Integration of Boundary Work Competencies

A particularly descriptive case study on the introduction of cardiology NPs in health care teams researched boundary work (defined as "crossing the boundaries between the nursing and medical professions") at two academic hospitals in Quebec (Kilpatrick et al., 2013). Findings revealed that boundary work is a micro-level process that includes creating space, loss of valued function, trust, interpersonal dynamics, and time. The development of trust between key members and co-location of team members for projects and medical and nursing leadership were revealed to be highly important, and NPs were found to improve communication and collaboration among team members. Kilpatrick et al. (2013) insightfully highlighted the significant and shifting boundaries concerning the power of NPs with privilege to write prescriptions. The transfer of prescribing authority to NPs facilitates the development of medical activities that are included in the NP scope of practice (Kilpatrick et al., 2012a). The loss of an exclusive and unique prescriptive authority for physicians narrows the competence gap that sets the medical profession apart from other health care groups. Overlapping activities and evolving scopes of practice in health care are necessary to provide safe and innovative care to patients (Kilpatrick et al., 2013). NP roles that share both medical and nursing activities may result in some boundary turf wars before they are fully integrated (Acorn, 2015a, 2015b).

Legislative and Regulatory Integration

Policy initiatives have reduced many practice barriers in an equitable effort to improve access, contain costs, and enable integration. NP care provision has resulted in significant care improvements though autonomous and accountable practice (CNO, 2013a). On a provincial level, legislative and regulatory changes have been phased in to enable and empower NPs to improve access to quality care, as well as in an effort to capitalize on our human resources for health (Acorn, 2015a).

On 1 July, 2011, Ontario Bill 179 of the Regulated Health Professions Act (RHPA), as well as Regulation 965 of the Public Hospital Act, were proclaimed, enabling treatment and discharging of in-patients by NPs. In July 2012, NPs were authorized to admit in-patients to Ontario hospitals. Other components of this newer legislation led to celebratory archiving of the majority of medical directives originally required to support NP care delivery. Before, an authorizing physician delegated specific directives in an effort to facilitate daily NP practice acts. Final proclamation of a remaining component of Bill 179, related to ordering broad diagnostic tests including CTs, MRIs, X-rays, and ultrasounds was anticipated announced late in 2015 (Acorn, 2015b). Full implementation of Bill 179 continues to be an issue, as Ontario NPs are still not authorized to order CTs or MRIs, and now remain the last jurisdiction in North America unable to prescribe controlled substances.

The Nurse Practitioner as Most Responsible Provider/ Practitioner (MRP) for Patient Care

The role of the MRP must be clearly established and communicated. Responsibilities for patient care upon hospital admission include taking a comprehensive patient history, ordering diagnostics tests, prescribing medications and treatments, rendering provisional diagnosis, regular care monitoring, keeping documentation during hospital care, ensuring on-call coverage, and thorough dictation and completion of medical records. These responsibilities conclude only with linking patients to relevant community primary care providers and resource services, as well as making referrals to specialists for transfer of accountability and responsibility (Acorn, 2015b, 2015c; OHA, 2012; RNAO, 2012).

There exists a range of APN care delivery models. NPs may function in a short-term consultative model, similar to clinical nurse specialists. In this role, NPs may support admission and treatment in a shared care dyad with a physician colleague. Those involved in shared care may also discharge patients with prescriptions, necessary referrals, and linkages to community resources (Acorn, 2015a, 2015b).

To date, only a few Ontario hospital organizations are leading early adopters designating NPs as the formal MRP. The Lakeridge Health NP-Led Hospital Model of Care in Whitby is the first pioneering hospital to showcase senior care delivered by NPs designated as the

MRP, and has granted full admitting rights through organizational supports since July 2012 (RNAO, 2012). Hospital gate keeping influences are being realized through cultural shifts, increased awareness, and championing leadership for access for professional equity in fully supporting integrated patient care (Acorn, 2015a, 2015b).

Evidence that hospital-based NP roles positively impact patient care does exist. Insightful information on NPs acting as MRP in primary health care in Canada is also available, although this type of NP hospital role has only been evaluated in the context of consultation and shared care. A mixed methods pilot study in Ontario examined qualitative NP satisfaction surveys, as well as quantitative data related to the total number of admissions and discharges in a community hospital. The staff worked with NPs for an average of four years and found that NPs were able to function as an MRP in hospitals, from admission through discharge. Those acting in the MRP role had high patient, family, and staff satisfaction, in addition to providing quality care. Embracing the full scope of practice for NPs, contributing as the MRP was seen as valuable for full integration (Acorn, 2015a, 2015b). By and large, NPs functioning in the MRP role strive for patient-centred care, quality, experience, and favourable outcomes. Enabling and empowering APNs to be champions of change for optimal patient and organizational success leverages their knowledge and leadership capacity. It is not about NP trailblazing; rather, it is about capitalizing on APNs as health human resource care champions. Nor is it about the transference of power and authority (namely in important prescriptive, diagnostic, and admission privileges). Capitalizing on the APN role is about the power to deliver safe, quality care and to optimize care accountabilities. Ulitimately NP competence and population needs should be the drivers of meaningful change (Acorn, 2015a, 2015b).

Integration of Title Protection for Advanced Practice Nurses in Canada

Transforming health care through professional education and experience is paramount for advanced practice nurses' integration in Canada. APN continues to evolve to meet complex health care system needs, yet doctorally prepared CNSs and NPs are limited in using the title of "doctor" when practicing due to professionally restrictive statutes. The Nursing and Regulated Health Professions Acts in 1991 restricted those who may use this title when providing health care in Ontario. For doctoral-prepared nurses to communicate their education credentials, they only have to write out the degree granted as it appears on their diploma (Acorn, 2015c; CNO, 2013b).

Those APNs registered with the CNO are required to use their protected titles to identify themselves in their practice. (Protected titles include RN or NP.) To date, lobbying efforts to protect the title of the CNS role have been unsuccessful. NPs may add their specialty certifications to their titles, such as NP–PHC, NP–Adult, NP–Pediatrics, or NP–Anesthesia (CNO, 2011). According to the CNO, there are 63 nurses who are registered with a doctorate education; 29 of those are NPs (CNO, 2013b). While APNs are denied the privilege to use their obtained doctoral educational titles, momentum and professional equality will be the driver for recognition and change (Acorn, 2015c).

According to the CNA (2008), the minimum educational preparation for APNs is a graduate degree. One paper put out in 2004 by the American Association of Colleges of Nursing (AACN) advocated for those entering APN roles to be changed from a graduate degree to the **Doctor of Nursing Practice (DNP)** (or equivalent) by 2015. Although the Doctor of Philosophy (PhD) is recognized as the highest distinction in scholarship, academic achievements, and research across all disciplines (including nursing), the DNP is considered the highest degree for the nursing profession, concentrating on direct care, research utilization, improved delivery of care, patient outcomes, and clinical systems management (AACN, 2004, 2014; Acorn, 2015c).

A unified American coalition from seven professional organizations, including the American Association of Nurse Practitioners (AANP), the American College of Nurse Practitioners (ACNP), and the National Organization of Nurse Practitioner Faculties (NONPF), convened regarding DNP education and titling recommendations. This coalition determined that utilization of the title of "doctor" represents an academic credential, and is not limited to a professional program. It was determined that all programs that confer academic degrees permit graduates to be "doctors" and no one discipline owns the title (NP Roundtable, 2008). In the health arena, the term *doctor* is no longer limited to medicine. Recognition of doctoral-educated nurses facilitates parity within the health care system (NP Roundtable, 2008), furthering credibility and legitimacy (Acorn, 2015c).

In 2003, Ontario's Regulated Health Professions Act (RHPA) proclaimed that the title of "doctor" may be used by an RN or NP in academic and social circles, or in conjunction with the delivery of nursing practice. The titles of "nurse, nurse practitioner, and doctor" are protected under the RHPA (Acorn, 2015c).

Parity with other professional disciplines that have established practice doctorates as the standard entry into practice is the desired equitable outcome. Enabling APNs to be champions of change for optimal patient and organizational success leverages their knowledge and leadership practice, and can be both a driver and the solution for delivering safe, quality care. Care should not be defined by geography, profession, or title restrictions. Legally recognizing nurses that have obtained doctorate degrees by authorizing the title of "doctor" for health provider parity, value, and respect is another key step in advancing health care integration. Removing the barriers for professional title protection is key for transforming professional change (Acorn, 2015c).

Conclusion

Implications for practice and scholarship reveal that enabling, empowering, and embracing advanced practice nurses to function at their maximal scope of practice can be highly valuable across the Canadian health care system. Full implementation, integration, and sustainability for models of care is a rich area of exploration through research, utilizing both clinical nurse specialists and nurse practitioners. Experiences and lessons learned require dissemination to enrich the building body of advanced nursing knowledge, and to further inform and leverage full system integration. Full integration, however, is dependent on the desire and ability to practice to full scope, as well as realizing the value-add of APN roles.

Critical Thinking Questions

1. What have been the key facilitators and barriers to full APN integration in Canada?
2. Do you feel that both CNSs and NPs have equally integrated into the Canadian health care system?
3. Identify three strategies to facilitate further integration and how these would be beneficial.

References

Acorn, M. (2015a). How does the nurse practitioner as the most responsible provider affect care in seniors age 65 and older admitted to hospitals in Ontario, Canada? *International Journal of Nursing & Clinical Practices, 2*(158). Retrieved from http://dx.doi.org/10.15344/2394-4978/2015/158

Acorn, M. (2015b). Nurse practitioners as most responsible providers: Impact on care for seniors admitted to an Ontario hospital. *International Journal of Nursing & Clinical Practices, 2*(126). Retrieved from http://dx.doi.org/10.15344/2394-4978/2015/126

Acorn, M. (2015c). Title protection policy for doctoral nursing education in Ontario, Canada. *International Journal of Nursing & Clinical Practices, 2*(116). Retrieved from http://dx.doi.org/10.15344/2394-4978/2015/116

American Association of Colleges of Nursing (AACN). (2004). *AACN position statement on the practice doctorate in nursing, October 2004.* Retrieved from http://www.aacn.nche.edu/publications/position/DNPpositionstatement.pdf

AACN. (2014). *DNP fact sheet: The doctor of nursing practice (DNP).* Retrieved from https://www.aacn.nche.edu/media-relations/fact-sheets/dnp

Bryant-Lukosius, D., Carter, N., Kilpatrick, K., Martin-Misener, R., Donald, F., Kaasalainen S., & DiCenso, A. (2010). The clinical nurse specialist role in Canada. *Nursing Leadership, 23*(Special Issue December), 140–166.

Canadian Institute for Health Information (CIHI). (2013) *Regulated nurses: Canadian trends, 2007 to 2011.* Retrieved from https://secure.cihi.ca/free_products/Regulated_Nurses_EN.pdf

CIHI. (2014). *Regulated nurses, 2013*. Retrieved from https://secure.cihi.ca/free_products/ Nursing-Workforce-2013_EN.pdf

Canadian Nurses Association (CNA). (2008). *Advance nursing practice: A national framework.* Ottawa, ON: CNA. Retrieved from http://www.cna-aiic.ca/~/media/cna/page-content/ pdf-en/anp_national_framework_e.pdf

CNA. (2011). *Collaborative integration plan for the role of nurse practitioners in Canada: 2011– 2015*. Ottawa, ON: CNA. Retrieved from http://www.npnow.ca/docs/Integration_Plan_for_ the_Nurse_Practitioner_Role-En.pdf

CNA. (2012). *2010 workforce profile of nurse practitioners in Canada*. Ottawa, ON: CNA. Retrieved from http://www.cna-aiic.ca/~/media/cna/page-content/pdf-en/2010_np_pro-files_e.pdf

Carter, N., Martin-Misener, R., Kilpatrick, K., Kaasalainen, S., Donald, F., Bryant-Lukosius, D., & DiCenso, A. (2010). The role of nursing leadership in integrating clinical nurse specialists and nurse practitioners in health care delivery in Canada. *Nursing Leadership, 23*(Special Issue December), 167–185.

College of Nurses of Ontario (CNO). (2011). *Practice standard: Nurse practitioner.* Retrieved from http://www.cno.org/Global/docs/prac/41038_StrdRnec.pdf

CNO. (2013a). *FAQ: Bill 179*. Retrieved from http://www.cno.org/en/what-is-cno/regula-tion-and-legislation/legislation-governing-nursing/faq-bill-179/

CNO. (2013b). *Membership totals at a glance*. Retrieved from http://www.cno.org/what-is-cno/ nursing-demographics/membership-totals-at-a-glance/

DiCenso, A., Bryant-Lukosius, D., Martin-Misener, R., Donald, F., Bourgeault, I., Kilpatrick, K., … Harbman, P. (2010). Factors enabling advanced practice nursing role integration in Canada. *Nursing Leadership, 23*(Special Issue December), 211–238.

Dierick-van Daele, A.T., Metsemakers, J.F., Derckx, E.W., Spreeuwenberg, C., & Vrijhoef, H.J. (2008). Nurse practitioners substituting for general practitioners: Randomized controlled trial. *Journal of Advanced Nursing, 65*(2), 391–401.

Donald, F., Bryant-Lukosius, D., Martin-Misener, R. Kaasalainen, S., Kilpatrick, K., Carter, N., & DiCenso, A. (2010a). Clinical nurse specialist and nurse practitioners: Title confusion and lack of role clarity. *Nursing Leadership, 23*(Special Issue December), 189–201.

Donald, F., Martin-Misener, R., Bryant-Lukosius, Kilpatrick, K., Kaasalainen, S., Carter, N., DiCenso, A. (2010b). The primary health care nurse practitioner role in Canada. *Nursing Leadership, 23*(Special Issue December), 88–113.

Government of Manitoba. (2015). *Primary care*. Winnipeg, MB: Gov.MB. Retrieved from http:// www.gov.mb.ca/health/primarycare/providers/index.html

Government of Ontario. (1991). *Regulated Health Professions Act, 1991, S.O. 1991, Chapter 18*. Toronto, ON: MOHLTC. Retrieved from http://www.e-laws.gov.on.ca/html/statutes/english/ elaws_statutes_91r18_e.htm#BK30

Hurlock-Chorostecki, C., Forchuk, C., Orchard, C., van Soeren, M., & Reeves, S. (2013). Hospital-based nurse practitioner roles and interprofessional practice: A scoping review. *Nursing & Health Sciences, 16*(3), 403–410.

Hurlock-Chorostecki, C., van Soeren, M., & Goodwin, S. (2008). The acute care nurse practi-tioner in Ontario: A workforce study. *Nursing Leadership, 21*(4), 100–116.

Integration (2014). In Merriam-Webster Encyclopedia Online. Retrieved from http://www. merriam-webster.com/dictionary/integration

Irvine, D., Sidani, S., Porter, H., O'Brien-Pallas, L., Simpson, B., McGillis Hall, L., ... Nagel, L. (2000). Organizational factors influencing nurse practitioners' role implementation in acute care settings. *Canadian Journal of Nursing Leadership, 13*(13), 28–35.

Jones, M.L. (2005). Role development and effective practice in specialist and advanced practice roles in acute care hospital settings: Systematic review and meta-synthesis. *Journal of Advanced Nursing, 49*(2), 191–209.

Kilpatrick, K., DiCenso, A., Bryant-Lukosius, D., Ritchie, J. A., Martin-Misener, R., & Carter, N. (2013). Pratice patterns and perceived impact of clinical nurse specialist roles in Canada: Results of a national survey. *International Journal of Nursing Studies, 50*(11), 1524–1536. doi:http://dx.doi.org/10.1016/j.ijnurstu.2013.03.005

Kilpatrick, K., Harbman, P., Carter, N., Martin-Misener, R., Bryant-Lukosius, D., Donald, F., ... DiCenso, A. (2010). The acute care nurse practitioner role in Canada. *Nursing Leadership, 23*(Special Issue December), 114–139.

Kilpatrick, K., Lavoie-Tremblay, M., Ritchie, J.A., Lamothe, L., & Doran, D. (2012a). Boundary work and the introduction of acute care nurse practitioners in healthcare teams. *Journal of Advanced Nursing, 68*(7), 1504–1515.

Kilpatrick, K., Lavoie-Tremblay, M., Ritchie, J.A., Lamothe, L., Doran, D., & Rochefort, C. (2012b). How are acute care nurse practitioners enacting their roles in healthcare teams? A descriptive multi-case study. *International Journal of Nursing Studies, 49*(7), 850–862.

Ministry of Health and Long-Term Care (MOHLTC). (2010). *Excellent Care for All Act.* Toronto, ON: MOHLTC. Retrieved from http://www.health.gov.on.ca/en/pro/programs/ecfa/legislation/

MOHLTC (2014). *Nurse practitioner-led clinics.* Toronto, ON: MOHLTC.

Mundinger, M., Kane, R., Lenz, E., Totten, A., Tsai, W., Cleary, P., & Shelanski, M. (2000). Primary care outcomes in patients treated by nurse practitioners or physicians: A randomized trial. *Journal of the American Medical Association, 238*(1), 59–86.

Nurse Practitioner Roundtable. (2008). Nurse practitioner DNP education, certification, and titling: A unified statement. Retrieved from http://c.ymcdn.com/sites/www.nonpf.org/resource/resmgr/imported/DNPUnifiedStatement0608.pdf

Ontario Hospital Association (OHA). (2012). *Enabling nurse practitioners to admit and discharge: A guide for hospitals.* Toronto, ON: OHA. Retrieved from http://www.oha.com/CurrentIssues/keyinitiatives/PhysicianandProfessionalIssues/Physicians/Resources/Documents/Final%20-%20NP%20Guide.pdf

Registered Nurses' Association of Ontario (RNAO). (2012). *Nurse practitioner utilization toolkit.* Toronto, ON: RNAO. Retrieved from http://rnao.ca/resources/toolkits/np-toolkit

Sackett, D.L., Spitzer, W.O., Gent, M., & Roberts, R.S. (1974). The Burlington randomized trial of the nurse practitioner: Health outcomes of patients. *Annals of Internal Medicine, 80*(2), 137–142.

van Soeren, M., & Hurlock-Chorostecki, C. (2009). *The integration of specialty nurse practitioners into the Ontario healthcare system.* Toronto, ON: NPAO. Retrieved from http://npao.org/nursepractitioners/specialty-project/

van Soeren, M., Hurlock-Chorostecki, C., & Reeves, S. (2011). The role of the nurse practitioners in hospital settings: Implications for interprofessional practice. *Journal of Interprofessional Care, 25*(4), 245–251.

van Soeren, M., & Micevski, V. (2001). Success indicators and barriers to acute nurse practitioner role implementation in four Ontario hospitals. *AACN Clinical Issues, 12*(3), 424–437.

Chapter 3

Understanding Regulatory, Legislative, and Credentialing Requirements

Lynn Miller

Lynn Miller is a Consultant in Policy, Practice, and Legislative Services at the College of Registered Nurses of Nova Scotia (CRNNS) in Halifax. She has acted in the past as an NP educator and is currently an NP–Family/All Ages at her practice in rural Nova Scotia.

KEY TERMS

competencies
legislation
regulation
self-regulation
standards

OBJECTIVES

1. Explore the evolution of advanced practice nursing (APN) legislation and regulation in Canada.
2. Explore the concepts of regulation and self-regulation in APN.
3. Examine the regulation and legislation of clinical nurse specialists (CNS) and nurse practitioners (NP).
4. Explore the concept of Right Touch Regulation.

Introduction

Registered nurses (RNs), including advanced practice nurses (APN), are self-regulated professionals. This privilege, granted by government through legislation, is grounded in the regulatory mandate of public protection. This chapter will explore the regulatory, legislative licensure, and credentialing of APNs in Canada. The principles and processes of self-regulation are explored as they apply to nursing in general, and then to the clinical nurse specialist (CNS) and nurse practitioner (NP) roles. It concludes with a look at Right Touch Regulation, an evolving approach that more proactively manages risk within the regulatory mandate of public protection.

What is Self-Regulation?

Public protection is a basic principle of our federal and provincial governmental structure; whether an individual is purchasing food or electronics at a local store, negotiating a mortgage at their bank, or seeking public or private health care services. Self-regulation is defined as

> a regulatory model which enables government to have some control over the practice of a profession and the services provided by its members but without having to maintain the special in-depth expertise required to regulate a profession that would be required under direct regulation. (Balthazard, 2010, p. 2)

This approach is widely used by Canadian health care regulators, including nursing regulators, to fulfill the public protection mandate delegated to them by both federal and provincial legislation (Balthazard, 2010).

Nursing has been accorded the privilege of self-regulation through provincial legislation, as it meets the definition of a profession; namely "it holds its practitioners accountable, possesses a specialized body of knowledge, emphasizes the competent application of knowledge, follows a code of ethics, has a tradition of the provision of service to the public, and engages in self-regulation" (Uhlich, Giblin, & Michaud, 2007, p. 4). Self-regulation of nurses in Canada is also guided by the International Council of Nurses' (ICN) principles of professional regulation, originally adopted as a list of 10 in 1985 and revised in 2013 with the addition of three statements (ICN, 2013).

The privilege of self-regulation is a dual responsibility of the regulatory body and its members; in this case nursing regulators and RNs (Balthazard, 2010; Canadian Nurses Association [CNA], 2007; Randall, 2000). Individual nurses must follow their professional standards and code of ethics no matter where they practice, while the regulator is accountable to ensure that its members' activities are in the public interest at all times (College of Nurses of Ontario [CNO], 2012; College of Registered Nurses of Nova Scotia [CRNNS], 2011). While accomplished differently across jurisdictions, the primary role of regulatory bodies in self-regulation includes "promoting good nursing practice, preventing poor nursing practice [and] intervening when practice is unacceptable" (CRNNS, 2011, p. 5). To achieve their mandate, regulators establish requirements for initial entry to practice, registration and licensure, approve education programs based on competencies, develop standards of practice, provide continuing competence resources for their members, and develop professional conduct processes when practice concerns are identified (CRNNS, 2014; Randall, 2000).

Understanding Nursing Regulation

Advanced practice nurses were not part of the nursing landscape until the mid-20th century, although there are historical accounts of APNs working in Newfoundland and Labrador and the Northwest Territories in the 1890s due to a lack of available physicians (Kaasalainen et al., 2010) (see Chapter 1). Because both the CNS and NP roles are grounded in nursing, they have been and are subject to the same legislation and regulations that apply to the profession as a whole; with additional legislation and regulations being enacted to define the NP scope of practice as the role evolved.

To better grasp the regulation of these advanced practice roles, it is essential to first lay the foundation for registered nurse regulation in Canada; specifically defining concepts such as legislation, regulations, registration, licensure, competencies, standards and scope of practice, and the differences between the college and association models of regulation. While these concepts are presented sequentially, they are better envisioned as the interwoven threads of the fabric of nursing regulation. In addition, unless otherwise specified, the term *nurse* will be used throughout the chapter to denote registered RNs, CNSs, and NPs.

Federal and Provincial Legislation and Regulation

First, legislation is another term for a law or statute, both of which may be created and passed at the federal, provincial, and/or territorial level to define the rights and responsibilities of government and citizens to govern individual and societal conduct, as well as to guide the delivery of services such as health care and justice (Government of Canada, 2001). Whereas the federal government enacts legislation that applies to the entire country, provincial or territorial governments enact laws that define how health, education, local resources, and municipal services are delivered within their individual jurisdictions (Government of Canada, 2001). For example, the Canada Health Act (R. S. C., 1985, c. C-6) outlines the federal government's obligations with respect to the funding of health services for Canadians, while the Canadian Constitution Act gives authority and accountability for administration of health care, including the regulation of professionals such as nurses, to the provincial/territorial governments (Department of Justice, 2015; Jackman, 2000; McMillan, 2010).

For the purposes of regulating health professionals, including RNs and APNs, provincial/territorial governments have created their own acts and regulations. These share a common purpose but take very different approaches across jurisdictions depending on population needs, stakeholder input, and governmental mandates and philosophies. One of the most important aspects of self-regulation is the legislated privilege of title protection, which restricts the use of "RN" (for registered nurses) and "NP" (for nurse practitioners) to members of a nursing regulatory body (CNA, 2007).

In governmental legislative parlance, **regulation** is both an entity and an action. As the former, a regulation is a type of law made to further define how legislation is interpreted, applied, and enforced. While an act or legislation is made at the broader federal or provincial government level, the responsibility for creating regulations is delegated to a ministry, department, or agency operating within that level of government. Regulations can only be developed when there is authority to do so in the related Act (Government of Canada, 2001). As an action, regulation is a responsibility of a provincial ministry or department, or is designated by legislation to another body such as a professional college or association, which is how self-regulation of the nursing profession is enabled (Balthazard, 2010; Randall, 2000).

Governance of Regulatory Bodies

In fulfilling their mandate of public protection, regulators face a two-fold accountability: the regulation of their members as well as regulation of their own activities. In Canada, most regulators have adopted a council or board structure to meet their self-monitoring obligations. This approach, often referred to as *policy governance*, is grounded in the assumption that the council or board is responsible for providing governance in the interest of the organization's owners, which for nursing is the public. Comprised of nursing and non-nursing members, the council/board is responsible for determining the strategic direction and accountabilities of the regulatory body, but is not involved with making decisions on how the work is done (Carver & Carver, 2001). Through the development of the policies and bylaws that define how the regulatory body carries out its day-to-day business, the council/board can ensure the public protection mandate is upheld, which is a cornerstone in professional self-regulation (CNA, 2006; CNO, 2013).

College and Association Regulatory Structures

There are currently two structures or models of nursing regulatory bodies in place in Canada: the college model and the association model. Under the college model, the regulatory body's legislated mandate and raison d'être is public protection through regulation of its members (College of Registered Nurses of Manitoba [CRNM], 2015b; RN Network of BC, 2010). Conversely, professional associations focus on the interests of their members through advocacy for their professional efforts and contributing to public policy development (College and Association of Registered Nurses of Alberta [CARNA], 2015b; CRNNS, 2009b; Nurses Association of New Brunswick [NANB], 2015b; RN Network of BC, 2010). Those who support the college model argue that professional associations could place themselves in a conflict of interest situation if forced to choose between representing their members or protecting the public; specifically, "the underlying premise of self-regulation dictates that public interest must prevail" (CRNNS, 2009b, p. 14). Both colleges and associations are recognized in Canada, although the latter is actually a blended model by virtue of provincial/territorial legislation that mandates their regulatory role in public protection (RN Network of BC, 2010; CNA, 2007). Table 3.1 summarizes the current regulatory model in place in each jurisdiction and enabling legislation.

TABLE 3.1: Regulators by Province and Enabling Legislation	
Province/Territory	**Name of Legislation**
Association of Registered Nurses of Newfoundland and Labrador (ARNNL)	Registered Nurses Act
Association of Registered Nurses of Prince Edward Island (ARNPEI)	Nurses Act
College of Registered Nurses of Nova Scotia (CRNNS)	Registered Nurses Act
Nurses Association of New Brunswick (NANB)	Nurses Act
L'Ordre des infirmières et infirmiers du Québec (OIIQ)	Nurses Act
College of Nurses of Ontario (CNO)	Regulated Health Professions Act
College of Registered Nurses of Manitoba (CRNM)	Registered Nurses Act
Saskatchewan Registered Nurses' Association (SRNA)	Registered Nurses Act
College and Association of Registered Nurses of Alberta (CARNA)	Public Health Act/Health Professions Act
College of Registered Nurses of British Columbia (CRNBC)	Health Professions Act
Yukon Registered Nurses Association (YRNA)	Registered Nurses Profession Act
*Northwest Territories Registered Nurses Association (NWTRNA)/**Registered Nurses Association of Northwest Territories and Nunavut (RNANT/NU)	*Nursing Profession Act/ **Nunavut Nursing Profession Act

Source: Adapted from Elliott, Rutty, & Villeneuve, 2013.

Regulatory Concepts

Nursing regulators rely on several key terms to define their structures and processes. While the definition of these terms may differ across jurisdictions and although they are sometimes used interchangeably, the intent of the concepts is fairly consistent across Canada: a critical requirement for mobility of professionals under the Agreement on Internal Trade (Internal Trade Secretariat, 2009).

Registration and Licensure

The term *registration* is used by some jurisdictions to encompass licensure and certification; however, it specifically defines the presence of a nurse's name on their regulatory body's membership list or register. Registration is considered the broadest, and potentially weakest, form of regulation (Balthazard, 2010; Randall, 2000). Licensure is considered more restrictive and not only defines the requirements for those who wish to practice nursing, but also restricts this privilege to those who have an active license (Balthazard, 2010). Criteria for registration and licensure vary across provinces but may include the completion of an education program approved by the regulator, successful completion of appropriate licensure examinations, proof of a minimum number of hours in active practice, jurisprudence examinations, and completion of continuing competency activities, as well as character or criminal record checks (Balthazard, 2010; CNO, 2013; CRNNS, 2014). Differences in registration and licensure for CNSs and NPs will be discussed later in this chapter.

In some jurisdictions, including Manitoba, New Brunswick, and Prince Edward Island, nurses may practice once their name appears on their regulatory body's register (Government of Manitoba, 2015; Government of New Brunswick, 2002; Government of Prince Edward Island, 2014), while in others registration alone does not grant a member the authority to practice nursing. In Nova Scotia, Saskatchewan, Newfoundland and Labrador, and the Yukon, a nurse must be listed on the provincial/territorial register in order to be granted a license to practice (Government of Newfoundland and Labrador, 2009; Government of Saskatchewan, 1988; Registered Nurses Act, 2006; Yukon Legislative Council Office, 2009). The terms *practice permit* and *certificate of registration* are used elsewhere, including Alberta, Ontario, the Northwest Territories, and Nunavut (Government of the Northwest Territories, 2010; Province of Alberta, 2013; Government of Ontario, 1991) to denote the authority to practice granted by the regulator in that province.

Competencies

Competencies are statements describing the knowledge, skills, and judgment expected of a nurse in order to provide competent, safe, and ethical care to their clients (CNA, 2010; CRNNS, 2011). Competency statements serve many purposes, including guiding content for education programs and entry to practice examinations required for registration/licensure, acting as a framework for competence assessment by regulatory bodies, supporting self-reflection and direction for the nurse continuing competence activities, and informing government, employers, clients, and other stakeholders about the services in which the nurse is educated and competent to provide (Canadian Council of Registered Nurse Regulators [CCRNR], 2015; CNA, 2007, 2010; CARNA, 2011; CRNNS, 2011).

In 2010, the CNA released the *Canadian Nurse Practitioner Core Competency Framework*, an updated version of the original 2005 document that arose from the Canadian Nurse

Practitioner Initiative, a national research project examining NP practice and role integration in Canada (CNA, 2010). Many regulators adapted or adopted this competency framework to guide NP practice in their jurisdiction. In 2014, the CNA released the *Pan-Canadian Core Competencies for the Clinical Nurse Specialist*, which similarly outlines the expectations for CNS services across various practice settings. No matter their role, however, CNSs and NPs are expected to integrate registered nurse competencies with their own in providing client care (Black et al., 2008; CRNNS, 2013). CNS and NP competencies will be addressed later.

Standards

Standards are authoritative statements that define the expected behaviours and professional and legal accountabilities for individual nursing practice. They serve to guide practice and provide benchmarks for assessing provider performance in their interactions with clients and the public (CRNNS, 2009a). Once again, there are jurisdictional differences in the application of the term *standards*, with the College of Registered Nurses of British Columbia (CRNBC) referring to standards as limits and conditions while the Saskatchewan Registered Nurses Association (SRNA) combine standards and core competencies (CRNBC, 2015a; SRNA, 2011). Currently, CNS practice in Canada is measured against RN standards of practice while NPs must adhere to these as well as their own standards of practice established within each jurisdiction.

Scope of Practice

Scope of practice is an intricate relationship between the context of practice (which involves the nurse, the client, and the practice setting), the competencies and standards of practice, and jurisdictional legislation and regulations; it must be considered from the lens of both the profession and the individual nurse. The scope of the nursing profession delineates "the outer limits of practice for all members at the same time retaining flexibility so that establishing rigid boundaries does not threaten the ability of the profession to grow and develop" (CRNNS, 2009a, p. 8). Individual scope of practice is shaped by the needs of the individual nurse's client population, the practice setting, education, and regulatory and employer policies that permit or limit specific interventions (CRNM, 2010; CRNNS, 2009a). In addition to regulations and legislation, British Columbia, Ontario, and Alberta further define scope of practice for all nurses using controlled or restricted acts (CNO, 2011; Schiller, 2015). This model identifies procedures or interventions that are considered high risk and require additional educational preparation before a nurse is authorized to perform then (Schiller, 2015). As health care providers' roles evolve, there is some overlap of scope, making it critical for nurses to understand and work within their professional and individual boundaries.

Nursing Regulation in Canada: Then and Now

In the late 19th century, nursing as a profession was in its infancy; it lacked the ability to control who could profess to be a nurse and was without consistent requirements for education or training. Two groups, the American Society of Superintendents of Training Schools for Nurses of the United States and Canada (formed in 1893) and the Associated Alumnae of the United States and Canada (formed in 1896), began the arduous process of developing registration processes and standardizing education to advance the profession and make nursing accountable to the public (McIntyre & McDonald, 2010). After recognizing that political differences between the two countries necessitated separate organizations, efforts continued in Canada to produce a national approach to regulatory legislation. However, even in the early 20th century, it quickly became apparent that regional and provincial interests would limit the viability of this national legislative framework (Elliot, Rutty, & Villeneuve, 2013). This marked the beginning of nursing regulation in Canada as provincial and territorial legislation gradually emerged that created nursing regulatory bodies. Provincial and territorial regulatory bodies and the year they were founded are shown in Figure 3.1; but it is important to note that some organizational names have changed as their governance models evolved, or through amalgamation (as with the Northwest Territories and Nunavut in 2004).

Opposition to this movement came from many fronts in the early stages, including physicians and politicians "who believed that their patients and constituents would be better served by an unregulated nursing marketplace [and] the fuss over legislation [would] put nurses in even greater danger of losing the womanly feelings of 'sympathy' and 'heart' so necessary ... to proper nursing service" (K. MacPherson, as cited in Elliot et al., 2013, p. 37).

From its inception in 1908, the CNA assumed a leadership role for nursing in Canada, including advocating for the nursing profession, policy development for nursing and health care, and nursing regulation. CNA's role in regulation expanded in 1970 when the need for a national registered nurse examination was recognized, and then further in 2005 when they introduced the Canadian Nurse Practitioner Examination (CNPE) for Primary Health Care or Family/All Ages NPs (Elliot et al., 2013). Throughout this tenure, the CNA supported the concept of a pan-Canadian regulatory framework (CNA, 2007) and developed the NP Core Competency Framework (CNA, 2010) and *Advanced Nursing Practice: A National Framework* (CNA, 2008). In addition, a literature review of NP legislation and regulation in Canada, the United States, the United Kingdom, Australia, and New Zealand was completed as part of the Canadian Nurse Practitioner Initiative (CNPI) to demonstrate the benefits of a national NP regulatory framework (Tarrant & Associates, 2005); however, this did not come to fruition.

The current approach to professional regulation is not without it challenges; despite sharing a similar mandate, the 12 nursing regulators have diverse processes to achieve it. Studies by Pulcini, Jelic, Gul, and Loke (2010) and Kleinpell et al. (2014) suggest that the variations in provincial/territorial legislation and regulation have contributed to existing barriers to CNS

FIGURE 3.1: Provincial and Territorial Regulatory Bodies and Year Founded

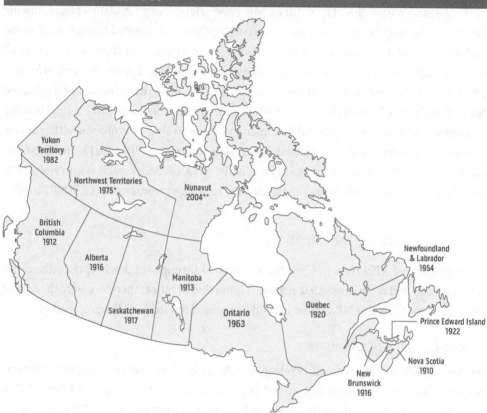

Source: Adapted from Elliott, Rutty, & Villeneuve, 2013. Reprinted with permission.

* Registered Nurses Association of Northwest Territories 1975-2004
** Registered Nurses Association of Northwest Territories and Nunavut after 2004

and NP role implementation and scope of practice. McDonald, Herbert, and Thibeault (2006) blamed this situation on "a patchwork of legislations and regulations governing all types of advanced practice nursing" (p. 176); however, given the differences in provincial legislation and nursing regulatory models, national consensus would be challenging.

In addition, amendments to federal and provincial legislation and regulations, while reflective of evolution of the system to meet population need and expanded scope of APN roles, can create inconsistencies and barriers to practice due to delays in enacting the changes (Calnan & Fahey-Walsh, 2005). One example is the ongoing process of authorizing NPs to prescribe controlled drugs and substances (CDS) across Canada. While the New Classes of Practitioners Regulations (Department of Justice, 2013), passed in November 2012, amended the federal Controlled Drugs and Substances Act (Department of Justice, 2012) to include NPs as authorized CDS prescribers, changes are still pending to both provincial governmental legislation and regulations and regulatory standards and policies in some jurisdictions.

In the early part of the 21st century, some provincial nursing regulators began moving away from the association model toward the college model, prompted by increased public and governmental scrutiny of existing self-regulation practices and processes across all professions (Lahey, 2011). Recognizing their legislated mandate of public protection as their priority, Canada's twelve nursing regulators formed the Canadian Council of Registered Nurse Regulators (CCRNR) in 2011. CCRNR "promotes excellence in professional nursing regulation and serves as a national forum and voice regarding interprovincial/territorial, national, and global regulatory matters for nursing regulation" (2014, p. 1). The organization's priorities include some previously under the CNA umbrella, such as entry-level RN and NP examinations and developing a national regulatory framework (CCRNR, 2014).

APN Regulation in Canada

The regulation of APN roles in Canada, as discussed throughout this chapter, falls within the same acts and regulations that regulate all nursing practice; therefore only the salient differences for CNS and NP regulation will be pointed out in the following section.

Clinical Nurse Specialists

As pointed out by DiCenso and colleagues (2010) in their decision support synthesis research, "CNS practice does not extend beyond the scope of the registered nurse (RN), regulation is not required for this role" (p. 217), and as such the term *CNS* is not a protected title. This lack of a CNS-specific credential has been recognized as a barrier to the sustainability of the CNS role, but falls outside the regulators' mandate (Bryant-Lukosius et al., 2010). In an effort to promote the CNS role, the CNA led a panel of advanced practice nurses (CNSs and NPs), nurse educators, and a regulatory representative to develop the *Pan-Canadian Core Competencies for the Clinical Nurse Specialist* (CNA, 2014). While this document is not likely to have an immediate impact on changes to CNS regulation, it will serve to clarify the CNS role for clients, colleagues, employers, and government.

Nurse Practitioners

As the NP role evolved across Canada, provincial governments and regulatory bodies recognized the need for legislation and regulation to authorize the expanded scope of practice and associated accountability of NP practice (Canadian Institute for Health Information [CIHI], 2006; DiCenso et al., 2010; Donald et al., 2010). Most regulators adopted or adapted the *Canadian Nurse Practitioner Core Competency Framework* (CNA, 2010) to develop and approve NP education programs, with graduate education recognized as the preferred minimum requirement for entry to practice (Kaasalainen et al., 2010). In addition, they developed NP standards of practice and continuing competency requirements for ongoing licensure. Table 3.2 summarizes NP provincial legislation and the year it was enacted, as well as the act providing the authority for NP practice.

There are currently four streams of NP practice recognized in Canada: primary health care or family/all ages, pediatrics, adult, and neonatal; however, not every province has NPs working in all streams. For example, New Brunswick registers only primary health care NPs while Quebec certifies primary care, neonatal, and NP–nephrology and NP–cardiology (NANB, 2015a). In addition, while some regulators license NPs by their practice stream or specialty (Association of Registered Nurses of Newfoundland and Labrador [ARNNL], 2014; CARNA, 2015a), others do so under a single NP category and regulate specialty practice through statutory committees and other internal regulatory mechanisms (CRNNS, 2009a).

An important defining element of NP legislation is title protection; similar to restrictions on use of the title RN, only those who have met the regulatory requirements for NP registration and/or licensure in a jurisdiction may use the title of NP or one of the accepted variants including RN(EC) in Ontario, RN(NP) in Saskatchewan, or RN(EP) in Manitoba (CNO, 2011; CRNM, 2015a; SRNA, 2011).

TABLE 3.2: Nurse Practitioner Legislation by Province and Year of Initial Legislation

Province/Territory	Year	Name of Legislation
Newfoundland and Labrador	1997	Registered Nurses Act
Prince Edward Island	2006	Nurses Act
Nova Scotia	2002	Registered Nurses Act
New Brunswick	2002	Nurses Act
Quebec	2003	Nurses Act
Ontario	1997	Regulated Health Professions Act
Manitoba	2005	Registered Nurses Act
Saskatchewan	2003	Registered Nurses Act
Alberta	1996	Public Health Act
British Columbia	2005	Health Professions Act
Yukon	2009	Registered Nurses Profession Act
Northwest Territories/Nunavut	2004	Nursing Profession Act/Nunavut Nursing Profession Act

Source: Adapted from Canadian Institute for Health Information (CIHI), 2006; Kaasalainen et al., 2010.

Looking to the Future of APN Regulation

Relational Regulation and Right Touch Regulation

Professional regulators are often perceived negatively for their role in monitoring and policing their member's activities, a perception that may have been reinforced for some RNs with the move by some regulators from the association model to the college model. In addition, regulation has traditionally taken a reactive approach to addressing performance that falls below expectations and standards set by regulatory bodies; however, this trend has come into question as consumers, governments, and other stakeholders are encouraged to question a profession's self-regulatory practices (Casey, 2008; CRNBC, 2012; Penney, Bayne, & Johansen, 2014). A new approach to self-regulation, called "relational regulation," challenges regulators to find alternative ways to promote safe practice and improve the quality of care delivered in ways other than by imposing more stringent rules on health care providers through building relationships with their members and other stakeholders (Cayton & Webb, 2014). These relationships do not prevent regulators from meeting their mandate of public protection, but enables them to connect with their members in a way that encourages a collaborative approach to meeting the professional mandate.

CRNBC led the way in Canada for adoption of relational regulation, with Nova Scotia following shortly behind. In their strategic plan, CRNBC (2015b) outlines the basic principles upon which relational regulation is based, including the aforementioned relationship building, simplified communication that looks outward to serve the public rather than inward for the regulator, acceptance of mistakes and an approach to risk reduction that is collaborative and open, adoption of a *right touch* approach to regulation, and the use of principles to guide regulatory decisions.

Right Touch Regulation uses evidence-informed strategies to assess risk so as to more appropriately target resources to manage it (Peterson & Fensling, 2011). The same evidence-informed decision-making that CNSs and NPs use to deliver care can be employed by their regulatory bodies to proactively identify potential risks or problems before deciding on a solution (Bayne, 2012), which is the reverse of the more reactive approach to professional regulation that exists at the present time. Nursing regulators in British Columbia and Nova Scotia are actively pursuing the right touch philosophy (Bayne, 2012; Brennan, 2013); it will be interesting to see if the trend continues across Canada.

Just Culture

Just Culture is a risk management approach that is part of the relational regulation philosophy and is being explored by health care regulators. Just Culture acknowledges that errors can happen for both human and system reasons and the best way forward is not to assess blame; instead these are opportunities to learn and change. Just Culture calls for changing priorities from provider-centric adherence to rules that focus more on avoiding harm while working with patients to reach their desired health outcomes. This proactive rather than reactive approach calls providers to base decisions on best evidence, and to collaborate with patients and other health care providers to support safe, quality care (Bayne, 2012).

Conclusion

APNs enjoy the privilege of self-regulation, but with this privilege comes an obligation to ground their practice within the legislative and regulatory boundaries within their jurisdiction. As advanced practice roles continue to evolve and be integrated into Canada's health care system, it is incumbent upon CNSs and NPs to be active participants in the regulatory process in order to fulfill their single and shared responsibility for public protection. Groundbreaking approaches to regulation (including Just Culture) and relational regulation (including principles of Right Touch Regulation) must be explored as mechanisms to support the evolution of APNs and the nursing profession as a whole.

Critical Thinking Questions

1. What are the implications of granting title protection for CNSs for government legislators and professional regulations?
2. How does the concept of Right Touch Regulation differ from the current model being used by your professional regulatory body?
3. Can Right Touch Regulation be applied to health care providers who work in interprofessional or collaborative teams?
4. How do the principles of labour mobility outlined in the Agreement on Internal Trade impact movement of CNSs and NPs across jurisdictional boundaries?

References

Association of Registered Nurses of Newfoundland and Labrador (ARNNL). (2014). *Nurse practitioner: Streams of practice.* St. John's, NL: ARNNL. Retrieved from https://www.arnnl. ca/nurse-practitioner

Balthazard, C. (2010). *What does it mean to be regulated?* Human Resources Professionals Association. Toronto, ON: HRPA. Retrieved from http://www.hrpa.ca/RegulationandHRDesignations/ Documents/Apr11_2014_What_does_it_mean_to_be_regulated.pdf

Bayne, L. (2012). *Underlying philosophies and trends affecting professional regulation.* Vancouver, BC: CRNBC. Retrieved from https://www.crnbc.ca/crnbc/Documents/783_framework.pdf

Black, J., Allen, D., Redfern, L., Muzio, L., Rushowick, B., Balaski, B., ... Round, B. (2008). Competencies in the context of entry-level registered nurse practice: A collaborative project in Canada. *International Nursing Review, 55*(2), 171–178.

Brennan, M. (2013). *Regulatory excellence framework*. Halifax, NS: CRNNSR. Retrieved from https://crnns.ca/wp-content/uploads/2015/02/CRNNSRegulatoryExcellence FrameworkArticle2013.pdf

Bryant-Lukosius, D., Carter, N., Kilpatrick, K., Martin-Misener, R., Donald, F., Kaasalainen, S., ... DiCenso, A. (2010). The clinical nurse specialist role in Canada. *Nursing Leadership, 23*(Special Issue December), 140–166.

Calnan, R., & Fahey-Walsh, J. (2005). *Practice consultation initial report*. Ottawa, ON: CNA. Retrieved from http://www.npnow.ca/docs/tech-report/section3/02_Practice_AppendixA.pdf

Canadian Council of Registered Nurse Regulators (CCRNR). (2014). *2013–2014 highlights*. Beaverton, ON: CCRNR. Retrieved from http://www.ccrnr.ca/assets/2013-2014-ccrnr-high-lights---final.pdf

CCRNR. (2015). *Competencies in the context of entry-level registered nurse practice*. Beaverton, ON: CCRNR. Retrieved from http://www.ccrnr.ca/entry-to-practice.html

Canadian Institute for Health Information (CIHI). (2006). *The regulation and supply of nurse practitioners in Canada: 2006 update*. Ottawa, ON: CIHI. Retrieved from http://publications. gc.ca/collections/Collection/H115-34-2006E.pdf

Canadian Nurses Association (CNA). (2006). *Canadian nurse practitioner initiative technical report*. Ottawa, ON: CNA. Retrieved from http://www.npnow.ca/docs/tech-report/section2 /01_Legislation_Regulation.pdf

CNA. (2007). *Understanding self-regulation*. Ottawa, ON: CNA. Retrieved from http://www. nurseone.ca/~/media/nurseone/files/en/nn_understanding_self_regulation_e.pdf?la=en

CNA. (2008). *Advanced nursing practice; A national framework*. Ottawa, ON: CNA. Retrieved from http://www.nanb.nb.ca/PDF/practice/ANP_National_Framework_e.pdf

CNA. (2010). *Canadian nurse practitioner core competency framework*. Retrieved from http:// www.cno.org/Global/for/rnec/pdf/CompetencyFramework_en.pdf

CNA. (2014). *Pan-Canadian core competencies for the clinical nurse specialist*. Ottawa, ON: CNA. Retrieved from https://www.cna-aiic.ca/~/media/cna/files/en/clinical_nurse_specialists_ convention_handout_e.pdf?la=en

Carver, J., & Carver, M. (2001). *Carver's Policy Governance® model in nonprofit organizations*. Retrieved from http://www.carvergovernance.com/pg-np.htm

Casey, J. (2008). Key trends in professional regulation. *Fieldlaw, 5*, 1–3.

Cayton, H., & Webb, K. (2014). The benefits of a "right-touch" approach to health care regulation. *Journal of Health Services Research & Policy, 19*(4), 198–199. doi: 10.1177/1355819614546031

College and Association of Registered Nurses of Alberta (CARNA). (2011). *Nurse practitioner (NP) competencies*. Edmonton, AB: CARNA. Retrieved from http://www.nurses.ab.ca/ content/dam/carna/pdfs/DocumentList/Standards/NP_Competencies_Jan2011.pdf

CARNA. (2015a). *NP renewal: Renewal requirements*. Edmonton, AB: CARNA. Retrieved from http://www.nurses.ab.ca/content/carna/home/maintain-my-registration/nurse-practitioner-requirements/np-renewal.html

CARNA. (2015b). *Together with RNs we protect the public*. Edmonton, AB: CARNA. Retrieved from http://www.nurses.ab.ca/content/carna/home/learn-about-carna.html

College of Nurses of Ontario (CNO). (2011). *Practice standard: Nurse practitioner*. Toronto, ON: CNO. Retrieved from http://www.cno.org/Global/docs/prac/41038_StrdRnec.pdf

CNO. (2012). *Self-regulation*. Toronto, ON: CNO. Retrieved from http://www.cno.org/en/become-a-nurse/entry-to-practice-examinations/jurisprudence-examination/competencies/self-regulation/

CNO. (2013). *Regulation, legislation & by-laws*. Toronto, ON: CNO. Retrieved from http://www.cno.org/en/what-is-cno/regulation-and-legislation/

CNO. (2014). *Legislation and regulation RHPA: Scope of practice, controlled acts model*. Toronto, ON: CNO. Retrieved from http://www.cno.org/Global/docs/policy/41052_RHPAscope.pdf

College of Registered Nurses of British Columbia (CRNBC). (2012). *Regulation of nurses*. Vancouver, BC: CRNBC. Retrieved from https://www.crnbc.ca/crnbc/RegulationOfNurses/Pages/Default.aspx

CRNBC. (2015a). *Scope of practice for nurse practitioners: Standards, limits and conditions*. Vancouver, BC: CRNBC. Retrieved from https://www.crnbc.ca/Standards/Lists/StandardResources/688ScopeforNPs.pdf

CRNBC. (2015b). *2013–2015 strategic plan*. Vancouver, BC: CRNBC. Retrieved from https://www.crnbc.ca/crnbc/StrategicPlan/Pages/Default.aspx

College of Registered Nurses of Manitoba (CRNM). (2010). *Understanding scope of practice for licensed practical nurses, registered nurses, registered psychiatric nurses in the province of Manitoba*. Winnipeg, MB: CRNM. Retrieved from http://cms.tng-secure.com/file_download.php?fFile_id=10231

CRNM. (2015a). *What is an RN?* Winnipeg, MB: CRNM. Retrieved from http://www.crnm.mb.ca/aboutus-whatsanrnnp.php

CRNM. (2015b). *What we do*. Winnipeg, MB: CRNM. Retrieved from http://www.crnm.mb.ca/aboutus-whatwedo.php

College of Registered Nurses of Nova Scotia (CRNNS). (2009a). *A discussion paper on scope of nursing practice for registered nurses in Nova Scotia*. Halifax, NS: CRNNS. Retrieved from http://crnns.ca/documents/Scope%20of%20Practice%20Discussion%20Paper%20website Nov2009.pdf

CRNNS. (2009b). *Self-regulation: A privilege of responsibility*. Halifax, NS: CRNNS. Retrieved from http://www.crnns.ca/documents/Self%20Regulation%20-%20A%20Privilege%20of%20Responsibility_SelfLearning2009.pdf

CRNNS. (2011). *Nurse practitioner core competency framework*. Halifax, NS: CRNNS. Retrieved from http://www.crnns.ca/documents/NS_NP_Competency_Framework.pdf

CRNNS. (2013). *Entry-level competencies for registered nurses in Nova Scotia*. Halifax, NS: CRNNS. Retrieved from http://www.crnns.ca/documents/Entry-LevelCompetenciesRNs.pdf

CRNNS. (2014). *Nurse practitioner standards of practice 2014*. Halifax, NS: CRNNS. Retrieved from http://www.crnns.ca/documents/NPStandards2014-WEB.pdf

Department of Justice. (2012). *Controlled Drugs and Substances Act*. Ottawa, ON: GC. Retrieved from http://laws-lois.justice.gc.ca/PDF/C-38.8.pdf

Department of Justice. (2013). *New classes of practitioners regulations*. Ottawa, ON: GC. Retrieved from http://laws-lois.justice.gc.ca/PDF/SOR-2012-230.pdf

Department of Justice. (2015). *Canada Health Act* (R.S.C., 1985, c. C-6). Ottawa, ON: GC. Retrieved from http://laws-lois.justice.gc.ca/PDF/C-6.pdf

DiCenso, A., Bryant-Lukosius, D., Martin-Misener, R., Donald, F., Abelson, J., Bourgeault, I., … Harbman, P. (2010). Factors enabling advanced practice nursing role integration in Canada. *Nursing Leadership, 23*(Special Issue December), 211–238.

Donald, F., Martin-Misener, R., Bryant-Lukosius, D., Kilpatrick, K., Kaasalainen, S., Carter, N., … DiCenso, A. (2010). The primary healthcare nurse practitioner role in Canada. *Nursing Leadership, 23*(Special Issue December), 88–113.

Elliott, J., Rutty, C., & Villeneuve, M. (2013). *Canadian Nurses Association: One hundred years of service.* Ottawa, ON: CNA.

Government of Canada. (2001). *Guide to making federal acts and regulations* (2nd ed.). Ottawa, ON: GC. Retrieved from http://www.pco.gc.ca/docs/information/publications/legislation/pdf-eng.pdf

Government of Manitoba. (2015). *The Registered Nurses Act* (C.C.S.M. c. R40). Winnipeg, MB: Gov.MB. Retrieved from http://web2.gov.mb.ca/laws/statutes/ccsm/r040e.php

Government of New Brunswick. (2002). *An act respecting nurses and nurse practitioners.* Fredericton, NB: GNB. Retrieved from https://www.gnb.ca/legis/bill/editform-e.asp?ID=113&legi=54&num=4

Government of Newfoundland and Labrador. (2009). *Registered nurse regulations under the Registered Nurses Act.* St. John, NL: Gov.NL. Retrieved from http://assembly.nl.ca/Legislation/sr/regulations/rc130066.htm

Government of the Northwest Territories. (2010). *Nursing Profession Act and Regulation.* Yellowknife, NT: Gov.NT. Retrieved from https://www.justice.gov.nt.ca/en/legislation/#gn-filebrowse-0:/n/nursing-profession/

Government of Ontario. (1991). *Nursing Act.* Toronto, ON: Gov.ON. Retrieved from http://www.e-laws.gov.on.ca/html/statutes/english/elaws_statutes_91n32_e.htm

Government of Prince Edward Island. (2014). *Registered Nurses Act.* Charlottetown, PE: Gov.PE. Retrieved from http://www.gov.pe.ca/law/statutes/pdf/R-08-1.pdf

Government of Saskatchewan. (1988). *The Registered Nurses Act* (2014, c.E-13.1). Regina, SK: Gov.SK. Retrieved from http://www.qp.gov.sk.ca/documents/English/Statutes/Statutes/R12-2.pdf

Internal Trade Secretariat. (2009). *Agreement on internal trade.* Ottawa, ON: GC. Retrieved from http://www.ait-aci.ca/index_en.htm

International Council of Nurses (ICN). (2013). *Nursing regulation.* Geneva, CH: ICN. Retrieved from http://www.icn.ch/images/stories/documents/publications/position_statements/B04_Nsg_Regulation.pdf

Jackman, M. (2000). *Constitutional Jurisdiction over Health in Canada.* Retrieved from http://ualawccsprod.srv.ualberta.ca/centres/hli/userfiles/jackmanfrm.pdf

Kaasalainen, S., Martin-Misener, R., Kilpatrick, K., Harbman, P., Bryant-Lukosius, D., Donald, F., … DiCenso, A. (2010). A historical overview of the development of advanced practice nursing roles in Canada. *Advanced Practice Nursing, 23*(Special Issue, December), 35–60.

Kleinpell, R., Scanlon, A., Hibbert, D., DeKeyser, F., East, L., Fraser, D., … Beauchesne, M. (2014). Addressing issues impacting advanced nursing practice worldwide. *The Online Journal of Nursing Issues, 19*(2). doi: 10.3912/OJIN.Vol19No02Man05

Lahey, W. (2011). Is self-regulation under threat? *Canadian Nurse, 107*(5), 7–8.

McDonald, J.A., Herbert, R., & Thibeault, C. (2006). Advanced practice nursing: Unification through a common identity. *Journal of Professional Nursing, 22*(3), 172–179.

McIntyre, M., & McDonald, C. (2010). *Realities of Canadian nursing: Professional, practice and power issues* (4th ed.). Philadelphia, PA: Wolters Kluwer.

McMillan LLP. (2010). *Health Law in Canada*. Retrieved from http://www.mcmillan.ca/files/Health_Law_in_Canada.pdf

Nurses Association of New Brunswick (NANB). (2015a). *Registration for NPs*. Fredericton, NB: NANB. Retrieved from http://www.nanb.nb.ca/index.php/registration/np

NANB. (2015b). *Vision, mission & public protection*. Fredericton, NB: NANB. Retrieved from http://www.nanb.nb.ca/about/nanb

Penney, C., Bayne, L., & Johansen, C. (2014). Developing a relational regulatory philosophy on a public protection mandate. *Journal of Nursing Regulation, 5*(3), 44–47.

Peterson, D., & Fensling, S. (2011). *Risk-based regulation: Good practice and lessons for the Victorian context*. Melbourne, VIC: State Government of Victoria. Retrieved from http://www.energyandresources.vic.gov.au/about-us/publications/economics-and-policy-research/2011-publications/risk-based-regulation-good-practice-and-lessons-for-the-victorian-context

Province of Alberta. (2013). *Health Professions Act*. Edmonton, AB: Alberta.ca. Retrieved from http://www.qp.alberta.ca/1266.cfm?page=h07.cfm&leg_type=Acts&isbncln=9780779748136

Pulcini, J., Jelic, M., Gul, R., & Loke, A.Y. (2009). An international survey on advanced practice nursing education, practice and regulation. *Journal of Nursing Scholarship, 42*(1), 31–39.

Randall, G.E. (2000). *Understanding professional self-regulation*. Retrieved from http://www.oavt.org/self_regulation/docs/about_selfreg_randall.pdf

Registered Nurses Act. (2006). *Statutes of Nova Scotia*. Halifax, NS: Government of Nova Scotia. Retrieved from http://nslegislature.ca/legc/statutes/regisnur.htm

RN Network of BC. (2010). *Differentiating the roles of regulatory bodies and associations for health professionals: A background document*. Vancouver, BC: CRNBC. Retrieved from http://www.nursing.ubc.ca/Scholarship/RNNetwork/documents/Differentiating%20the%20Roles%20of%20Regulatory%20Bodies%20and%20Associations%20%20-%20Feb%202010.pdf

Saskatchewan Registered Nurses Association (SRNA). (2011). *Registered nurse (nurse practitioner) RN(NP) standards & core competencies*. Regina, SK: SRNA. Retrieved from http://www.srna.org/images/stories/pdfs/communications/pdf/standards_and_comp_2011.pdf

Schiller, C.J. (2015). Self-regulation of the nursing profession: Focus on four Canadian provinces. *Journal of Nursing Education and Practice, 5*(1), 95–106.

Tarrant, F., & Associates. (2005). *Literature review of nurse practitioner legislation & regulation*. Ottawa, ON: CNA. Retrieved from http://www.npnow.ca/docs/tech-report/section2/02_LegReg_AppendixA.pdf

Uhlich, C., Giblin, C., & Michaud, S.L. (2007). *Nursing in Canada: An overview*. Retrieved from http://www.macewan.ca/web/services/ims/client/upload/Nursing%20in%20Canada.pdf

Yukon Legislative Counsel Office. (2009). *Registered Nurses Profession Act*. Whitehorse, YT: Gov. YK. Retrieved from http://www.gov.yk.ca/legislation/acts/renupr_c.pdf

Chapter 4

Advanced Practice Nursing Frameworks Utilized or Developed in Canada

Dana Edge and Rosemary Wilson

Dana Edge is an Associate Professor at Queen's University, School of Nursing in Kingston, Ontario. She has practiced nursing across North America (including Alaska and Labrador), and her ongoing research interests include rural health, population health, and primary care.

Rosemary Wilson is an Assistant Professor at Queen's University, School of Nursing in Kingston, Ontario. She is also an NP–Adult in chronic pain management at Kingston General and Hotel Dieu Hospitals.

KEY TERMS

advanced nursing practice (ANP)
advanced practice nursing (APN)
nursing frameworks

OBJECTIVES

1. Appreciate the development of advanced practice nursing (APN) frameworks.
2. Identify the APN frameworks most commonly utilized in Canada.
3. Explore current trends and future development of APN frameworks.

Introduction

Nursing frameworks or models provide structure and guidance to clinical practice, and are also used by nursing educators to formulate curriculum. This chapter will provide an overview of the development of advanced practice nursing (APN) frameworks and their use within Canada. In particular, frameworks developed or advanced by Canadian researchers, professional bodies, and educators are highlighted chronologically; early frameworks and models are discussed first, followed by more recently developed conceptualizations.

Definitions

The current definition of **advanced nursing practice (ANP)** in Canada (Canadian Nurses Association [CNA], 2007) emerged from the national consensus work of the Canadian Nurse Practitioner Initiative (CNPI) that began in 2004 and culminated with the publication of *Advanced Nursing Practice: A National Framework* in 2008 (CNA, 2008) (see Chapter 5). In Canada, *APN* is an umbrella term used to describe an advanced level of clinical nursing practice of registered nurses (RNs) who possess graduate-level education and clinical expertise to address the health of the population, including individuals, families, groups, and communities (CNA, 2007). Embedded in the definition is the ability to use evidence and research to guide practice and influence policy. The position statement also delineates 10 characteristics of advanced nursing practice, including the ability to explicate and apply theoretical foundations of nursing practice. In Canada, APN roles currently include the clinical nurse specialist (CNS), primary health care nurse practitioner (PHCNP), and acute care nurse practitioner (ACNP).

It is important to note that in the United States (US), the umbrella term developed by the American Nurses Association (ANA, 2004) that is equivalent to the CNA definition is *APN*. The terms *APN* and *ANP* are often used interchangeably in Canada, as noted with the title of the Canadian Association of Advanced Practice Nurses (CAAPN-ACIIPA), a national organization of Canadian CNSs, ACNPs, and PHCNPs (CAAPN, 2015). For the remainder of this chapter, the term *APN* will be used.

Significance of Nursing Frameworks in Practice

Individual theoretical perspectives and worldviews of nurses continue to influence how nursing practice is conceived, implemented, and practiced (Jansen, 2010). Understanding the collective view of APN is important to the discipline of nursing. Not only must we be able to articulate what advanced practice is to those within the profession, it is also incumbent upon nursing to describe the nature of advanced practice to others. Conceptual frameworks and models assist in "conveying the reality of ANP through symbolic representation that often takes the form of words, pictures, or diagrams" (Chinn & Kramer, 2015, p. 159).

Advanced Practice Nursing Frameworks Utilized in Canada

Canadian nursing initially drew upon literature and research from other jurisdictions, most notably the US, to shape APN curriculum and roles in advanced practice. Four models are central to the development of APN in Canada: the Shuler Nurse Practitioner Practice Model, the National Organization of Nurse Practitioner Faculties (NONPF) domains of practice, Hamric's Model of Advanced Practice Nursing, and the Strong Model of Advanced Practice Nursing. Each is briefly discussed, with a synopsis of current use and including Canadian models of APN (see Table 4.1).

TABLE 4.1: Overview of APN Models Utilized or Developed in Canada

Model Name	Year	Country	Classification of Model*	Key Elements
Shuler Nurse Practitioner Practice Model	1993	United States	Clinical practice model	• Person • Health • Nursing • NP role • Environment
Hamric's Model of Advanced Practice Nursing	1996	United States	Nature of advanced practice nursing	• Primary criteria • Central competency–practice • Core competencies • Critical environmental elements
The Strong Memorial Hospital Model of APN	1996	United States	Administrative or organizational	Five domains: • Direct comprehensive care • Support of systems • Education • Research • Publication and leadership
National Organization of Nurse Practitioner Faculties (NONPF); Family Nurse Practitioner (FNP) Competencies	2002	United States	Regulatory	FNP competencies: • Health promotion, health protection, disease prevention, and treatment • Nurse practitioner–patient relationship • Teaching-coaching function • Professional role • Managing and negotiating health care delivery systems • Monitoring and ensuring the quality of health care practice • Cultural competence
The Nature of Nursing Model	2001	Canada	Differentiation between basic and advanced practice	• Theory • Pattern recognition • Practical knowledge • Practical wisdom • General to the particular

Framework	Year	Country	Component	Details
The Ottawa Hospital Advanced Practice Nurse Role Components	2001	Canada	Administrative or organizational	• Clinical practice • Consultation • Research • Education • Leadership/Administration
Participatory, Evidence-based, Patient-focused Process, for guiding the development, implementation, and evaluation of APN (PEPPA) Framework	2004	Canada	Role implementation and evaluation	Nine steps: • Define patient population and model of care • Identify stakeholders • Determine need for new model of care • Identify priority problems and goals to improve care • Define new model of care and APN role • Plan implementation • Initiate role implementation • Evaluate APN role and model of care • Determine future needs
University Health Network (UHN) Framework for APN	2004	Canada	Administrative or organizational	Core competencies: • Clinical practice • Leadership • Research • Change agent • Collaboration
Conceptual Model for NP Practice in Canada (CNPI)	2005	Canada	Nature of advanced practice nursing	• Vision of health • Client • Discipline • Context • Nurse practitioner • Inquiry/EBP • Health care system • Greater society

continued

TABLE 4.1: Overview of APN Models Utilized or Developed in Canada *(cont.)*

Model Name	Year	Country	Classification of Model*	Key Elements
Advanced Nursing Practice: A National Framework	2008	Canada	Regulatory	• Evolution of advanced nursing practice • Definition and characteristics • Educational preparation • Roles • Regulation • Competencies • Impact of advanced nursing practice • Support for advanced nursing practice
APN Practice at SickKids	2010	Canada	Administrative or organizational	Five domains: • Pediatric clinical practice • Research and scholarly activities • Interprofessional collaboration • Education and mentorship • Organizational and systems management
The Acute Care Nurse Practitioner Conceptual Framework	2012	Canada	Nature of advanced practice nursing	Process: • Boundary work • ACNP role enactment • Perceptions of team effectiveness Structure: • Patient-level • ACNP-level • Team-level • Organization-level • Health care system–level Outcomes: • Quality • Safety • Cost • Team

The SNAP Conceptual Framework	2013	Canada	Administrative or organizational	Five domains: • Direct comprehensive care • Support of systems • Educative practice • Evidence-informed practice • Professional leadership

*Based on characterizations developed by Spross (2014)

Source: Spross, 2014.

The Shuler Nurse Practitioner Practice Model

Salient nursing components of nurse practitioner (NP) practice are explicated in the model developed by Shuler and Davis (1993a). The authors intended to articulate a model that could be used by clinicians, as well as educators and researchers, to demonstrate how nursing and medicine are blended in practice. The nursing paradigm of person, health, nursing, and environment, as well as the nursing process, are clearly evident in the model. Preventive measures and health promotion activities also form key components of the model. Although Shuler's model is lengthy and extensive, the authors provided an expanded explanation of the model's clinical application in an accompanying article shortly after the publication of the original article (Shuler & Davis, 1993b).

Despite its complexity, the practice model gained wide appeal and use in Canadian PHCNP programs since the 1990s and is the only APN framework to incorporate the competency of diagnosing, which makes it very specific to NP practice. While other models for the most part have supplanted the Shuler model, references to the model are found in the current advanced health assessment curriculum in Ontario's Primary Health Care Nurse Practitioner Program (PHCNP Program, 2015).

Hamric's Model of Advanced Nursing Practice

In the first edition of the book, *Advanced Practice Nursing: An Integrative Approach* (1996), Hamric described the nature of APN using concentric circles to represent the characteristics of the model (Hamric, 1996). The model initially arose from Hamric's work with CNSs, but evolved over time to be inclusive of all APN roles (Spross, 2014).

In the current model, primary criteria (i.e., graduate education, certification, and practice focused on patient/family) comprise the centre of the circle. The central competency of direct clinical practice encircles the primary criteria, and is surrounded by core competencies of leadership, collaboration, ethical decision-making, guidance and coaching, consultation, and evidence-based practice (Spross, 2014). Graduate nursing education in Canada has utilized the work of Hamric extensively in classroom discourse on the nature of advanced practice.

Strong Model of Advanced Practice Nursing

In the early 1990s at the Strong Memorial Hospital in Rochester, New York, APNs developed an organizational model to depict the five domains that characterized their advanced practice: direct comprehensive care, support of systems, education, research, and publication and professional leadership (Ackerman, Norsen, Martin, Wiedrich, & Kiztman, 1996). The model is in a pentagonal shape with the patient at the centre, and the five domains each occupy a "slice" of the pentagon. Scholarship, collaboration, and empowerment are necessary threads that cross through the domains. Embedded in the model is the concept of the APN transitioning from novice to expert, depicted by shading of the pentagon (see Figure 4.1).

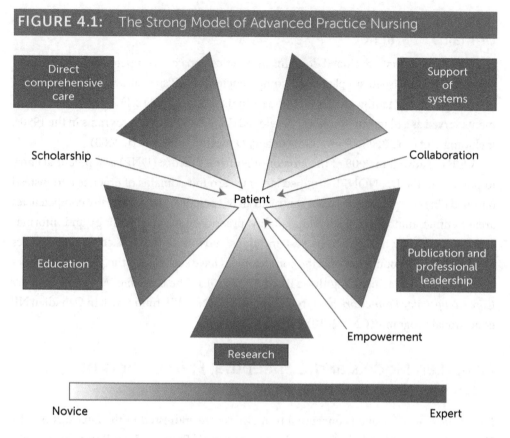

FIGURE 4.1:   The Strong Model of Advanced Practice Nursing

Source: Adapted from Mick & Ackerman, 2000. Reprinted with permission.

In a pilot study (*n* = 18) that aimed to differentiate roles of ACNPs and CNSs, Mick and Ackerman (2000) asked participants to self-rank individual expertise and relative importance of tasks using the five domains of the Strong Model. While the sample was small, clear differences in mean ranking scores were found between ACNP and CNS respondents, with CNSs self-ranking their expertise higher in all domains compared to ACNPs. Certain task aspects of direct clinical care were ranked higher among ACNPs than CNSs (e.g., history-taking, initiating diagnostic tests, performing specialized procedures). From their pilot work, the authors concluded that the Strong Model better described CNS practice than ACNP. It is critical to note, however, that not all of the 12 participating ACNPs had formal NP education or had taken the ACNP certification examination when the survey was conducted.

Several tertiary hospitals in Canada adopted the Strong Model to guide APN in their institutions, including the Winnipeg Health Authority (2015) and the Hospital for Sick Children (SickKids) in Toronto (LeGrow, Hubley, & McAllister, 2010). While the original Strong Model continues to guide practice in Winnipeg, modifications occurred in several Ontario institutions and are discussed later in the chapter.

National Organization of Nurse Practitioner Faculties' (NONPF) Domains of Practice

NONPF (2002a) first developed domains of practice and core competencies in 1990, and subsequently published supplemental competencies for NP specialties (NONPF, 2002b), including those for family nurse practitioners in the US (see Table 4.1). The NONPF documents served as a blueprint for newly developed Canadian PHCNP programs in the 1990s, including Ontario's PHCNP program (Cragg, Doucette, & Humbert, 2003).

With the advent in 2008 of the Doctor of Nursing Practice (DNP) as a potential entry to practice in the US, NONPF dropped language around domains of practice and instead outlined nine competencies that are central to all NP practice. These nine core competencies are: scientific foundation, leadership, quality, practice inquiry, technology and information literacy, policy, health delivery system, ethics, and independent practice competencies (NONPF, 2014). Population-specific competencies have superseded the previous NP specialty competencies, including those listed in Table 4.1. The *Canadian Nurse Practitioner Core Competency Framework* has largely replaced the NONPF framework in Canadian NP educational programs (CNA 2010).

Canadian Models and Conceptual Frameworks of Advanced Practice Nursing

Nine Canadian-developed conceptual frameworks are addressed in the next section: the Nature of Nursing Model; the Ottawa Hospital Advanced Practice Nurse Role Components; the Participatory, Evidence-based, Patient-focused Process, for guiding the development, implementation, and evaluation of APN (PEPPA) Framework; the University Health Network (UHN) Framework for APN; Conceptual Model for NP Practice in Canada; the National Framework for APN; Advanced Practice Nursing (APN) Practice at SickKids; the Acute Care Nurse Practitioner Conceptual (ACNP) Framework; and the Saskatchewan Nursing Advanced Practice (SNAP) Conceptual Framework. These Canadian practice frameworks and models have evolved from education, practice, and professional bodies, most notably the Canadian Nurses Association (CNA).

The Nature of Nursing Model

In 2001, two nurse educators from Alberta—Kathleen Oberle and Marian Allen—explored the theoretical and philosophical literature in nursing to untangle confusion surrounding expert versus advanced practice, and to clarify the linkages between existing conceptual models and advanced practice. Their conceptualization of advanced practice articulates that an APN is first an expert practitioner, who is characterized by having well-developed pattern recognition skills and practical knowledge (Oberle & Allen, 2001). What separates the APN from the expert practitioner, according to the authors, is the theoretical knowledge base of the APN gained from graduate education. The educational process, along with reflection, leads to transformation of practice. At the time of the Oberle and Allen (2001) publication, not all advanced practice educational programs in Canada were at the graduate level; their work propelled the debate and provided a theoretical basis for all APN preparation to be delivered through graduate educational programs.

The Ottawa Hospital Advanced Practice Nurse Role Components

A merger of three tertiary hospitals in 1998 was the impetus for clarification of APN in the new amalgamated entity, The Ottawa Hospital (TOH). Nursing leadership established a task force and over a six-month period of time, a literature review was completed, focus groups were held, and input was sought from nurses, physicians, administration, and nursing faculty members from the University of Ottawa (De Grasse & Nicklin, 2001). The output was an ANP job description and framework, as well as assessment, implementation, and evaluation recommendations. Graduate education was considered to be "imperative" (De Grasse & Nicklin, p. 9). The role components within the framework include: clinical practice, consultation, research, education, and leadership/administration. The model remains in use at The Ottawa Hospital with 21 APNs currently profiled on the hospital website (TOH, 2015).

PEPPA Framework

Classified as a role implementation and evaluation model, the PEPPA Framework was developed by a CNS/researcher at McMaster University (Byrant-Lukosius & DiCenso, 2004). The nine steps in the framework provide a logical template for engaging stakeholders in the process of designing, implementing, and evaluating an APN role within an agency or institution (see Figure 4.2).

Uptake of the PEPPA Framework has been extensive; the framework gained national attention and distribution in 2008 with its inclusion in the CNA publication on advanced nursing practice (CNA, 2008). The PEPPA Framework has guided research investigations studying role implementation and evaluation throughout Canada (see Box 4.1).

University Health Network (UHN) Framework for APN

Role ambiguity at the UHN sites in Toronto prompted a subcommittee of NPs to undertake a critical review of existing literature and to consult within the network in the early 2000s; the aim was to develop a comprehensive conceptual framework to promote role clarity (Miceviski et al., 2004). After reviewing four conceptual models for APN, including the Strong Model (Ackerman et al., 1996), the group decided to use components from several models to construct its own framework: the UHN Framework for Advanced Nursing Practice (Miceviski et al., 2004).

FIGURE 4.2:   The PEPPA Framework

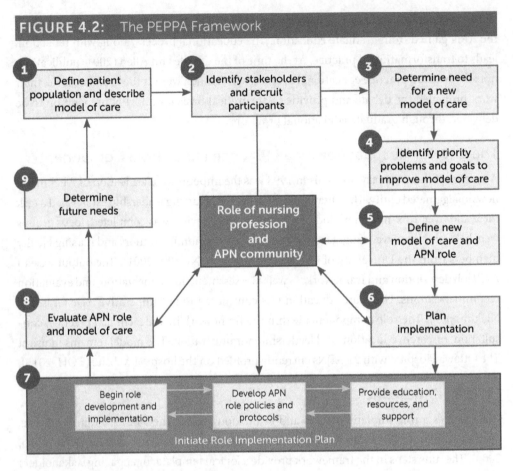

Source: Bryant-Lukosius & DiCenso, 2004. Reprinted with permission.

At first glance, the UHN framework has visual features similar to the Strong Model; however, there are important distinctions. First, the model reads from left to right, starting with inputs into the central circle with five spokes and ending with an arrow with outcomes, and thus depicting the structure, process, and outcome elements of the framework. The inputs represent individual, organizational, professional, and societal variables that can affect APN practice; these inputs could include such variables as patient acuity, educational preparation of the APN, entry to practice regulations, and societal values. Advanced practice is conceptualized as having five core antecedents necessary for APN practice: advanced knowledge, scholarship, experience, communication, and compassion for others. These five antecedents make up the spokes or pillars of the central circle. Five APN competencies are identified as wedges between the spokes and include clinical practice, leadership, research, change agent, and collaboration (Miceviski et al., 2004). These vary from the Strong Model domains in that education and support of systems are missing. Collaboration, which is

---

BOX 4.1

Use of the PEPPA Framework in Studying
Rural Nurse Practitioners

The PEPPA Framework formed the conceptual framework for a 2004 study to define the role of rural nurse practitioners (NPs) in Nova Scotia. A mixed methods research design was employed using interviews and mailed questionnaires. Stakeholders were identified as per steps outlined in the PEPPA Framework. Nine rural health board chairpersons were interviewed by telephone. The questionnaire was distributed to NPs, public health nurses, family practice nurses, and family physicians ($n = 51$). Findings demonstrated congruence between the health board chairpersons and the health care providers on the health care needs of rural Nova Scotians, the holistic nature of NP practice, and gaps in the current service model for primary health care. Further, the study identified a vision for NPs in rural communities as well as the steps that required attention to optimize successful employment and integration of the NP role.

Source: Martin-Misener, Reilly, & Vollman, 2010.

a thread in the Strong Model, forms a competency in the UHN framework. The model also incorporates a systems approach, as the inner circle is encompassed by the larger environment and has an interface of the following optimal characteristics: empowerment, autonomy, respect, inquiry, and advocacy. The output categories mirror those of the input: individual, organizational, professional, and societal. The authors infer that the model positions APNs at the point of care to engage in and contribute to clinical scholarship.

Conceptual Model for Nurse Practitioner Practice in Canada

In 2004, CNA launched the CNPI to develop a sustainable and integrated national framework to incorporate NPs into the Canadian health care system (CNPI, 2006). Funding for the project was provided by Health Canada as part of a larger initiative of primary health care renewal in the country. One of the outputs of the two-year project was the development of a conceptual model for NP practice within the Canadian context (CNPI, 2006) (see Figure 4.3).

The vision of health forms the inner circle of the model, surrounded by four "commonplaces" defined as the ordinary, everyday components that assist in conceptually organizing topics (Robinson Vollman & Martin-Misener, 2005). The commonplaces identified as central to nurse practitioner practice are: client, from individual to communities; discipline, from narrow

FIGURE 4.3:   Conceptual Model for Nurse Practitioner Practice in Canada

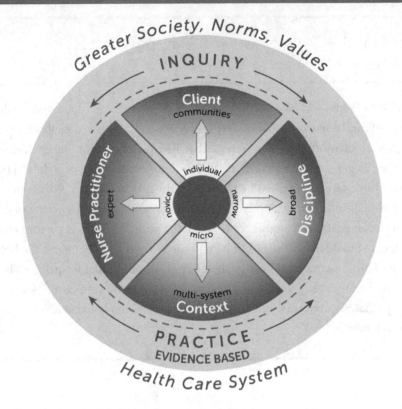

Source: Robinson Vollman & Martin-Misener, 2005. Reprinted with permission.

to broad; context, from micro- to multi-system; and nurse practitioner, from novice to expert (which signifies a fifth commonplace, time). These commonplace elements are encircled by evidence-based practice and inquiry, which make up the final ring around the model circle. Finally, the model as described is situated in the broader contexts of the health care system and the greater society, norms, and values. Despite the national exposure of the model in 2006, it is not widely represented in current literature or in NP educational program curricula.

The National Framework for Advanced Nursing Practice

Building upon the work of the CNPI, the Board of Directors of the CNA endorsed a national framework to guide provincial jurisdictions, educational institutions, and others in the evolution of APN (CNA, 2008). The framework was deliberately broad to allow for variation across the country. In the document, the CNA elaborates on eight elements of the national framework, including: evolution of APN, definition and characteristics, educational preparation, roles, regulation, competencies, impact of APN, and support for APN. Of note, the board reiterated its endorsement of graduate education as a minimum requirement and identified four overarching competency categories for APNs: clinical practice, research, leadership, and collaboration and consultation (ibid.). As previously mentioned, the document also endorsed the PEPPA Framework (see Figure 4.2) for use in the implementation and evaluation of APN roles. The national framework provides cohesion in the approach to APN definitions, roles, and educational preparation, and remains central to discussion about APN practice in Canada.

Advanced Practice Nursing at SickKids

The tertiary children's hospital in Toronto, SickKids, has utilized CNSs at their institution since the late 1960s (LeGrow, Hubley, & McAllister, 2010). When the Strong Model was published, SickKids initially endorsed the model to guide their APN practice. Several years following the adoption of the Strong Model at SickKids, the APNs realized that inconsistency in its use was a problem. In analyzing the issues around the lack of uptake of the Strong Model, the APN council concluded that they needed to develop a conceptual model that represented their vision, would guide APN practice, and address the unique aspects of their practice with ill children and their families.

To do this, they spent three months using innovative exercises and leadership techniques to capture the essence of the APN vision at SickKids. The effort was based on existing frameworks to invoke change and was deliberate in its approach. In the end, the APN council achieved a vision to guide practice and fashioned a conceptual model with tenants rooted in the Strong Model (Ackerman et al., 1996). The framework has similar features to the UHN-FAPN model (Miceviski et al., 2004), but despite the attributes that appear comparable to those put forward at the UHN, the APN practice at SickKids model has decidedly different components (see Figure 4.4).

Rather than "inputs," the model begins at the left with acknowledgement of theories that are considered to be foundational elements. These include the Strong Model (Ackerman et al., 1996), the CNA APN standards and competencies, the Illness Beliefs Model (Wright, Watson, & Bell, 1996), and the Leadership Practice Model (Kouzes & Posner, 2002). The central circle, which is fashioned like the UHN-FAPN's model, has the child and family at the centre. Five small circles make spokes to the child and family and represent the SickKids APN core domains; interestingly, four of these domains are identical to those found in the Strong Model. The one Strong Model domain that is absent is leadership; in its place, the SickKids APN model identifies interprofessional collaboration as a key domain. Holistic care that encompasses the family is represented by the area between the spokes and represents the context of communication, family-centred care, partnerships, human relationships, and collaboration. The various settings (such as the home, community, hospital, or ambulatory clinics) where holistic care is delivered by APNs are depicted by an encircling

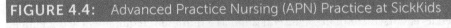

FIGURE 4.4:   Advanced Practice Nursing (APN) Practice at SickKids

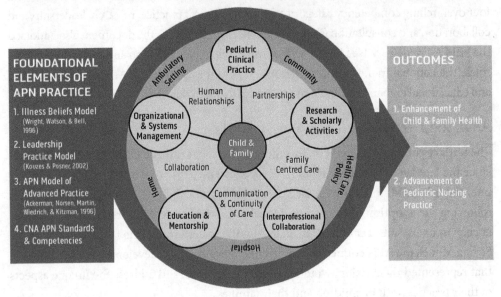

Source: LeGrow, Hubley, & McAllister, 2010. Reprinted with permission.

ring. Like the UHN-FAPN model, an arrow leads to the right from the circle to outcomes. Unlike the UHN-FAPN model, outcomes specific to child health and pediatric practice are expressed. A self-evaluation tool for the model is identified, but does not provide a timeline for formal, planned evaluation of the model at SickKids (LeGrow et al., 2010).

The Acute Care Nurse Practitioner Conceptual Framework

A conceptualization of APN practice (Kilpatrick, Lavoie-Tremblay, Lamothe, Ritchie, & Doran, 2012) was developed from theoretical literature and a multiple-case study implemented in Quebec that explored role enactment by acute care NPs (ACNPs). In particular, the researchers aimed to investigate role boundaries, team processes with the enactment of ACNP roles, and the perception of effectiveness by team members (Kilpatrick et al., 2012).

Using cross-case analysis from the case study findings, a new conceptual framework was constructed using identified process, structure, and outcome dimensions. In the centre, the three process dimensions of APN role enactment, boundary work, and team perception are shown with bivariate arrows to each other, showing the interconnectedness of the processes. Concentric circles around the process dimensions depict how structure dimensions can restrict or expand the process dimensions. These elastic, concentric circles include patient, ACNP, team, organizational, and health care system-level structural dimensions that influence and affect the ability of the ACNP to carry out the role, to define boundaries, and to promote team effectiveness (Kilpatrick et al., 2012). Outcome dimensions are represented to the right of the concentric circles with quality, safety, cost, and team outcomes identified as key indicators of ACNP practice. The work addressed a gap in the understanding of the underlying processes and structures that occur with the introduction of an ACNP to the health care team (Kilpatrick et al., 2012). As the model is relatively new, further elucidation of ACNP team interaction and boundary work in other settings is important. The research-driven model holds promise in assisting nurse managers, administrators, and researchers in clarifying the nature of role enactment by ACNPs.

SNAP Conceptual Framework

The most recently reported conceptualization of APN was developed from the partnership, known as the Collaborative Nurse Practitioner Program (CNPP), between Saskatchewan Polytechnic School of Nursing and the University of Regina's Faculty of Nursing. Initially, the CNPP team looked at a number of APN models and frameworks to guide the CNPP's curricular and program design. Identifying the Strong Model as a valid and reliable APN model, the team realized that the model's focus and language did not reflect a Saskatchewan or Canadian context of APN. Therefore, the CNPP team adapted the Strong Model and the Saskatchewan Nursing Advanced Practice (SNAP) Conceptual Framework was developed (Saskatchewan Collaborative Programs in Nursing, 2015) (see Figure 4.5).

The Strong Model's core principles and concepts were aligned to fit the context of the Saskatchewan health system, as well as reflect current literature and the expertise of the CNPP faculty. The SNAP Conceptual Framework depicts five domains of advanced nursing practice: direct comprehensive care, support of systems, educative practice, evidence-informed practice, and professional leadership. For consistency, these concepts were mapped against the core provincial RN(NP) competencies developed by the Saskatchewan Registered Nurses Association (SRNA), as well as the APN educational and practice competencies developed by the CNA.

In 2015, the SNAP Conceptual Framework was officially adopted to guide the CNPP's curricular and program design. The framework guides advanced practice, recognizes the expertise APN students bring to the program, and reflects APN from both national and provincial competencies and practice standards.

Conclusion

Within this sketch of APN conceptual models, several themes emerged. First, reliance on models from the US is decreasing as new Canadian models have emerged to address contextual nuances of our health care systems. Clearly, Hamric's Model of Advanced Nursing

FIGURE 4.5:   Saskatchewan Nursing Advanced Practice (SNAP) Conceptual Framework

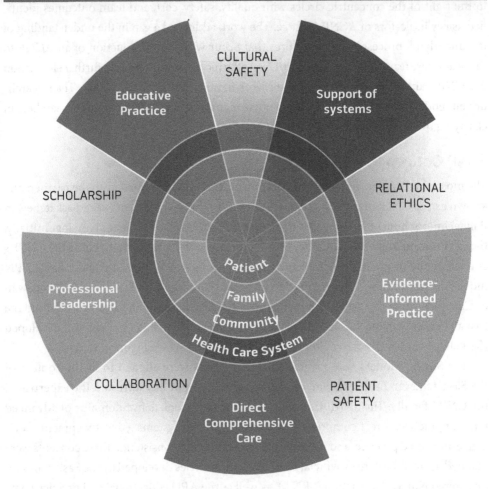

Source: Saskatchewan Collaborative Programs in Nursing, 2015. Reprinted with permission.

Practice (Hamric, 1996) continues to influence thinking surrounding the core elements of APN. Likewise, we can find the Strong Model (Ackerman et al., 1996) in use in Canadian acute care hospitals. However, the work of the CNPI in the early 2000s led to the development of a national competency framework that resulted in a better understanding of the nature of APN in Canada. Research and critical appraisal of APN roles paralleled the professional efforts to define and conceptualize APN.

Of the Canadian-developed frameworks presented, three are specific to NP practice and the remainder address APN generally; it is important to note that four of the Canadian models were strongly influenced by the Strong Model. Of equal importance is the initiative of three tertiary hospitals to undertake conceptual development of APN role definitions and conceptualizations. Only one model clearly arose from research findings, while the PEPPA Framework has been extensively used as a framework in research investigations.

Despite the search to identify all APN conceptual models used or developed in Canada, it is quite possible that other models are in use that have not yet been reported in the literature. An inventory of APN framework utilization in practice settings was beyond the scope of this overview. Yet, with increased development of Canadian models since 2000, we need to grasp the extent of their use by APNs and how effective the models will prove to be in providing guidance for role development, as well as in affecting APN-sensitive outcomes. Continued inquiry into role implementation will help refine current APN frameworks and more clearly define the crucial elements that characterize the various advanced practice roles.

Critical Thinking Questions

1. What were the major driving forces in Canada that led to the evolution of APN frameworks?
2. Compare and contrast the four Canadian models that were influenced by the Strong Model (i.e., UHN-FANP, SickKids, the ACNP Conceptual Framework, and SNAP Conceptual Framework). What contextual factors of the three settings might account for the different models?
3. How can APN models be used in nursing research? From your understanding of the models presented, which models could most easily be used to inform research?

References

Ackerman, M.H., Norsen, L., Martin, B., Wiedrich, J., & Kitzman, H.J. (1996). Development of a model of advanced practice. *American Journal of Critical Care, 5,* 68–73.

American Nurses Association (ANA). (2004). *Nursing: Scope and standards of practice.* Washington, DC: ANA.

Bryant-Lukosius, D., & DiCenso, A. (2004). A framework for the introduction and evaluation of advanced practice nursing roles. *Journal of Advanced Nursing, 48*(5), 530–540.

Canadian Association of Advanced Practice Nurses (CAAPN). (2015). *Vision, mission, values.* Kitchener, ON, Ontario: CAAPN. Retrieved from http://caapn-aciipa.org/index.htm

Canadian Nurses Association (CNA). (2007). *Position statement: Advanced nursing practice.* Ottawa, ON: CNA. Retrieved from www.cna-aiic.ca/~/media/cna/page-content/pdf-en/ps60_advanced_nursing_practice_2007_e.pdf?la=en

CNA. (2008). *Advanced nursing practice: A national framework*. Ottawa, ON: CNA. Retrieved from https://www.cna-aiic.ca/~/media/can/page-content/pdf-en/anp_national_framework_e.pdf

CNA. (2010). *Canadian nurse practitioner core competency framework*. Ottawa, ON: CNA. Retrieved from www.cna-aiic.ca/~/media/cna/files/en/competency_framework_2010_e.pdf?la=en

Canadian Nurse Practitioner Initiative (CNPI). (2006). *Nurse practitioners: The time is now*. Ottawa, ON: CNA. Retrieved from, http://www.npnow.ca/docs/tech-report/section1/01_Integrated_Report.pdf

Chinn, P.L., & Kramer, M.K. (2015). *Knowledge development in nursing: Theory and process* (9th ed.). St. Louis, MO: Elsevier Mosby.

Cragg, C.E., Doucette, S., & Humbert, J. (2003). Ten universities, one program: Successful collaboration to educate nurse practitioners. *Nurse Educator, 28*(5), 227–231.

De Grasse, C., & Nicklin, W. (2001). Advanced nursing practice: Old hat, new design. *Canadian Journal of Nursing Leadership, 14*(4), 7–12.

Hamric, A.B. (1996). A definition of advanced practice nursing. In A.B. Hamric, J.A. Spross, & C.M. Hanson (Eds.). *Advanced practice nursing: An integrative approach* (pp. 25–41). Philadelphia, PA: WB Saunders.

Jansen, M.P. (2010). Advanced practice within a nursing paradigm. In M.P. Jansen & M. Zwygart-Stauffacher (Eds.). *Advanced practice nursing: Core concepts for professional role development* (2nd ed.), (pp. 31–42). New York, NY: Springer.

Kilpatrick, K., Lavoie-Tremblay, M., Lamothe, L., Ritchie, J.A., & Doran, D. (2012). Conceptual framework of acute care nurse practitioner role enactment, boundary work, and perceptions of team effectiveness. *Journal of Advanced Nursing, 69*(1), 205–217.

Kouzes, J.M., & Posner, B.Z. (2002). *The leadership challenge* (3rd ed.). San Francisco, CA: Wiley & Sons.

LeGrow, K., Hubley, P., & McAllister, M. (2010). A conceptual framework for advanced practice nursing in a pediatric tertiary care setting: The SickKids' experience. *Nursing Leadership, 23*(2), 32–46. doi: 10.12927/cjnl.2013.21831

Martin-Misener, R., Reilly, S.M., & Vollman, A.R. (2010). Defining the role of primary health care nurse practitioners in rural Nova Scotia. *Canadian Journal of Nursing Research, 42*(2), 30–47.

Micevski, V., Korkola, L., Sarkissian, S., Mulcahy, V., Shobbrook, C., Belford, L., & Kells, L. (2004). University Health Network framework for advanced nursing practice: Development of a comprehensive conceptual framework describing the multidimensional contributions of advanced practice nurses. *Nursing Leadership, 17*(3), 52–64. doi: 10.12927/cjnl.2004.16231

Mick, D.J., & Ackerman, M.H. (2000). Advanced practice nursing role delineation in acute and critical care: Application of the strong model of advanced practice. *Heart & Lung, 29*(3), 210–221.

National Organization of Nurse Practitioner Faculties (NONPF). (2002a). *Domains and core competencies of nurse practitioner practice, 2002*. Washington, DC: NONPF. Retrieved from http://c.ymcdn.com/sites/www.nonpf.org/resource/resmgr/competencies/domainsandcorecomps2002.pdf

NONPF. (2002b). *Nurse practitioner primary care competencies in specialty areas: Adult, family, gerontological, pediatric, and women's health*. Washington, D.C.: NONPF. Retrieved from http://c.ymcdn.com/sites/www.nonpf.org/resource/resmgr/competencies/primarycarecomps02.pdf

NONPF. (2014). *Nurse practitioner core competencies with suggested curriculum content.* Washington, DC: NONPF. Retrieved from http://c.ymcdn.com/sites/nonpf.site-ym.com/resource/resmgr/Competencies/NPCoreCompsContentFinalNov20.pdf

Oberle, K., & Allen, M. (2001). The nature of advanced practice nursing. *Nursing Outlook, 49*(3), 148–153.

Ontario Primary Health Care Nurse Practitioner (PHCNP) Program. (2015). *Advanced health assessment and diagnosis (AHAD) I.* Toronto, ON: COUPN. Retrieved from http://np-education.ca

Robinson Vollman, A., & Martin-Misener, R. (2005). A conceptual model for nurse practitioner practice. In Canadian Nurse Practitioner Initiative (2006). *Practice framework for nurse practitioners in Canada* (Appendix A) (pp. 1–13). Ottawa, ON: CNA. Retrieved from www.npnow.ca/docs/tech-report/section3/05_PracticeFW_AppendixA.pdf

Saskatchewan Collaborative Programs in Nursing. (2015). *Nurse practitioners – Improving health care in communities.* Regina, SK: Saskatchewan Polytechnic and University of Regina. Retrieved from http://www.sasknursingdegree.ca/cnpp/vision-mission-values-and-the-snap model/

Shuler, P.A., & Davis, J.E. (1993a). The Shuler nurse practitioner practice model: A theoretical framework for nurse practitioner clinicians, educators, and researchers, part 1. *Journal of the American Academy of Nurse Practitioners, 5*(1), 11–18.

Shuler, P.A., & Davis, J.E. (1993b). The Shuler nurse practitioner practice model: Clinical application, part 2. *Journal of the American Academy of Nurse Practitioners, 5*(2), 73–88.

Spross, J. (2014). Conceptualizations of advanced practice nursing. In A.B. Hamric, C.M. Hanson, M.F. Tracy, & E.T. O'Grady (Eds.). *Advanced practice nursing: An integrative approach* (5th ed.), (pp. 27–66). St. Louis, MO: Elsevier Saunders.

The Ottawa Hospital (TOH). (2015). Advanced practice nurses. Retrieved from http://www.ottawahospital.on.ca/wps/portal/Base/TheHospital/OurModelofCare/ProfessionalTeam/Nursing/AdvancedPracticeNurses

Winnipeg Regional Health Authority. (2015). *Advanced practice.* Winnipeg, MB: Winnipeg Health Authority. Retrieved from http://www.wrha.mb.ca/professionals/nursing/practice-advanced.php

Wright, L.M., Watson, W.L., & Bell, J.M. (1996). *Beliefs: The heart of healing in families and illness.* New York, NY: Basic Books.

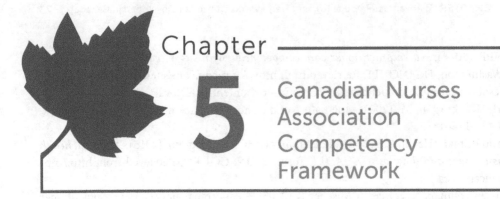

Chapter 5

Canadian Nurses Association Competency Framework

Josette Roussel

Josette Roussel is a Senior Nurse Advisor at the Canadian Nurses Association (CNA) in Ottawa, Ontario.

KEY TERMS

advanced nursing
    practice (ANP)
advanced practice
    nurses (APNs)
competencies
framework
core competencies

OBJECTIVES

1. Identify key elements of a competency framework.
2. Describe core competencies of advanced nursing practice (ANP).
3. Describe the history of the development of the nurse practitioner (NP) competency framework in Canada.
4. Describe the development of the clinical nurse specialist's (CNS) pan-Canadian competencies.

Introduction

This chapter describes the Canadian Nurses Association (CNA) competency framework as it relates to *Advanced Nursing Practice: A National Framework* (CNA, 2008) and the two **advanced nursing practice (ANP)** roles in Canada: the nurse practitioner (NP) and clinical nurse specialist (CNS). *ANP* is a broad term referring to an advanced level of nursing practice that maximizes a nurse's graduate education, "in-depth nursing knowledge, and expertise in meeting the health needs of individuals, families, groups, communities and populations" (CNA, 2008, p. 9). All NPs are "registered nurses (RNs) with additional education and experience, and are able to autonomously diagnose, order and interpret tests, prescribe medications, and perform specific procedures within their legislated scope of practice" (CNA, 2009a, p. 1). All CNSs are RNs with a graduate or doctorate degree in nursing, extensive nursing knowledge and skills, clinical expertise, and experience in a specialty area (CNA, 2009b).

This chapter will highlight key definitions of competencies and related concepts, as well as the overall framework of competencies for ANP. Then a review of the various steps in the development of a competency framework for the NP and the CNS is demonstrated, based on CNA's experience. These competencies serve as the basis for the overall practice of NPs and CNSs in Canada. The competency framework for the NP was designed to facilitate the development of a national NP examination. The CNS competency framework was developed to achieve greater clarity about this role in the Canadian health care landscape and to inform the development of standardized educational programs within Canada.

Definition of Competencies

Competencies have been defined as a means to identify the range of functions, skills, knowledge, personal attributes, and behaviours needed to effectively perform a role within an organization (Lucia & Lepsinger, 1999). They are linked to a specific job and the related knowledge, skills, abilities, attitudes, and judgment required for a professional to become competent (Raymond, 2001).

Competencies are highly relevant to today's health care context and are key enablers for nursing practice. Not only are they used to provide recognition of learning wherever it takes place, but they also enable links to be made between professional and organizational requirements (Storey, Howard, & Gillies, 2002). Competencies are required whenever specific nursing roles need to be further refined (CNA, 2000) in conjunction with the standards of nursing practice that nursing regulatory bodies develop to protect the public in their provinces or territories. As such, CNA depicts competencies as the knowledge, skills, and abilities of a nurse to perform a specific action in a given situation (2005). The International Council of Nurses (ICN) describes nurses' competence as the "effective application of a combination of knowledge, skill and judgement demonstrated by an individual in daily practice or job performance" (2009, p. 6).

Competency Development

While the development of competency is not something new in nursing, it has become more relevant in recent years (Windsor, Douglas, & Harvey, 2012). A core competency is often linked to strategic, future-oriented, collective functions at the organizational level and is therefore called upon to provide the basic knowledge, attitudes, and skills needed to perform one's role as a health care professional (Moingeon & Edmondson, 1996; Parhalad & Hamel, 1990; Taber's Cyclopedic Medical Dictionary, 2013). The developmental process of a competency framework includes identifying a set of **core competencies** required for proficiency in a specific role or job (Chen & Naquin, 2005). Since the number and the level of competencies depend on the complexity of the role, developing competencies can take various forms. Some organizations identify competencies in specific ways, such as in performance or behavioural indicators, while others describe competencies in more general terms (Chen & Naquin, 2005).

Competency Frameworks

Competencies and competency frameworks received increasing attention in the 1980s as a popular alternative to job analysis (Assessment Strategies Inc. [ASI], 2013). A number of factors need to be considered when choosing a competency framework. One is the usefulness or meaningfulness of the competency framework, since it is often based on the intended use and audience. Another consideration is whether to include observable components.

Even if a competency profile is not being used for testing (i.e., for a licensing examination), it must still be determined if a professional requires development of a particular competency. For this reason, competency statements are typically expressed as measurable behaviours (ASI, 2013).

Competency frameworks seek to provide a picture of the "whole individual at work," including key elements of the knowledge, skills, abilities, attitudes, judgments, and other attributes required to perform a job. Moreover, they allow for broader, more general depictions of jobs and occupations by including descriptions of the worker and the organizational context (Chinn & Hertz, 2010). As a result, competency frameworks have become widespread across the various health care professions (ASI, 2013).

A competency framework is essentially a method for arranging competencies into logical groupings, based on a common theme or context. As such, it provides an organized layout for selecting the appropriate competency areas for a particular role and setting, and it also helps to promote a common definition as well as more precise language for its users (Vargas, 2004). While a competency framework can take a number of forms, in the health care context it generally focuses on what people need to achieve in the workplace, based on work outcomes and standards, as opposed to the mere acquisition of knowledge or skills (Storey, Howard, & Gillies, 2002).

Advanced Nursing Practice Competency Framework

In 2008, CNA described the core competencies for ANP in its publication *Advanced Nursing Practice: A National Framework*. The competencies developed are based on "an appropriate depth, breadth and range of nursing knowledge, theory and research, enhanced by clinical experience" (CNA, 2008, p. 22). Further, it is the blend of nurses' knowledge, skills, judgment, and personal attributes in a variety of environments that specifically defines ANP. Therefore, the development of new ANP roles requires an integrated approach that takes into account the regulatory aspect, the competencies to fulfill the role, and the education needed to prepare nurses with those desired competencies (Bryant-Lukosius & DiCenso, 2005). The framework continues to be used in a variety of ways, including developing educational courses, outlining concepts for research, shaping government policy statements, and interpreting ANP to employers, the public, other health care workers, and policy-makers.

Development of the Advanced Nursing Practice Framework

CNA approved the key elements of an ANP national framework in June 1999. The framework was first published in May 2000, and was then revised in 2002 to reflect the educational preparation for ANP as a graduate degree in nursing. In 2006, other initiatives in Canada highlighted the need to revise the framework to reflect current ANP and the evolution of nursing roles, which were and are still changing to serve clients' best interests. These projects included the Canadian Nurse Practitioner Initiative's (CNPI) *The Time is Now: Technical Reports* (2006) and CNA's *Dialogue on Advanced Nursing Practice* (2006). For the ANP dialogue, CNA invited nursing leaders, ANP experts, and nurses in ANP roles to participate. The key messages that arose from this dialogue (CNA, 2006) guided CNA's collaborative work with other stakeholders in maximizing the contribution of nurses in existing ANP roles, as well as in new roles that may emerge.

With national consultation in 2007, a national advisory committee was involved in the subsequent revision of this national framework. Developed by members of a national working group from CNA's 11 jurisdictional member organizations, the framework describes four categories of ANP competencies: clinical, research, leadership, and consultation and collaboration; these resulted in *Advanced Nursing Practice: A National Framework* (2008) as a national consensus document. Other components, such as evidence on the benefits of ANP and future direction, were also included.

The clinical competencies, which the framework describes as key ANP components, include the integration of "extensive clinical experience with theory, research and in-depth nursing and related knowledge" (CNA, 2008, p. 22). These competencies are founded on a holistic and integrated approach, as well as on working in partnership with clients and interprofessional members of a health care team to provide comprehensive care.

The research competencies encompass the generation, synthesis, and use of research evidence, which are central to ANP. In leadership competencies, **advanced practice nurses** (APNs) are leaders in improving overall patient care, along with care in their own settings. APNs lead interprofessional teams in identifying clinical goals to improve care to individuals, groups, and/or populations, and are "agents of change, consistently seeking effective new ways to practice, to improve the delivery of care, to shape their organizations, to benefit the [client] and influence health policy" (CNA, 2008, p. 24). For the consultation and collaboration competencies, APNs are considered experts and consult, communicate, and collaborate with colleagues, clients, and others across all sectors (CNA, 2008, 2009a, 2009b).

Nurse Practitioner Competencies

In 2005, CNPI was established and tasked with developing a pan-Canadian framework to promote the sustained integration of the NP role in primary health care. There were five components of CNPI:

1. Practice and evaluation
2. Legislation and regulation
3. Health human resource planning
4. Education
5. Change management and communications (CNPI, 2006)

CNPI developed a number of tools, including the *Canadian Nurse Practitioner Core Competency Framework* (2005). In 2005, Canadian nursing regulatory bodies worked together to develop required competencies and standards of practice for NPs (CNPI, 2005). This was the first time a delineation and consensus on core competencies for NPs had been achieved. This work was needed to define entry-level requirements for the NP role and to develop the basis for ongoing competence requirements. Initial work on core competencies for Canadian NPs was led by CNA's member jurisdictions and the College of Nurses of Ontario (CNO). By developing a Canadian core competency framework, CNPI sought a pan-Canadian consensus on the competencies NPs needed to practice, as well as a basis for the design and content of educational programs and licensure/registration exams (CNPI, 2006). The framework was also meant to support greater role clarity and understanding both within and outside the nursing profession.

The development of the NP competency framework (CNPI, 2005) consisted of four distinct activities. The first was to compare and analyze the existing NP competency documents developed by Canada's jurisdictional regulatory bodies. The resulting master list of competencies across jurisdictions led to a report with common core competencies for NPs in Canada. The second activity was a committee review to compare and analyze these competencies. This process expanded the definition of a patient to include the family and the community. It also identified categories for the competencies, such as health assessment and diagnosis; health care management and therapeutic interventions; health promotion and the prevention of illness, injury, and complications; and professional roles and responsibilities. The third step was the validation phase, which consisted of an extensive survey asking NPs, educators, employers, physicians, RNs, and other key stakeholders to identify the competencies required for safe and effective practice of entry-level nurse practitioners in Canada. The final step, a national consensus document on NP competencies, was developed under CNPI in 2005.

The final competencies, outlined in the *Canadian Nurse Practitioner Core Competency Framework* (CNPI, 2005), are presented in four categories to encompass the NP's holistic approach to health care:

1. Health assessment and diagnosis
2. Health care management and therapeutic interventions
3. Health promotion and the prevention of illness, injury, and complications
4. Professional roles and responsibilities

Within the categories, the descriptions outlined the integrated knowledge, skills, judgments, and attributes required of an NP to practice safely and ethically in a designated role and setting, regardless of client populations or practice environments. These core competencies were understood as building on those required of an RN. The competencies and validation data made it possible to describe and develop the essential components of the Canadian NP: Family/All Ages (CNPE: F/AA) examination (CNPI, 2006), which are also based on the CNPI competencies and framework. In the end, CNA's work during the CNPI brought national agreement for the core competencies (CNPI, 2005).

In 2009, in collaboration with all Canadian nursing regulatory bodies (with the exception of Quebec), CNA led a revision of the 2005 core competencies for NPs in Canada. This work was the result of a request for review from the executive directors of the nursing regulatory bodies. Their representatives participated in all phases of this process, identifying, developing, and validating the comprehensive competencies expected of the entry-level NP. This was done in collaboration with the CNPE core competency review committee, led by a consultant at ASI (CNA, 2010). ASI, a subsidiary testing agency of CNA, developed psychometrically sound and legally defensible registration/licensure examinations (CNA, 2004). These competencies were further validated by an extensive survey that asked NPs, educators, employers, physicians, RNs, and other key stakeholders to identify the competencies required for the safe and effective practice of entry-level NPs in Canada. Most of the jurisdictions adopted CNPI's *Canadian Nurse Practitioner Core Competency Framework* (2005) as the basis for NP competencies in their respective province/territory, some adding competencies specific to NP practice within their particular jurisdictions and legislation. The core competencies are transferrable across NP settings, as well as the needs of various populations. They reflect the competencies developed for ANP and build on the competencies for RNs.

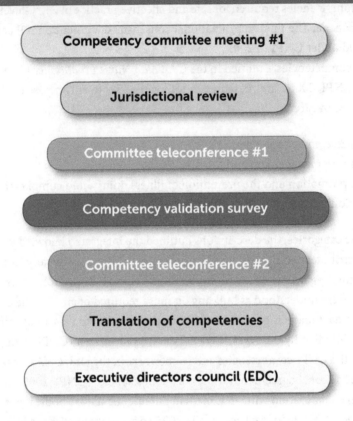

FIGURE 5.1:   An Overview of the Process and Work Plan for Reviewing the Canadian Nurse Practitioner Competencies

Competency committee meeting #1

Jurisdictional review

Committee teleconference #1

Competency validation survey

Committee teleconference #2

Translation of competencies

Executive directors council (EDC)

Source: Canadian Nurses Association (CNA), 2009c.

Clinical Nurse Specialist Competencies

The CNS role involves analyzing, synthesizing, and applying nursing knowledge, theory, and research evidence in order to foster system-wide changes, thereby advancing nursing care and the profession as a whole (CNA, 2008). Recently, Canadian researchers expressed the need for a pan-Canadian initiative to identify clear competencies for the CNS role in Canada (Bryant-Lukosius et al., 2010; Kilpatrick et al., 2011). To meet this need, the Pan-Canadian Competency Framework was created "to reflect the diversity of specialty areas and practice environments in which CNSs work and to support evolution of the CNS role to meet the changing needs of patients and the Canadian health care system" (CNA, 2014, p. 1). The purpose of the CNS framework is to

1. promote clarity of the CNS role;
2. facilitate understanding, and highlight the importance of the CNS role for improving health and the delivery of health care services;
3. guide the development of CNS education curricula and outcomes;
4. support CNSs in advancing their practice; and
5. support employers who are implementing CNS roles in their organizations. (CNA, 2014, p. 1)

CNA's development of CNS core competencies, in collaboration with ASI, began with a review of relevant literature. Assessing diverse competency profiles from ANP and other health care professions helped to create a framework for the pan-Canadian CNS competency profile. Each profile was examined according to scope (i.e., entry level vs. advanced, national vs. provincial/territorial), purpose, and general framework (including the types of competency categories used).

In this review, a number of CNS competencies and standards documents were discovered that were classified as "key" or "essential" competency categories. In many of the profiles, the CNS position is described in terms of functions. CNA's function-based recommendations for the CNS competency profile model, used by the national CNS competency task force, classifies the competencies around seven key functions: direct care, consultation, system leadership, collaboration, coaching, research, and ethical decision-making/advocacy.

Similar functions are reported in Canadian Clinical Nurse Specialists in Action—Standards (1997), and in the Framework for the Establishment of Clinical Nurse/Midwife Specialist Posts Intermediate Pathway (2007) from the National Council for the Professional Development of Nursing and Midwifery in Ireland. Interestingly, CNA also uses similar terms when describing the work of CNSs (CNA, 2009a), but instead of expressing these terms as functions, it frames their practice using key roles such as clinician, consultant, educator, researcher, and leader. No matter which of these descriptions is used, a fair degree of agreement exists on the CNS's role, even when other types of categorization are preferred.

While function and role-based models predominate in the CNS literature, some groups prefer to use variations of the general nursing process (i.e., assessment, diagnosis, intervention, and evaluation). For instance, the national CNS competency task force in the United States (US) categorizes competencies by the nursing process under three "spheres of influence" (2010), a phrase that refers to the areas impacted by the CNS's work: patients/clients, nurses and nursing practices, and organizational systems. In much the same vein, the ICN Framework of Competencies for the Nurse Specialist (2009), elements of which were considered when developing CNS competency standards in Canada, uses a modified nursing process model.

CNA also considered the emerging trends in CNS practice that were likely to impact the development of the competency profile. Examining these trends from several national and international publications highlighted the need to address three further issues: greater role clarity, the growing number of specialties within the CNS field, and the importance of interprofessional collaboration (Bryant-Lukosius et al., 2010; CNA, 2008, 2012). These fundamental elements formed the assumptions prior to developing the competencies.

The need for greater role clarity has occurred as health care has become more specialized and driven by outcomes. These changes are what gave rise to the development of new APN roles in Canada, namely the CNS and NP. As this process unfolded, however, some confusion arose about the distinct contribution of each role in the health care system. This lack of role clarity affects CNSs more than NPs, partly because the NP role in primary care has been more prominent over the past decade and also because of title protection for NPs in each province and territory. The lack of title recognition has been a key reason for greater confusion about the CNS role, as has a lack of consensus on entry-to-practice requirements (CNA, 2012). The many distinct specialties that the CNS works in (including pediatrics, oncology, and geriatrics, among others) have also added to the confusion over the CNS role. While all CNSs have a similar primary function to promote continuous improvement of patient outcomes and nursing care, the environments in which they operate vary considerably (CNA, 2009a). Thus, it was necessary that the competency framework for the CNS role easily communicate common practice elements while allowing for this variation in practice environments.

The need for collaborative relationships with other health care providers, for the purpose of setting goals and implementing care plans, was another issue to consider in establishing the CNS competency framework. Here, the framework needed to provide a clear road map not only for health care practitioners but also for the public and for those developing policies. At the same time, the framework had to remain broad enough to encompass the variety of environments the CNS operates in and to clearly express the strong interprofessional nature of the role.

To meet these challenges, the CNS competency framework adopted a five-step process. In the first step, CNA brought together a CNS steering committee and expert working group, representing CNSs and nurses from education, policy, management, and practice from each region of Canada. The CNS steering committee reviewed the practice of CNSs in Canada, and these elements were considered in the development of a draft framework. In step two, the project's steering committee and CNS expert working group solicited advice from another CNS working group, who participated in the design of competencies in a three-day workshop with ASI. Step three involved sending the resulting set of draft competencies to the steering committee for review, which would then become part of the document submitted for validation. In step four, a broad group of stakeholders reviewed and validated the competencies by means of an online ASI survey with guidance from CNA. Respondents were asked to rate each of the 59 competencies for its applicability to entry-to-practice, importance for safe and effective practice, frequency of use, and level of impact (i.e., client, practice setting, or organizational/system).

Using a snowball sampling approach, 93 surveys were completed (CNA, 2014). The responses were then analyzed to determine if the competencies were relevant to CNS practice. Both quantitative and qualitative results were reviewed; they showed a high level of applicability for the competencies that were developed. Once the CNS steering committee made its last adjustments and revisions based on feedback, some of the competencies were reviewed to verify relevance to safe and effective practice. During step five, CNA and the CNS steering committee made final decisions based on the survey results. In total, two competencies and sub-competencies were added while four were modified. The final profile consisted of 59 competencies, outlined in CNA's *Pan-Canadian Core Competencies for the Clinical Nurse Specialist* (2014).

The final CNS competencies expand on those required of an entry-level baccalaureate RN and reflect ANP by remaining consistent with CNA's *Advanced Nursing Practice: A National Framework* (2008), as well as by articulating competencies specific to the CNS role (CNA, 2014). The CNS core competencies in the national framework are grouped into four categories: clinical care, system leadership, advancement of nursing practice, and evaluation and research.

These competencies were developed as a means to learn more about the role of the CNS in Canada. They were created, reviewed, and validated using an evidenced-informed approach. The process relied heavily on the expertise of a diverse group of CNSs from across the country, who were part of more than 125 stakeholders that became involved. Moving forward, it is recommended the CNS competencies be reviewed in five years to ensure they are still relevant to Canadian CNS practice.

Conclusion

In 2012, the National Expert Commission, a Canadian consultation with health professionals and the public, recommended that an expanded scope of practice for nurses and other professionals be established to meet the country's growing health care needs. It also reinforced the importance of having competencies that are continually aligned with these evolving needs (National Expert Commission, 2012). The pan-Canadian competencies for CNS and NP roles are contributing to role clarity, public awareness, and nurse mobility, and are an important resource for many stakeholder groups such as nurses (RNs, CNSs, NPs), employers, educators, regulators, governments, and policy-makers. Several authors have suggested that nursing competencies serve a number of diverse purposes (ICN, 2003; Percival, 2004; Black et al., 2008). For example, as part of a framework for approving or recognizing nursing education programs in Canadian jurisdictions, competencies are used to describe what is expected of an entry-level graduate nurse in order to provide safe, competent, and ethical nursing care in a variety of practice settings. Competencies may also be used to develop practice standards, increase public and employer awareness of nurses' practice, facilitate the recognition of qualifications and skills required of internationally educated nurses, guide the development of definitions, clarify roles and responsibilities, facilitate the assessment of professional misconduct, and increase collaboration and communication (ICN, 2003; Percival, 2004).

Each set of competencies for nurses describe their unique and distinctive contributions to health care (ICN, 2008). Nursing competencies such as those in ANP roles are consistent with the scope of practice and requirements of nursing practice, as defined within the practice environment (ICN, 2008). The competencies for NPs and CNSs are progressive and build upon the competencies of the entry-level graduate nurse. While NPs and CNSs share some competencies, differences in the two roles emerge when these competencies are applied since the CNS and NP roles are distinct and have distinct competencies (DiCenso & Bryant-Lukosius, 2010). While the competency framework for APNs establishes clarity on the NP and CNS roles, it is the specific competency frameworks for NPs and CNSs that further delineate the differences and contributions of these roles in our health care system.

Critical Thinking Questions

1. What is the importance of developing competencies for advanced practice nurses (APNs)?
2. What are the steps for developing competencies for nurse practitioners (NPs)?
3. Why did the CNA develop competencies for NPs in Canada?
4. What is the purpose of developing separate competencies for CNS and NP roles in Canada?
5. Look at either the CNS or NP role within your organization, and consider if the respective competencies reflect the key aspects of their role? Why or why not?

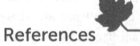

References

Assessment Strategies Inc. (ASI). (2013). *Report on suitable competency frameworks for the pan-Canadian clinical nurse specialist competency profile.* Unpublished.

Black, J., Allen, D., Redfern, L., Muzio, L., Rushowick, B., Balaski, B., ... Round, B. (2008). Competencies in the context of entry-level registered nurse practice: A collaborative project in Canada. *International Nursing Review, 55,* 171–178.

Bryant-Lukosius, D., Carter, N., Kilpatrick, K., Martin-Misener, R., Donald, F., Kaasalainen, S., … DiCenso, A. (2010). The clinical nurse specialist role in Canada. *Nursing Leadership, 23* (Special Issue December), 140–166. doi: 10.12927/cjnl.2010.22273

Bryant-Lukosius, D., & DiCenso, A. (2005). A framework for the introduction and evaluation of advanced practice roles. *Journal of Advanced Nursing, 48*, 530–540.

Canadian Nurses Association (CNA). (2000). *A national framework for continuing competence programs for registered nurses.* Ottawa, ON: CNA.

CNA. (2004). *The Canadian nurse practitioner competency project.* Ottawa, ON: CNA.

CNA. (2005). *Canadian nurse practitioner: Core competency framework.* Ottawa, ON: CNA.

CNA. (2006). *Report on the 2005 dialogue on advanced practice nurses.* Ottawa, ON: CNA.

CNA. (2008). *Advanced nursing practice: A national framework.* Ottawa, ON: Author.

CNA. (2009a). *Postion statement: The nurse practitioner.* Ottawa, ON: CNA.

CNA. (2009b). *Position statement: The clinical nurse specialist.* Ottawa, ON: CNA.

CNA. (2009c). *An overview of the process and work plan for reviewing the Canadian nurse practitioner competencies.* Unpublished manuscript. Ottawa, ON: CNA.

CNA. (2010). *Canadian nurse practitioner core competency.* Ottawa, ON: CNA.

CNA. (2012). *Strengthening the role of the clinical nurse specialist in Canada.* Ottawa, ON: CNA.

CNA. (2014). *Pan-Canadian core competencies for the clinical nurse specialist.* Ottawa, ON: CNA.

Canadian Nurse Practitioner Initiative (CNPI). (2005). *Canadian nurse practitioner core competency framework.* Ottawa, ON: CNA.

CNPI. (2006). *Nurse practitioners: The time is now. Technical reports.* Ottawa, ON: CNA.

Chen, H., & Naquin, S.S. (2005). *Development of competency-based assessment centers.* Retrieved from http://files.eric.ed.gov/fulltext/ED492404.pdf

Chinn, R.N., & Hertz, N.R. (2010). *Job analysis: A guide for credentialing organizations.* Lexington, KY: CLEAR.

Core competency. (2013). In D. Venes (Ed.). *Taber's cyclopedic medical dictionary* (22nd ed.). Philadelphia, PA: F.A. Davis.

Dicenso, A., & Bryant-Lukosius, D. (2010). *Clinical nurse specialists and nurse practitioners in Canada: A decision support synthesis.* Ottawa, ON: CHSRF.

International Council of Nurses (ICN). (2003). *An implementation model for the ICN framework of competencies for the generalist nurse.* Geneva, CH: ICN.

ICN. (2008). *Nursing care continuum: Framework and competencies.* Geneva, CH: ICN.

ICN. (2009). *ICN regulation series: ICN framework of competencies for the nurse specialist.* Geneva, CH: ICN.

Kilpatrick, K., DiCenso, A., Bryant-Lukosius, D., Ritchie, J.A., Martin-Misener, R., & Carter, N. (2011). Practice patterns and perceived impact of clinical nurse specialist roles in Canada: Results of a national survey. *International Journal of Nursing Studies, 50*, 1524–1536.

Lucia, A.D., & Lepsinger, R. (1999). *The art and science of competency models: Pinpointing critical success factors in organizations.* San Francisco, CA: Jossey-Bass/Pfeiffer

Moingeon, B., & Edmonson, A. (1996). *Organizational learning and competitive advantage.* Thousand Oaks, CA: Sage.

National CNS Competency Task Force. (2010). *Clinical nurse specialist core competencies* [Executive summary]. Philadelphia, PA: NACNS.

National Council for the Professional Development of Nursing and Midwifery (NCNM). (2007). *Framework for the establishment of clinical nurse/midwife specialist posts intermediate pathway*. Dublin, Ireland: NCNM.

National Expert Commission. (2012). *A nursing call to action: The health of our nation, the future of our health system*. Ottawa, ON: CNA.

Prahalad, C.K., & Hamel, G. (1990). The core competence of the corporation. *Harvard Business Review, 68*(3), 79-91. Retrieved from http://papers.ssrn.com/sol3/papers.cfm?abstract_id=1505251

Percival, E. (2004). *Common competencies for registered nurses in Western Pacific and South East Asian Region (WPSEAR)*. Dickson, ACT: ANMAC.

Raymond, M.R. (2001). Job analysis and the specification of content for licensure and certification examinations. *Applied Measurement in Education, 14*, 369–415.

Storey, L., Howard, J., & Gillies, A. (2002). *Competency in healthcare: A practical guide to competency frameworks*. Retrieved from http://www.myilibrary.com?ID=85788

Vargas, F. (2004). *40 questions on labour competency* (Technical office papers, 13). Montevideo, Uruguay: CINTERFOR.

Windsor, C., Douglas, C., & Harvey, T. (2012). Nursing and competencies — a natural fit: The politics of skill/competency formation in nursing. *Nursing Inquiry, 19*, 213–222. doi: 10.1111/j.1440-1800.2011.00549.x

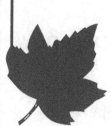

SECTION II

Advanced Practice Nursing Competencies in Canada: A Case Study Approach

This section applies the Canadian Nurses Association's (CNA) advanced practice nursing (APN) framework for clinical, research, leadership, consultation, and collaboration competencies, using a variety of case studies developed by clinical nurse specialists (CNSs) and nurse practitioners (NPs) to demonstrate how each APN contributor enacts the role competency presented. In this section, there may appear to be some repetition between chapters, but, as a whole, each competency discussion demonstrates consistency in practice approaches between APNs, and further informs and substantiates the competency discussion.

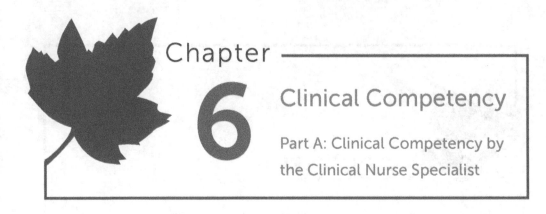

Chapter 6

Clinical Competency

Part A: Clinical Competency by the Clinical Nurse Specialist

Patricia A. McQuinn

Patricia A. McQuinn is a CNS-Palliative Care, Extra-Mural Program at Horizon Regional Health Authority in Moncton, New Brunswick.

> ### KEY TERMS
>
> advanced practice
> nurses (APNs)
> clinical competency
> clinician

> ### OBJECTIVES
>
> 1. Explore the clinical competency of the CNS role.
> 2. Discuss the importance of the CNS's clinical competency in Canada's complex health care environment.
> 3. Explore the application of the CNS clinical role competency in practice.

Introduction

The Canadian Nurses Association's (CNA) *Advanced Nursing Practice: A National Framework* (2008) established the competency requirements that define and clarify clinical nursing practice for **advanced practice nurses (APNs)**. APNs require in-depth nursing knowledge and expertise to meet the health care needs of clients, which include individuals, families, organizations, groups, and specific populations. In addition to focusing on the needs of clients, APNs possess a graduate degree in nursing, providing them with the ability to analyze, synthesize, and apply nursing knowledge, theory, and evidence-informed research in order to facilitate changes and build on expertise within all levels of health care (CNA, 2008).

APNs utilize leadership skills, educational opportunities, clinical expertise, and understanding of organizations, health policy, and decision-making to play an important role in client and health care system outcomes in combination with an integration of knowledge from other disciplines (CNA, 2008).

This chapter will explore the CNA core clinical competency for the CNS role, including discussion of a CNS-led case study that demonstrates application of the competency.

Clinical Nurse Specialist

Globally, a goal of the CNS role is to advance nursing care and the profession as a whole (CNA, 2008). As a domain of advanced practice, the clinical competency of a CNS influences a diverse number of specialty areas and environments. The environments for application of the CNS competencies may be within an area of practice or subspecialty, a disease, a type of care or health problem, a specific patient population, or a specific facility (CNA, 2014).

Key to the CNS role is autonomy and flexibility in responding to the evolving needs of clients—whether they be individuals, patients, nursing staff, clinical settings, and/or health care organizations—with consideration to associated economic variability, population groups, geographic locations, and other attributing factors. The goal of the CNS is to ensure safety, quality of care, and positive health outcomes. In the clinical environment, the CNS fills a critical role in reaching these goals for clients/patients, nursing professionals, other health care providers, and health care organizations. CNSs may be hospital- or community-based, practicing in collaborative private practices, or in industry or business organizations. CNSs may deliver care across different clinical environments; for example, a CNS may follow a patient through the trajectory of the illness (including from home to hospital).

Clinical Competency

This section focuses on the clinical competency that is outlined in the recently developed *Pan-Canadian Core Competencies for the Clinical Nurse Specialist* (CNA, 2014). The clinical role of the CNS usually revolves around complex or difficult patient or nursing situations. When CNSs strategize to improve and resolve challenging situations, they draw on an in-depth knowledge of nursing and other relevant sciences (CNA, 2009). Integral to this facilitation and resolution, the CNS assesses, develops, or contributes to the plan of clinical care and provides information or education throughout the various stages as the situation evolves. The level of direct clinical involvement a CNS has with the client—whether nursing staff, other health care professionals, community care workers, or even the patient—may fluctuate.

The role of a CNS as a clinician involves the other defining characteristics of the CNS competencies (i.e., research, leadership, consultation, collaboration). These aspects of the professional responsibilities or attributes of the CNS competencies cannot be separated from each other; rather, these attributes are interwoven into clinical practice situations.

Due to the increasing acuity and complexity of care delivery, the CNS as a clinician is integrally involved in work with health care providers to assess, plan, implement, and evaluate care of patients/clients. Many CNSs in clinical situations assist to facilitate and help coordinate care of complex patient/client situations during their hospital stays, and prepare them for discharges to their homes or to other care facilities. Interesting to note is that the coordination of care by CNSs had resulted in fewer readmissions of certain populations of patients (Jansen & Zwygart-Stauffacher, 2010).

To prepare for management of complex situations, the CNS utilizes proficiency in the nursing process, communication strategies, collaboration techniques, and knowledge of the workings of partnerships and relationships. However, evaluation, assessment, professional accountability, and awareness of the availability of information or resources, along with current advanced clinical knowledge (such as evidence-informed practice), help the CNS better understand and resolve issues related to clinical situations. Often, the goal of the CNS is to gather as much information from the team concerning the clinical situation, issue, or presenting problem. After gathering all the relevant information, the CNS endeavours to bring the clinical team together in order to clarify and establish desired outcomes.

More often than not, the situations that the CNS is consulted for are unexpected, troublesome to the individuals involved, have a complicated nature, and are at a critical or crisis level for the individual, team, or organization. By completing a thorough assessment, the CNS is able to elaborate and illuminate the multiple perspectives of the situation, issue, or concern to the players who may be involved in the situation. This will often include the perspectives of the nursing staff, the interprofessional team, the patient, and the family (as individuals and a combined unit). The organization's perspective cannot be forgotten and often becomes part of the process because of the need to consider economic realities and resource availability. The literature reports that the CNS in the clinical setting has an impact on outcomes of care and has led to reduced risks of patient injuries and financial loss (DeNisco & Barker, 2013). Involvement of the CNS brings a holistic view of all interactions and the dynamics of the situation.

Clinical Practice Development

Development of procedures, techniques, and protocols for nurses is a clinical aspect the CNS works to enhance. Nurses require knowledge to guide their performance of tasks and institutes require protocols to coordinate care. The CNS utilizes access, credibility, understanding, and interpretation of the relevant literature findings to implements changes in practice. The development of practices and protocols requires an in-depth knowledge and review of current evidence and research; this is often initiated by the CNS. The CNS facilitates this process by asking critical questions, and uses this opportunity to ensure participation for all involved. Ultimately the CNS, during the development of clinical practices and protocols, must engage all stakeholders who will be impacted as this will also help educate and disseminate information throughout the clinical setting.

In addition, the inquiries and research information provided by the CNS is useful to patients/individuals/clients, teams, and decision-makers for planning resources and approaches to care, as well as the management of complex situations. This may manifest as training documentations, flow diagrams, and/or educational or informational brochures.

CNSs can effectively "demonstrate clinical expertise and mentor individuals through role modelling key behaviours, especially in complex patient/family situations" (Fulton, Lyon, & Goudreau, 2010, p. 123). The CNS may mentor staff by directly providing care, educating the patient/family, or supporting other health care providers. The education or guidance the CNS provides to the nursing and interprofessional teams assists in enhancing and applying these abilities to manage similar complex situations in the future.

In the clinical environment, the CNS often offers situation-reviewing formats (such as debriefing and reflection) that encourage understanding of care provided, facilitates opportunities for staff to communicate with peers and other colleagues, and assists in building a foundation of collaborative care. Debriefing can bring challenging practice situations back to the clinical environment for review and ongoing learning. The use of reflection in clinical practice assists in team development by re-evaluating care practices, critically analyzing a care situation in detail, brainstorming alternative practice behaviours, as well as preparing for and anticipating potential future situations.

Communication Team Player

Fundamental to clinical competency is the CNS's ability to critically analyze the complex interaction of sociological, psychological, and physiological processes, including the determinants of health and understanding the client's lived experience (CNA, 2008). A key component of the CNS role is the ability to positively affect complex situations through actions, behaviours, and information or learning sessions, which will eventually impact outcomes. Adapting to changes, coordinating and balancing availability, developing protocols, attending meetings, conducting research, and dealing with paperwork are a necessary part of the CNS role and tend to consume precious time. The skills of balancing workload, flexibility, multitasking, and collaborative team partnerships are key to the success of the CNS clinician role.

The following case study illustrates the clinical competency of the CNS role at a level of direct involvement with the patient and family, as well as with front-line caregivers in different care environments.

CASE STUDY

The Story of Sandy

Sandy was a 42-year-old married female who had been a palliative patient in the hospital for three weeks. She lived with her husband, Ethan, and their two children aged six and ten. She was diagnosed with breast cancer four years ago and underwent a modified radical mastectomy, aggressive chemotherapy, and radiation. Sandy developed metastases to her brain, liver, and bone, and her condition deteriorated to the point where she experienced mild confusion and physical symptoms (including back pain, nausea, anorexia, constipation, and weakness), yet continued to ambulate with assistance.

On admission to the hospital, the CNS was consulted to assist with the patient's physical symptoms, determine the patient's goals, and facilitate the coordination of care with the interprofessional team. Through collaboration, priority-setting, and using best practice guidelines related to medical options, Sandy's symptoms were soon managed. The CNS quickly and efficiently followed up to help manage any setbacks to Sandy's physical care, including consulting with the occupational therapist (OT) and physiotherapist (PT) to assist with safety, skin integrity, and mobility, including home arrangements for Sandy's potential discharge.

Sandy and her husband expressed concern related to how their children were going to handle their mother's death. Coordinating information and resources, the CNS and social worker on the case found books related to death and dying that were age appropriate for the children.

Sandy wanted to go home to spend time with her children and prepare them for her death. The nursing staff, however, felt that her care could not be managed at home. Her husband, Ethan, and her mother, Eileen, were prepared to do what they could to make this happen. The CNS guided and facilitated the transfer of care to the community care partners, including discussing the do-not-resuscitate (DNR) order of the patient with family. Ethan appeared to understand the gravity of Sandy's condition and, after discussion, agreed to a DNR order and together with the CNS made funeral arrangements. At the family's request, a social worker and child life specialist continued to help guide the children in understanding the situation and helping them voice concerns about the changes they saw in their mother. The CNS also participated in family discussions of where Sandy wanted to die, if readmission to hospital was an option, and how these decisions would affect her care and impact the children.

Anticipatory plans were discussed and put in place for end-of-life care in the home. Initially, Sandy's condition allowed her to participate in family life and talk with her children; she made memory boxes and knitted special items for her children with her mother. The child life specialist followed up with the family and reviewed how the children were coping with the situation. Once Sandy was home, the CNS continued her supportive relationship with the family, and provided guidance and support related to any concerns or care issues for the home care team.

Sandy's condition progressed and gradually she became semi-conscious. Ethan and the children adapted to the change, and continued to spend time in Sandy's room doing activities and talking to her about their daily accomplishments. The children talked about having a "Mommy angel" around them and this seemed to give them comfort. During discussions with the CNS, Ethan was able to confide his concern related to how he would cope after his wife's death. Following Sandy's death at home, the CNS followed up with the family, the hospital, and community caregivers, encouraging all to reflect on and discuss the experience.

Discussion

In Sandy's case study, the CNS initially collaborated with the in-hospital care team and helped to identify the major symptoms associated with the patient's palliative condition, as well as identify the probable cause of each symptom. Guidance by the CNS was needed to establish priorities in symptom management, and to provide insight for therapeutic interventions to manage the symptoms Sandy was experiencing. The CNS helped guide the development of an in-patient care plan with Sandy and the care team. Education and information on current practices provided support to the nursing staff providing Sandy's care.

Many professionals had different perspectives and information in relation to Sandy's care. The CNS coordinated, engaged, and involved the different disciplines in a case conference to share information among members and plan Sandy's care. This was paramount as it was instrumental in facilitating a smooth plan of care, of which Sandy and her family's goals were an integral part. While the patient stayed in hospital, the CNS, with the family's permission, arranged for the children to spend time with the child life specialist.

Leadership, interprofessional collaboration, communication strategies, evidence-informed symptom management, and evaluation of outcomes are evident from the CNS. The CNS worked alongside and followed up with the in-hospital care and interprofessional teams to facilitate a safe and seamless transition home. The CNS guided the care team in preparing for discharge by contacting the discharge planner, arranging for home care supplies, and coordinating an OT in conjunction with Sandy's husband. The volunteer hospice organization was contacted to arrange support, companionship, and respite for the family; a homemaker agency was contacted to assist with Sandy's physical care and household needs.

The CNS monitored and supported the community-based interprofessional team in symptom management, care coordination, education, and support of Sandy's family. The CNS communicated with the team about the patient's and family's goals of care, and helped modify the plan of care to adapt to changes in Sandy's condition and the needs of her caregivers. The CNS worked within both the in-hospital and in-home care environments, and kept the hospital team apprised of the Sandy's condition, the family's coping ability, possible readmission, and end-of-life care.

The case study further illustrates the CNS role in planning and collaboration to facilitate transition from one setting to another in complex care. An example of this was the request to have a do-not-resuscitate (DNR) order prior to Sandy's discharge home. In this situation, the CNS facilitated informed decision-making by initiating discussion with the family related to this difficult topic and assessing their spiritual needs. As the family felt increasingly anxious and sought reassurance regarding Sandy's condition, the CNS and community care team provided continued support.

The story of Sandy illustrates the clinical competency of a CNS role. The CNS was involved in Sandy's care from beginning to end, through evaluation and follow-up. The CNS influenced the patient and family, as well as health care teams and various organizations and institutions. The CNS endeavoured to provide best practices, as well as efficient and effective care, with measurable outcomes that are critical when timelines are short and the patient and family are vulnerable. The case study also demonstrated how CNSs use evolving best care practices to meet both care team and patient/family needs through consultation, mentoring, education, evaluation, and advocacy by identifying symptoms, establishing priorities, and providing education as needed.

Conclusion

The CNS as clinician expertise is outlined in the CNA *Pan-Canadian Core Competencies for the Clinical Nurse Specialist*. CNSs are involved in complex health care situations that are often not predictable and require flexibility, resourcefulness, and expertise. These are but a few of the strengths of the CNS role.

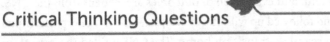

Critical Thinking Questions

1. Describe different clinical situations where the CNS influences patient and organizational outcomes.
2. In a hypothetical situation, consider a practice change and outline the way that the CNS would lead the change.
3. Identify how theory and research-based sources can contribute to, or enhance, day-to-day nursing clinical practices.

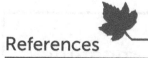

References

Canadian Nurses Association (CNA). (2008). *Advanced nursing practice: A national framework.* Ottawa, ON: CNA. Retrieved from http://www.cna-aiic.ca/~/media/cna/page-content/pdf-en/anp_national_framework_e.pdf

CNA. (2009). *Position statement: Clinical nurse specialist.* Ottawa, ON: CNA. Retrieved from https://www.cna-aiic.ca/~/media/cna/page-content/pdf-en/clinical-nurse-specialist_position-statement.pdf?la=en

CNA. (2014). *Pan-Canadian core competencies for the clinical nurse specialist.* Ottawa, ON: CNA. Retrieved from http://cna-aiic.ca/en/news-room/news-releases/2014/canadian-nurses-association-launches-core-competencies-for-clinical-nurse-specialists

DeNisco, S., & Barker A. (Eds.). (2013) *Advanced practice nursing: Evolving roles for the transformation of the profession* (2nd ed.). Burlington, MA: Jones and Bartlett.

Fulton, J.S., Lyon, B.L., & Gaudreau, K.A. (Eds.). (2010). *Foundations of clinical nurse specialist practice.* New York, NY: Springer.

Jansen, M., & Zwygart-Stauffacher, M. (Eds.). (2010) *Advanced practice nursing: Core concepts for professional role development* (4th ed.). New York, NY: Springer.

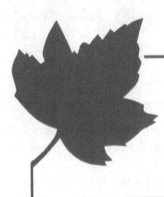

Clinical Competency

Part B: Clinical Competency by the Nurse Practitioner

Margaret (Marnee) Wilson

Marnee Wilson is an NP–Adult and Professional Practice Leader for NPs, NP Cardiovascular Surgery at St. Michael's Hospital in Toronto, Ontario. She holds an appointment as Adjunct Lecturer at the Lawrence Bloomberg Faculty of Nursing, University of Toronto, and has acted as Director of Professional NP Practice for the Nurse Practitioners' Association of Ontario (NPAO).

KEY TERMS

clinical competencies
direct patient care
nurse practitioner (NP)
    practice competencies

OBJECTIVES

1. Describe how the nurse practitioner (NP) enacts the Canadian Nurses Association (CNA) clinical competencies in practice.
2. Compare and contrast CNA's advanced nursing practice and NP clinical competencies.
3. Identify how the NP competencies are actualized in NP practice.

Introduction

Advanced practice nursing (APN) is an umbrella term that describes an advanced level of clinical nursing practice, and usually refers to either clinical nurse specialists (CNSs) or nurse practitioners (NPs) (CNA, 2008). Both roles are recognized as providing expert nursing care to patients that involve an advanced level of analysis and synthesis of information, utilization of existing research, and contribution to the advancement of the nursing profession.

The clinical competencies in advanced practice are characterized by the provision of clinical care to patients that is grounded in specialty nursing knowledge in a particular field. It is, in particular, the application of theoretical, research-based, and experiential concepts that guide complex nursing assessments, decision-making, and intervention strategies for patients, families, and communities. **NP practice competencies** extend this practice to include specific, scope-related responsibilities for diagnosis and therapeutic planning.

Accountability for direct clinical care and autonomous decision-making typically comprises a greater proportion of the NP role than that of the CNS role. For NPs in both primary and acute care settings, most of the time spent in the NP role is involved in **direct patient care** (Donald et al., 2010; Kilpatrick et al., 2010). The clinical role of the NP is built upon, and extends, the APN clinical competencies. NPs provide care that utilizes these clinical competencies to enhance continuity, communication, comprehensiveness of care, and collaboration with the interprofessional team (see Table 6.1).

TABLE 6.1: Comparison of APN and NP Clinical Competencies

APN Clinical Competencies	NP Clinical Competencies
• Develop multiple advanced assessment and intervention strategies within a client-centred framework for individual clients, communities, and populations. • Use qualitative and quantitative data from multiple sources, often in ambiguous and complex situations, when making clinical decisions and initiating and managing change. • Analyze the complex interaction of sociological, psychological, and physiological processes, with determinants of health and clients' lived experience. • Anticipate and explain the wide range of client responses to actual or potential health problems and recommend action. • Guide decision-making in complex clinical situations. • Engage clients and other team members in resolving issues at the individual, organizational, and health care system levels. • Identify and assess trends or patterns that have health implications for individuals, families, groups, or communities. • Generate and incorporate new nursing knowledge and develop new standards of care, programs, and policies. • Plan, initiate, coordinate, and conduct educational programs based on needs, priorities, and organizational resources.	• Practice in accordance with federal and provincial/territorial legislation, professional and ethical standards, and policy relevant to nurse practitioner practice. • Understand the changes in scope of practice from that of a registered nurse, and the ways that these changes affect responsibilities and accountabilities when assuming the reserved title and scope of practice of a nurse practitioner. • Incorporate knowledge of diversity, cultural safety, and determinants of health in the assessment, diagnosis, and therapeutic management of clients, as well as in the evaluation of outcomes. • Incorporate knowledge of developmental and life stages, pathophysiology, psychopathology, epidemiology, environmental exposure, infectious diseases, behavioural sciences, demographics, and family processes when performing health assessments, making diagnoses, and providing overall therapeutic management. • Incorporate knowledge of the clinical manifestations of normal health events, acute illness/injuries, chronic diseases, comorbidities, and emergency health needs, including the effects of multiple etiologies in the assessment, diagnosis, and therapeutic management of clients and in the evaluation of outcomes. • Integrate the principles of resource allocation and cost-effectiveness into clinical decision-making. • Provide client diagnostic information and education that are relevant, theory-based, and evidence-informed using appropriate teaching/learning strategies.

continued

TABLE 6.1: Comparison of APN and NP Clinical Competencies *(cont.)*	
APN Clinical Competencies	**NP Clinical Competencies**
• Manage a wide range of patient responses to actual and potential health problems.	• Promote safe client care by mitigating harm and addressing immediate risks for clients and others affected by adverse events and near misses. • Disclose the facts of adverse events to clients and reports adverse events to appropriate authorities, in keeping with relevant legislation and organizational policies. • Document clinical data, assessment findings, diagnoses, plans of care, therapeutic interventions, client responses, and clinical rationale in a timely and accurate manner. • Adhere to federal and provincial/territorial legislation, policies and standards related to privacy, documentation, and information management. • Engage in ongoing professional development and accept personal responsibility for maintaining nurse practitioner competence.

Source: Adapted from Canadian Nurses Association (CNA), 2008, 2010.

A case study example from hospital-based, NP–Adult practice will be used to describe and compare APN and NP clinical competencies.

CASE STUDY

The Story of Jim

Chief Complaint: Jim was a 68-year-old male who managed a small plumbing business in a remote community in Ontario. He was discharged 10 days ago following coronary artery bypass graft surgery (CABG), but presented again for readmission because of shortness of breath.

History of Present Illness: Jim had been experiencing exertional chest tightness for several months. He recently had a prolonged episode of chest pain and presented to the emergency department (ED) of the local hospital. Jim was diagnosed with a non ST-elevation acute coronary syndrome (NSTE-ACS) and admitted to hospital where he received supportive care and underwent cardiac diagnostics to delineate his risk for further cardiac events. A coronary angiography identified critical left main coronary artery disease and Jim was transferred to an urban cardiac centre. On that admission, he underwent uncomplicated CABG and his hospital care was led by a nurse practitioner (NP). He was discharged several days later with careful support, including an escort to a commercial aircraft, an attendant while on the flight, and family to meet him at the airport close to home.

After being discharged from the hospital, Jim did not participate in any of the recommended components of the discharge plan. He did not get his prescriptions filled, did not want to participate in the walking program, shower, or observe dietary restrictions. He missed his follow-up appointment with his primary care provider, NP Jones. Jim became progressively more short of breath and grew fearful, finally presenting to the ED of the local hospital at his fiancée's urging. He was transferred back to the urban centre for further evaluation, under the care of the NP.

Past Medical History: BMI 40, hypertension, dyslipidemia, moderate left ventricular dysfunction and heart failure syndrome, osteoarthritis.

Social History: Jim had been divorced for many years, had one daughter aged 32, and was engaged to Eleanor. He was financially independent. He was dyslexic and had only completed a grade-three education. Jim was unable to read signs or numbers (information not volunteered by him but disclosed by family). He had not allowed any family members to accompany him, or visit him while in hospital.

Family History: Non-contributory.

Relevant Physical Examination Findings:
Afebrile
Cardiac: BP 130/72; heart rate 102 (sinus tachycardia); JVP 9, 3+ edema (up to sacrum); noted weight gain of 7 kg since discharge; S1 and S2 regular; no extra heart sounds or murmurs.
Respiratory: RR 24; O2 saturation 94% with 4L/minute oxygen via nasal prongs; breath sounds diminished halfway up posterior lung fields with bibasilar crackles. Dull to percussion, no wheezes. Noted use of intercostal muscles.
Psycho-emotional: Anxious and tearful; states not sleeping.
Integumentary: Skin intact; surgical incision healing well with no signs of infection. Sternal incision well healed; bone solid.
Pain: None.
All other systems within normal limits.

Review of Systems:
No fevers, chills, or night sweats.
Cardiac: Two-pillow orthopnea, no paroxysmal nocturnal dyspnea (PND). Jim has not been following fluid or sodium restriction. No chest pain.
Respiratory: Progressive shortness of breath with activity; no cough/sputum.
Integument: Wound intact; no redness or drainage.

GI/GU: Within normal limits.
All other systems within normal limits.

Relevant Diagnostic Tests:
Blood Work: Electrolytes, complete blood count (CBC), D-dimer within normal limits.
Recent Echocardiogram: Normal valvular function; left ventricular ejection fraction 37%; no pericardial effusion.

Allergies: None.

Oral Medications: ASA 81 mg daily; Bisoprolol 5 mg daily; Ramipril 7.5 mg daily; Rosuvastatin 20 mg daily; Furosemide 80 mg daily. Acetaminophen 325-650 mg Q4H prn, Hydromorphone 2 mg q4h prn for incisional pain.

Discussion

An analysis of Jim's case illustrates that the NP provided care that was grounded in a nursing role, with the aim of supporting Jim through the experience of cardiovascular illness to attain/regain optimal function (CNO, 2011). His care was enhanced by specialty knowledge relevant to cardiovascular disease on the part of the NP.

In this case, the NP demonstrated many of the APN competencies outlined in the APN competency framework (CNA, 2008). The NP provided advanced assessment and intervention strategies developed appropriately for Jim's age, body size, educational/literacy background, emotional state, and family circumstances. Additionally, the practice demonstrated the integration of data from multiple sources (Jim, his daughter, and his fiancée, as well as the sending hospital and provider) and analysis of the complex interaction of processes to understand Jim's unique experience of illness. Further, the NP understood and explained Jim's response to his health problems and demonstrated an understanding of common patient needs and trends. For example, the NP assessed that Jim's response to his first discharge was a result of his unique experience and limitations, but not a problem with the discharge decision or process.

The NP also engaged the client and other team members in resolving issues by working with Jim and his family to find a solution that would meet his unique needs, while balancing the need for system efficiency. The NP engaged other members of the interprofessional team including the RN staff, physiotherapist, and occupational therapist to facilitate communication about Jim's needs and experiences, as well as to incorporate discipline-specific recommendations into the plan of care. Finally, the NP generated new nursing knowledge, policies, and education programs by integrating lessons learned from Jim's experience into unit and policy around the approach to patient communication, values, and needs related to discharge.

NP Clinical Competency

NP competencies build and expand upon APN competencies, and allow the APN to provide guidance and make recommendations for care (CNA, 2010). The NP competencies permit the NP to lead care by using the expanded scope of practice to make autonomous diagnoses and treatment decisions. NPs' care decisions are based on an analysis of health information obtained though utilization of APN competencies, and by obtaining additional information via the NP clinical competencies of advanced health assessment, diagnostic reasoning, and therapeutic planning. This section will analyze the NP's utilization of the NP clinical competencies in the provision of Jim's care.

The NP integrated information from Jim's comprehensive assessment to formulate differential diagnoses for the presenting symptom of shortness of breath. The NP also incorporated complex information about the patient and disease process, and recognized abnormal responses and multiple etiologies to develop a list of differential diagnoses, which included pleural effusion, atelectasis, heart failure, pneumonia, pneumothorax, and pulmonary embolus. The NP's impression was that Jim was in moderate respiratory distress, but not in any immediate danger (promoting safe client care by mitigating harm) of respiratory failure. The NP confirmed this by ordering and interpreting arterial blood gases.

The NP also ordered and reviewed a chest X-ray, which showed large bilateral pleural effusions, atelectasis, and mild pulmonary edema but no pneumothorax or pneumonia. They also conducted a risk score, based on research evidence that indicated that Jim's likelihood for pulmonary embolus was low. The NP ordered blood work along with an electrocardiogram to differentiate heart failure from non-cardiac pulmonary edema and to rule out cardiac ischemia. Investigations for cardiac ischemia were negative, but confirmed heart failure.

Diagnostic information and education was provided to Jim that explained the diagnoses of pleural effusion, atelectasis, and heart failure in simple terms, using pictures as needed. With permission (adhering to privacy legislation) the information was also discussed with Jim's fiancée and daughter, who were very fearful because they had been told that Jim was critically ill. The NP took the time to listen to their concerns and clarified Jim's condition and the plan of care.

The NP documented the clinical data, assessment findings, diagnoses, plan of care, therapeutic interventions, client responses, and clinical rationale in the patient's chart and developed a therapeutic plan that included medication reconciliation to assure that Jim was receiving his usual heart failure regimen, increased diuresis, and reinforced fluid and dietary sodium restriction to achieve euvolemia. The NP obtained Jim's consent and provided orders for thoracentesis, ensuring they ordered appropriate fluid analysis to identify the nature of the pleural effusion. To assist in resolving the atelectasis, the NP collaborated with nursing staff and a physiotherapist to demonstrate techniques for lung expansion to Jim, as well as provide coaching to help build Jim's confidence in working with the team to improve his mobilization (which was somewhat limited by his large body size and poor conditioning). Jim's respiratory status improved quickly with diuresis, careful titration of his heart failure regimen, thoracentesis, and mobilization.

Recalling that Jim had been euvolemic and was at normal "dry" weight prior to discharge on a stable dose of diuretic as part of his heart failure regimen, the NP sought to understand what had happened at home to contribute to the fluid retention. The NP investigated the cause for Jim's respiratory problems and confirmed that Jim had received post-operative health teaching about recovery from surgery and heart failure self-management prior to discharge. They also learned that Jim had been able to articulate key concepts using a *teach back* method (relevant, theory-based, and evidence-informed using appropriate teaching/ learning strategies). Unfortunately, Jim's anxiety severely impaired his ability to self-manage and, once home, was unable to participate in self-care activities.

Further, the NP incorporated knowledge of diversity, cultural safety, and determinants of health in discussing reasons for readmission with Jim and developing and strategies to prevent further readmission. The NP listened to Jim's account of his unsuccessful discharge; he had been significantly traumatized by the experience of the commercial flight home, and as a result he described feeling overwhelmed and intimidated and lost confidence in his ability to recover. The NP acknowledged Jim's experience and although the previous discharge plan had been appropriate with respect to safety and utilization of resources (resource allocation and cost-effectiveness), it had not been successful for him given his particular needs. The NP then worked further with Jim to arrange a discharge plan that would be successful.

Once Jim was stable and his care requirements could be met at a hospital close to his home and family, the NP made the autonomous decision to discharge him as per provincial hospital legislation and institutional policy. In working with the interprofessional team to provide care to Jim, the NP understood and demonstrated the differences between their role and that of the RNs they collaborated with. The NP also successfully worked with team members to provide a broad framework and understanding of the NP roles and accountabilities within the team.

Conclusion

NP clinical practice is deeply rooted in advanced nursing competencies that provide the foundation for the values, knowledge, and theories of professional nursing practice. NP clinical practice must also include utilization of expanded skills and scope to provide care to patients that pertains to health promotion and illness and injury prevention, as well as rehabilitative, curative, supportive, and palliative care (CNA, 2010).

Legislation has now been passed in all Canadian jurisdictions that extends the scope of practice of NPs (NPAO, 2014), with the intention of increasing access to care for patients, increasing interprofessional collaboration, and maintaining safety (Wakulowsky & Chaiet, 2010). Graduate education prepares NPs to use these expanded clinical competencies to place an individual's experience of illness at the centre of the plan of care and engage in high levels of care coordination that improves patient satisfaction and demonstrates improved physical and social function (Sidani & Doran, 2010). Importantly, the NP role also allows for better and improved continuity of care post discharge (Robles et al., 2011) and enables quality, safe, and timely patient care (Hurlock-Chorostecki, Forchuk, Orchard, van Soeren, & Reeves, 2013).

Further, the NP clinical role improves team functioning and interprofessional care (van Soeren, Hurlock-Chorostecki, Goodwin, & Baker, 2009; van Soeren, Hurlock-Chorostecki, & Reeves, 2011), in addition to collaboration, team dynamics, efficiencies, quality of care, enhanced job satisfaction, and nursing professionalism (Searle, 2008). The NP serves as a lynchpin for the team, promoting enhanced communication and practice that facilitates a patient's journey (Williamson, Twelvetree, Thompson, & Beaver, 2012), enhances knowledge and efficiency of team members, and improves patient flow through the system (Hurlock-Chorostecki, Forchuk, Orchard, van Soeren, & Reeves, 2014).

Challenges still exist in terms of successful implementation and integration of the NP role. Central to these barriers is role confusion, both between the CNS and NP roles and other role titles within the clinical environment (e.g., physician assistant, hospitalist, resident physician, and case manager). Improved clarity of roles will help facilitate role integration, as it is the clinical domain in particular—and the access to the expanded scope of practice—that delineates the NP from the CNS and other nursing roles (Donald et al., 2010).

On the other hand, it is the advanced nursing roots of the NP that differentiates the role from other medically based roles that share similar scopes of practice. It is crucial that NPs themselves understand and can clearly articulate the synergy of the APN and NP clinical competencies; the advanced nursing knowledge, coupled with the expanded scope of practice that distinguishes the NP role from other similar roles, is key in contributing to the benefits of the role in terms of patient outcomes, satisfaction, and team functioning.

Critical Thinking Questions

1. How do the NP and CNS roles differ in terms of clinical accountability?
2. Which of the NP clinical competencies would be the most challenging to initiate? Why?
3. What supports are available to an NP to implement or develop clinical competencies?

References

Canadian Nurses Association (CNA). (2008). *Advanced nursing practice: A national framework.* Ottawa, ON: CNA. Retrieved from www.cna-aiic.ca/~/media/cna/page-content/pdf-en/anp_national_framework_e.pdf

CNA. (2010). *Canadian nurse practitioner core competency framework.* Ottawa, ON: CNA. Retrieved from www.cna-aiic.ca/~/media/cna/files/en/competency_framework_2010_e.pdf

College of Nurses of Ontario (CNO). (2011). *Practice standard: Nurse practitioner. Revised 2011.* Toronto, ON: CNO. Retrieved from http://www.cno.org/Global/docs/prac/41038_StrdRnec.pdf

Donald, F., Bryant-Lukosius, D., Martin-Misener, R., Kaasalainen, S., Kilpatrick, K., Carter, N., ... DiCenso, A. (2010). Clinical nurse specialists and nurse practitioners: Title confusion and lack of role clarity. *Nursing Leadership, 23*(Special Issue December), 189–201.

Hurlock-Chorostecki, C., Forchuk, C., Orchard, C., van Soeren, M., & Reeves, S. (2013). The value of the hospital-based nurse practitioner role: Development of a team perspective framework. *Journal of Interprofessional Care, 27*(6) , 501–508. doi:10.3109/13561820.2013.796915

Hurlock-Chorostecki, C., Forchuk, C., Orchard, C., van Soeren, M., & Reeves, S. (2014). Labour saver or building a cohesive interprofessional team? The role of the nurse practitioner within hospitals. *Journal of Interprofessional Care, 28*(3), 260–266. doi: 10.3109/13561820.2013.867838

Kilpatrick, K., Harbman, P., Carter, N., Martin-Misener, R., Bryant-Lukosius, D., Donald, F., ... DiCenso, A. (2010). The acute care nurse practitioner role in Canada. *Nursing Leadership, 23*(Special Issue December), 114–139.

Nurse Practitioners' Association of Ontario (NPAO). (2014). *A pan-Canadian environmental scan scope of practice for nurse practitioners.* Toronto, ON: NPAO.

Robles, L., Slogoff, M., Ladwig-Scott, E., Zank, D., Larson, M.K., Aranha, G., & Shoup, M. (2011). The addition of a nurse practitioner to an inpatient surgical team results in improved use of resources. *Surgery, 150*(4), 711–717. doi: 10.1016/j.surg.2011.08.022

Searle, J. (2008). Nurse practitioner candidates: Shifting professional boundaries. *Australasian Emergency Nursing Journal, 11*(1), 20–27. Retrieved from http://dx.doi.org/10.1016/j.aenj.2007.06.003

Sidani, S., & Doran, D. (2010). Relationships between processes and outcomes of nurse practitioners in acute care: An exploration. *Journal of Nursing Care Quality, 25*(1), 31–38. doi: 10.1097/NCQ.0b013e3181b1f41e

van Soeren, M., Hurlock-Chorostecki, C., Goodwin, S., & Baker, E. (2009). The primary health-care nurse practitioner in Ontario: A workforce study. *Nursing Leadership, 22*(2), 58–72. Retrieved from http://www.longwoods.com/content/20798

van Soeren, M., Hurlock-Chorostecki, C., & Reeves, S. (2011). The role of nurse practitioners in hospital settings: Implications for interprofessional practice. *Journal of Interprofessional Care, 25*(4), 245–251. doi: 10.3109/13561820.2010.539305

Wakulowsky, L., & Chaiet, L. (2010). *A prescription for better access: Bill 179 receives royal assent.* Toronto, ON: McMillan LLP. Retrieved from http://www.mcmillan.ca/Files/Bill179_ReceivesRoyalAssent_0110.pdf

Williamson, S., Twelvetree, T., Thompson, J., & Beaver, K. (2012). An ethnographic study exploring the role of ward-based advanced nurse practitioners in an acute medical setting. *Journal of Advanced Nursing, 68*(7), 1579–1588. doi: 10.1111/j.1365-2648.2012.05970.x

Chapter 7

Research Competency

Part A: Research Competency by the Clinical Nurse Specialist

Cheryl Forchuk

Cheryl Forchuk is a Distinguished Professor and Associate Director of Nursing Research at the Arthur Labatt Family School of Nursing, Scientist and Assistant Director of the Lawson Health Research Institute, and Professor in the Department of Psychiatry, Schulich Medicine & Dentistry, Western University, in London, Ontario. She also holds an appointment as Associate Clinical Professor at McMaster University, School of Nursing in Hamilton, Ontario. Previously, Cheryl practiced as a CNS–Mental Health in Hamilton.

KEY TERMS

evidence informed
continuous
   improvement
knowledge translation
research competency

OBJECTIVES

1. Describe the differences between being a user of research findings and a generator of research findings.
2. Summarize key reasons for advanced practice nurses (APN) to actively engage in research.
3. Identify strategies for implementing the research competency in practice.

Introduction

Advanced practice nurses (APN) have often described the **research competency** as one of the more challenging roles to enact (Fitzgerald et al., 2003). Part of the problem relates to differences in role timelines and perceived priorities. Clinical issues are often urgent and immediately apparent. Research is a much slower, more drawn-out process, with potentially fewer tangible outcomes. However, there is a risk of being so caught up with various everyday crises that questions about why these crises occur, how they can be prevented, and how they can best be addressed when they do occur don't get framed as researchable questions. There might also be a perception of not having enough time to engage in research. The situation is similar to the seminal paper on upstream-downstream thinking in nursing (Butterfield, 1990); people may be so busy pulling others from the bottom of the stream that they forget to send someone upstream to find out why they are falling in.

The Research Competency

As part of the CNS role, the research competency can be described as having different levels of intensity. At the most basic level, an APN is expected to be able to be an educated consumer of research. However, since baccalaureate education as the entry level for registered nurses (RN) has become a reality in Canada, this level is expected of all RNs. Generally, all nurses need to know how to critically appraise the literature to decide whether or not to change practices. Yet the sheer volume of new research impedes nurses being able to do this in a timely fashion. Core competencies for the evaluation and research role of the clinical nurse specialist (CNS) across Canada have recently been set out by the Canadian Nurses Association (CNA) (2014), which includes the CNS role expectation of dissemination and integration of evidence. A CNS will frequently receive consultations or requests for education on issues that are often well covered in the literature. The research dissemination role in these situations is fairly straightforward. Literature can be retrieved, summarized, and discussed with colleagues and staff. Copies of research findings can be left to read and referenced in the consultation report, or developed further as an educative handout. With best practice guidelines, such as those available from the Registered Nurses' Association of Ontario's (RNAO) website, or other research synthesis sites such as the Cochrane Library, the hard work is often already done (see Table 7.1).

TABLE 7.1: Websites for Gathering Best Practices

Organization	Summary	Web Address
Registered Nurses' Association of Ontario (RNAO)	Provides best practices in nursing that includes common nursing concerns.	http://www.rnao.ca/bpg/guidelines http://rnao.ca/bpg
The Cochrane Library	A collection of databases in medicine and other health care specialties.	http://www.cochranelibrary.com
Joanna Briggs Institute	Provides examples of nursing best practices.	http://joannabriggs.org

For example, in the process of developing a particular RNAO Best Practice Guideline (BPG), "Establishing Therapeutic Relationships," team members identified and reviewed over 2,000 research papers related to the topic. Now that this guideline has been developed, all of the relevant information, fully synthesized and interpreted from a nursing perspective, can be easily accessed.

It is a different level of involvement to be engaged in actually producing research knowledge (rather than simply retrieving and sharing such knowledge) and it is this level of involvement that APNs are more likely to struggle with. Before discussing the struggles, it is first useful to consider why it is necessary for an APN to take on this challenge. Consider who else would be expected to be in an ideal situation to identify and generate knowledge about the clinical aspects of nursing? Are academics in a position to do this? Without input from nurses working directly in clinical practice, there might well be gaps between what academics identify as clinical nursing issues and what practitioners actually struggle with. Table 7.2 provides an example of how a CNS can take an issue from practice to research, and how the research can impact future practice.

TABLE 7.2:   Example of Taking an Issue from Practice to Research and Back to Practice

Phase of Process	Issues and Activities	Products
Problem identification	Some mental health patients were being discharged from psychiatric wards to no fixed address.	Task group with mental health, housing, shelters, and income support.
Review of literature	Very little literature on subject; academic literature at times called this a myth.	Decided on the need to look at local data.
Baseline data	Looked at hospital and shelter administrative data to see how frequently this actually happened (almost 200 times a year).	Forchuk, C., Russell, G., Kingston-MacClure, S., Turner, K., Lewis, K., & Dill, S. (2006). From psychiatric wards to the streets and shelters. *Journal of Psychiatric and Mental Health Nursing*, 13(3), 301–308.
Pilot project to address	Piloted an intervention, partnering with income support agencies and housing supports.	Forchuk, C., MacClure, S.K., Van Beers, M., Smith, C., Csiernik, R., Hoch, J., & Jensen E. (2008). Developing and testing an intervention to prevent homelessness among individuals discharged from psychiatric wards

Phase of Process	Issues and Activities	Products
		to shelters and "no fixed address." *Journal of Psychiatric and Mental Health Nursing, 15*(7), 569–575.
Large-scale implementation of intervention	Incorporated pilot approach, including Internet access to income support agency data and housing data on vacancies at both city hospitals.	Forchuk, C., Godin, M., Hoch, J., Kingston-MacClure, S., Jeng, M., Puddy, L., Vann, R., & Jenson, E. (2013). Preventing psychiatric discharge to homelessness. *Canadian Journal of Community Health, 32*(3), 31–42.

CASE STUDY

The Story of Saad

Saad is a clinical nurse specialist (CNS) on a busy orthopedic unit of a large health sciences centre. The unit has experienced a significant turnover of nursing staff over a short period of time. Recently, there have been a number of incidents related to post-operative delirium that have impacted patient outcomes and led to prolonged hospitalization, increased health care costs, and high stress levels.

The orthopedic surgeons approached Saad and the nurse manager, concerned that there may be knowledge gaps related to the risk factors for and presentation of delirium post-operatively and requested Saad address this concern.

In responding to the request, Saad began by performing a literature search related to post-operative delirium. In critically appraising the literature, Saad found that some researchers indicated that education programs for nurses can improve outcomes for patients experiencing delirium. Many studies identified a lack of nursing knowledge in recognizing and managing delirium, but Saad could only find one research study that specifically assessed nurses' knowledge of delirium.

In response to this finding, Saad, in consultation with the nurse manager, decided to conduct a research study to examine delirium knowledge levels before and after delivering a tailored educational intervention that he would develop for the orthopedic nursing staff.

Utilizing evidence-informed research on delirium, Saad developed and delivered an educational program for the orthopedic nursing staff and administered the Nurses' Knowledge of Delirium Questionnaire (Hare, Wynaden, McGowan, Lancisborough, & Speed, 2008), using a pre/post-test study design.

The pre-test scores found nurses' knowledge of delirium to be poor, and that they were unaware of the fluctuating nature of delirium and its clinical presentation. Post-test scores suggested the educational program had a positive impact on the orthopedic nurses' knowledge level of delirium, especially in the area of cognitive assessment and delirium specifically.

In response to the study, plans were incorporated to provide ongoing in-service education to increase and reinforce team members' knowledge levels, as well as to increase the identification of delirium, reduce the potential for negative outcomes, and improve health outcomes for patients experiencing delirium, and, ultimately, cost efficiencies.

Discussion

CNSs, in their clinical role, are aware of the concerns of practicing nurses. They receive nursing consultations for input on issues that nurses or other members of the health care team find challenging, requests for education on areas where current practice is perceived as not working well enough, and requests from leadership in hospital or health care agencies related to systemic issues that need to be resolved. In everyday practice, a CNS may come across uncertainties, which, in themselves, provide insight into where further knowledge is needed. As a critical appraiser of research, the CNS can determine where knowledge already exists to address issues of concern or interest. Unfortunately, there are occasions when it will be realized that the required information is either not available at all, or was available but had not been systematically evaluated. Canada has been depicted as a country of perpetual pilot projects (Bégin, Eggertson, & Macdonald, 2009). However, if these projects are never evaluated and published they cannot easily be built upon to add to the pool of knowledge. Even within one hospital or health care organization the CNS may observe similar projects taking place without researchers being aware of each other's work, and therefore unable to build upon what has already been achieved.

Nurses, in general, are now being asked to make decisions that are **evidence informed** and include the preferences of their patients within their own practice settings (Yost et al., 2014). However, the extent to which research findings are incorporated into practice remains questionable (Squires et al., 2011). In this context, the APN is well positioned to act as a mentor to others by providing **knowledge translation** interventions that aim to enhance their research utilization (Abdullah et al., 2014).

What prevents CNSs from generating new knowledge? Two possible belief systems may be involved: the belief that they lack the required training or expertise to undertake research; and the belief that they do not have either the time or material resources to do research.

Addressing Expertise to Conduct Research

One factor why APNs' level of expertise related to research varies is because the amount of course work on research methods often differs substantially between academic programs. Programs also vary on whether or not a thesis, or even a major project, is required. It is not uncommon for APNs to feel they are experts in clinical practice but novices in research. The most practical solution to amend this deficit is to collaborate with others who possess greater research expertise.

Multiple people could be potential collaborators for the CNS. These may include the following:

1. Partnering with other APNs who have more research experience can help with confidence in building skills. When meeting with other APNs, it is beneficial to use this opportunity to identify common areas of concern that could be mutually addressed. For example, healthy sexual function can be adversely affected by a history of sexual abuse, as well as by the use of psychiatric medications. As these issues are commonly encountered in mental health settings, assessment of sexual health is an important mutual concern. One example is a collaborative initiative on this topic that was undertaken across a number of mental health clinical areas as part of a quality improvement project. A small research project was established and this work also succeeded in producing a publication from the process (Dorsay & Forchuk, 1994).

2. Partnering with academics can also be a useful strategy. In particular, beginning academics often struggle with identifying issues of importance to the profession, and also struggle with gaining access to clinical populations for research purposes. An APN, with access to the clinical area, is ideally situated to be a research partner for academics. An alternative place for the APN to start is with clinically based educators or in-service trainers who may also be aware of other resources or partners. For example, a CNS in oncology and an oncologist collaborated with a CNS in psychiatric and mental health nursing about helping to evaluate a telephone support program for women undergoing chemotherapy for breast cancer. Although this specialism was not the primary area of expertise of the CNS in psychiatry and mental health nursing, the methodology lent itself to providing assistance with this particular aspect of the research process, and again, as well as completing the initial evaluation of the initiative, a publication resulted (Smithies, Bettger-Hahn, Forchuk, & Brackstone, 2009).

3. Partnering with colleagues from different disciplines, especially those with more active research portfolios, should not be overlooked. Within the clinical setting,

other members of the interprofessional team may have more background in research and could be approached to partner. If the researcher has a planned or funded project it can be a simple matter of adding an additional tool to address supplemental issues. This would be much easier than doing a completely separate project, and allows for the opportunity to learn research skills by active participation in research rather than pure theory.

4. Working with staff nurses and others as a collaborative learning project to evaluate something is already happening. The CNS can take advantage of this strategy to integrate the research, educator, and change agent role competencies. This is also an excellent way to boost staff morale as they consequently have increased opportunities to present the results and/or co-author papers.

Strategies to Address Lack of Time and Resources

The most fundamental, and simplest, way to address the perception of the lack of time is not to view research as separate from the other roles, but rather entwined with them. If research is seen as a separate activity to be completed when there is time, it simply will not happen. Examples of how the CNS can address perceived lack of time or resources include the following:

1. Building in an evaluation component to everyday activities. Part of the Accreditation Canada certification process requires the self-evaluation of continuous improvement and/or quality assurance standards. Evaluation may often be done without the rigour demanded of the research process. What is the purpose of evaluation that does not meet research criteria? (For example, if it uses "homemade" as opposed to valid and reliable tools, or doesn't use pre- and post-test assessments, or a comparison group.) What is its purpose if it doesn't consider the sampling strategy? For just a little more effort, a valid evaluation can be completed that might also contribute to advancing nursing knowledge. (Table 7.3 includes a list of what is needed for a quality assurance project, as well as what extra steps are needed to convert this work into a research project.)

2. Setting aside time for evaluation and research. This can be achieved by making self-appointments or appointments with others where time is blocked off in the calendar. Ideally, negotiating to have time away from the clinical area or program reduces possible distractions and the risk of being recalled to deal with emerging clinical issues as they arise.

3. Looking at what could be delegated to others in order to reduce the workload. For example, could a student do a literature review as part of an assignment, or

retrieve data as part of a project? An underused resource that directly relates to time is the opportunity for employing staff who are working on modified job duties. Employers often struggle to find suitable activities for staff on modified job duties, which can often be frustrating for the staff member and doesn't help with the recovery process or the staff member's self-image. Staff have the ability to assist with literature reviews, collating data, and chart reviews. Furthermore, this can be an incentive for staff to make positive career changes, including going back to graduate school after the experience of a modified job duty placement.

4. A CNS with an academic appointment may be eligible to take work-study students. These students work for faculty as part of a financial assistance program and are paid by the government, not the academic faculty. Work-study students could potentially be nursing students, but could also be any university students with an interest in the work. For example, depending on the needs of specific research projects, the author has offered computer science, engineering, and law students the opportunity to be actively involved in the research process. It is here that the issue of time and resources overlap, since the more resources that can be identified, the less personal time it will take from the CNS to participate in the research.

TABLE 7.3:   Moving from Continuous Improvement to Research

Issue	Continuous Improvement/ Quality Assurance	Research
Purpose	• To understand problem or solution in local context	• To understand problem or solution
Ethics approval	• Local approval or inferred if part of program evaluation	• Local approval and communication with Research Ethics Board (if using data already accessed by virtue of role, formal ethics approval may not be necessary)
Measurement tools/scales	• Often use own instruments • Questionnaires designed in-house • Often interested in patient satisfaction	• Use standardized tools where possible • Often interested in outcome measures
Qualitative approaches	• Open-ended responses on questionnaires that would have a basic summary or content analysis	• More in-depth, open-ended items or focus groups and formal qualitative analysis method employed
Dissemination of results	• Usually an in-house purpose • May be used for accreditation or as part of a quality process • Primarily shared with clinical team and management	• Can be used for presentation locally, regionally, nationally, or internationally • Can be published in academic literature

Other strategies for resources include the following:

1. Identifying financial resources of support, such as hospital or community foundations, and organizations that address the specific clinical area of concern. (Small seed grants for projects are often available.)
2. If an administrative request for a project is being made, negotiating resources (such as funds to support statistical analysis or the creation of a summer student position to help with writing a research report) upfront is a useful strategy.
3. Depending on the nature of the project being proposed, potential industry partners could be considered; however, there may be administrative policies on this possibility that need to be consulted first.

Conclusion

The research role is an important and necessary competency of any CNS's professional practice. Collaborating with others is one useful strategy to develop confidence and skills in this area, but specific strategies to address time and resource factors may also be helpful in fully implementing this role. Most important is the ongoing need to incorporate the research competency into all of the other APN roles, rather than seeing research as a separate stand-alone activity.

Critical Thinking Questions

1. What are some of the potential strategies that might assist CNSs to disseminate research findings or to promote evidence-informed practice?
2. How might collaborating with others on clinical questions enhance the research-related skills of the CNSs and improve patient outcomes?
3. Time and resource issues are often identified as barriers to engaging in research-based activities. In what ways can this perception be altered to fully integrate the research role of CNSs into their everyday practice?

References

Abdullah, G., Rossy, D., Ploeg, J., Davies, B., Higuchi, K., Sikora, L., & Stacey, D. (2014). Measuring the effectiveness of mentoring as a knowledge translation intervention for implementing empirical evidence: A systematic review. *Worldviews on Evidence-Based Nursing, 11*(5), 284–300.

Bégin, M., Eggertson, L., & Macdonald, N. (2009). A country of perpetual pilot projects. *Canadian Medical Association Journal, 180*(12), 1185.

Butterfield, P.G. (1990). Thinking upstream: Nurturing a conceptual understanding of the societal context of health behavior. *Advances in Nursing Science, 12*(2), 1–8.

Canadian Nurses Association (CNA). (2014). *Pan-Canadian core competencies for the clinical nurse specialist.* Ottawa, ON: CNA. Retrieved from http://cna-aiic.ca/~/media/cna/files/en/clinical_nurse_specialists_convention_handout_e.pdf

Dorsay, J., & Forchuk, C. (1994). Assessment of the sexuality needs of individuals with psychiatric disability. *Journal of Psychiatric and Mental Health Nursing, 1*(2), 93–97.

Fitzgerald, M., Milberger, P., Tomlinson, P.S., Peden-McAlpine, C., Meiers, S.J., & Sherman, S. (2003). Clinical nurse specialist participation on a collaborative research project. Barriers and benefits. *Clinical Nurse Specialist, 17*(1), 44–49.

Forchuk, C., Godin, M., Hoch, J., Kingston-MacClure, S., Jeng, M., Puddy, L., Vann, R., & Jensen, E. (2013). Preventing psychiatric discharge to homelessness. *Canadian Journal of Community Mental Health, 32*(3), 17–28.

Forchuk, C., MacClure, S.K., Van Beers, M., Smith, C., Csiernik, R., Hoch, J., & Jensen E. (2008). Developing and testing an intervention to prevent homelessness among individuals discharged from psychiatric wards to shelters and "no fixed address." *Journal of Psychiatric and Mental Health Nursing, 15*(7), 569–575.

Forchuk, C., Russell, G., Kingston-MacClure, S., Turner, K., Lewis, K., & Dill, S. (2006). From psychiatric wards to the streets and shelters. *Journal of Psychiatric and Mental Health Nursing, 13*(3), 301–308.

Hare, M., Wynaden, D., McGowan, S., Landsborough, I., & Speed, G. (2008). A questionnaire to determine nurses' knowledge of delirium and its risk factors. *Contemporary Nurse, 29*(1), 23–31.

Smithies, M., Bettger-Hahn, M., Forchuk, C., & Brackstone, M. (2009). Telephone contact intervention in women undergoing treatment for breast cancer. *Canadian Oncology Nursing Journal, 19*(3), 122–128.

Squires, J.E., Hutchinson, A.M., Boström, A.M., O'Rourke, H.M., Cobban, S.J., & Estabrooks, C.A. (2011). To what extent do nurses use research in clinical practice? A systematic review. *Implementation Science, 6*(21), 1–17. Retrieved from http://www.implementationscience.com/content/pdf/1748-5908-6-21.pdf

Yost, J., Thompson, D., Ganann, R., Aloweni, F., Newman, K., McKibbon, A., … Ciliska, D. (2014). Knowledge translation strategies for enhancing nurses' evidence-informed decision making: A scoping review. *Worldviews on Evidence-Based Nursing, 11*(3), 156–167.

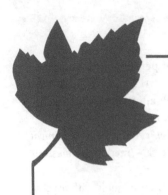

Research Competency

Part B: Research Competency by the Nurse Practitioner

Kathleen F. Hunter

Kathleen F. Hunter is an Associate Professor and Coordinator for MN Entry to Practice as an NP in the Faculty of Nursing, as well as Assistant Adjunct Professor, Faculty of Medicine, Division of Geriatric Medicine, at the University of Alberta in Edmonton. She has acted in both the CNS role and currently is an NP–Adult in a continence clinic.

KEY TERMS

competencies
critical appraisal
knowledge translation
patient outcomes

OBJECTIVES

1. Identity key research activities embedded in the Canadian Nurses Association (CNA) nurse practitioner (NP) competencies.
2. Discuss the concept of knowledge translation, and the role of the NP in changing practice.
3. Discuss the NP role of researcher, as a research team member or as a lead researcher.
4. Identify challenges and strategies to address enacting the NP research competency.

Introduction

As advanced practice nurses (APNs), it is imperative that nurse practitioners (NPs) integrate evidence-informed practice into client care. The Canadian Nurses Association (CNA) NP **competencies** identify activities including: **critical appraisal** and application of relevant research and best practice guidelines, development and evaluation of processes that address client outcomes and contribute to the development of knowledge, identification and implementation of research-based innovations, evaluation of NP practice, collaboration in research, and assuming the role of change agent through dissemination of research findings (CNA, 2010). NP education programs must include in their curriculum course work that supports role development in meeting research competencies, but must also prepare graduates to be lifelong learners (Canadian Association of Schools of Nursing [CASN], 2012). The competent NP is expected to act as an ongoing consumer of research, working toward improvements in client care at both the individual and systems levels, a researcher or member of a research team, and an instrument of practice change. The main focus of the research competencies is validating improvement of **patient outcomes**.

Development of critical appraisal and critical thinking skills to support evidence-based practice has been one of the central factors underscoring the necessity of graduate preparation of APNs, including NPs. Central to APN in Canada is the expectation of analysis and synthesis of knowledge; an ability to understand, interpret, and apply nursing theory and research; and the development and advancement of nursing knowledge (CNA, 2007). Although the focus of the NP is predominantly clinical, a key component of clinical client care is the integration of new knowledge into practice (CNA, 2009). At times, the NP can also act as a researcher, generating new knowledge to support evidenced-based care. This chapter will explore the research role expectations and competencies for NPs from the perspectives of knowledge translation and researcher, moving from the novice to a more experienced NP. As well, challenges that NPs face in meeting the research competencies will be identified, and strategies to address these challenges will be proposed.

Meeting the Research Competencies

Knowledge Translation: Changing Practice

In Canada, **knowledge translation** has been defined as a process that is both iterative and dynamic (Tetroe, 2007). Components of knowledge translation include synthesis of research findings, dissemination tailored to the target audience, mutual learning through the exchange of knowledge between researchers and knowledge users, and ethically sound activities aimed at application of knowledge (Tetroe, 2007). Aspects of knowledge translation can be seen as a thread across many of the NP research competencies. Effective knowledge translation draws on the ability of the NP to critically appraise literature, synthesize research findings, and thoughtfully apply these to the patient population and practice setting.

Maintaining currency of knowledge is an essential first step to best practice and utilization of research. The ability to synthesize evidence and translate knowledge to the care setting supports achievement of the best possible client outcomes, and also in building a positive relationship with clients. A study of NP practice in a rural area of Ontario found that rural women were extremely satisfied with their care, and valued the collaborative relationship with the NP (Leipert, Delaney, Forbes, & Forchuk, 2011). In addition, the knowledge base of NPs is valuable to the care team, leading to changes in practice. In a study of long-term care settings, Sangster-Gormley and colleagues (2013) reported that managers valued the NP role for the expertise in care of complex residents, as well as their potential for capacity building and staff development. All of these factors require that the NP maintain a current base of knowledge related to best practices in client care.

APNs move through a process of development throughout their careers, moving from novice to a more experienced and expert practitioner (Brykcaynski, 2014). Development of expertise in fulfilling the expectations for NP research competencies support the need to be a change agent over time to facilitate and support growth into the role. For the novice NP focused on gaining clinical experience, assuming the role of change agent may seem daunting. One starting point would be to systematically build on critical appraisal skills learned in the NP education program by reviewing current research and appraising best practice guidelines relevant to the practice area. These can be discussed with colleagues and mentors on the care team to identify potential areas of practice change. As experience is gained, the NP might select a component of a practice guideline that addresses an aspect of patient care where a practice gap exists or care approaches require updating. It is a reasonable starting point for the novice and intermediate NPs to begin with quality improvement approaches to evaluate patient outcomes for local use, rather than a formal research project. Focusing on local practice, the developing NP may elect to present information on guideline recommendations formally or informally to unit staff, identify the practice gaps with them, and develop procedures or patient education materials focused on closing the gaps and improving client outcomes.

As the NP gains experience and confidence in the role, opportunities to participate in more structured and formal research appraisal within the team or other groups such as professional or special interest associations may present themselves. This could include participation in scoping or systematic reviews of literature for the development of best practice guidelines. The experienced NP would be well situated to lead or share leadership within the interprofessional team in the practice setting with regards to practice change initiatives, quality improvement projects and, potentially, research projects that involve evaluation of patient outcomes and best practice.

The Nurse Practitioner as Researcher

Today, more Canadian NPs are seeking doctoral education to develop their research skills and knowledge. These NPs may assume positions that involve joint academic and clinical roles, enabling more sophisticated research studies to be undertaken, and have a key role to play in mentoring students or practicing NPs in research.

The involvement of the NP in research initiatives for knowledge translation, practice change, and development of new knowledge must evolve over time as experience is gained in the role. At the entry to practice level, NPs should seek opportunities to identify potential research questions and join research collaborations in their area of practice in order to gain confidence and skill in research. For early career NPs, one strategy is to take advantage of opportunities to participate in research initiatives being undertaken by their team. This could include working with the team to identify research questions stemming from practice, participating in data collection, and participating in knowledge translation strategies.

CASE STUDY

The Story of Kathy

Kathy is an NP who holds a joint academic/practice appointment with a university. She works in an outreach falls management clinic that takes place in client homes. Kathy recognizes, from her experience in gerontology and continence nursing, that few falls risk tools or approaches include continence assessment in spite of the falls risk assessment guidelines recommending assessment of continence status (Panel on Prevention of Falls in Older Persons, 2011).

Kathy conducted a literature review on the association of falls risk and continence in older adults. The search also included assessment tools. The falls risk management team, which included two occupational therapists (one was the clinic coordinator) and a physical therapist, reviewed the literature and selected a screening tool to use as a trial for interprofessional falls risk assessment. Clinic clients who identified bothersome lower urinary tracts were referred to Kathy for further assessment of continence status. The team undertook evaluation of client outcomes from the clinic (Hunter, Voaklander, Hsu, & Moore, 2013).

As part of the findings, the initial continence tool trialed was identified as lengthy and better suited to research than to clinical practice. Kathy recommended an alternate screening tool, which was incorporated into the current falls risk assessment. When the new continence service opened at the local hospital, any patients screened and found to have lower urinary tract symptoms using the new falls risk assessment tool had the opportunity to be referred. This had a two-fold improvement in patient outcomes, namely falls and continence. Kathy was able to work with the clinic and advocate for these patients who directly benefited from the clinic's practice change.

Discussion

The case study demonstrates how the NP brings discipline and specialty knowledge to the interprofessional team that can be useful in the identification of practice gaps. Using knowledge and skills from graduate nursing education to search for and critically appraise the literature, NPs can support knowledge translation and introduce practice changes to address these gaps. Practice changes present opportunities to formally and informally evaluate client-focused outcomes, which is the focus of the research competency.

Challenges to Enacting the Research Competencies

Although there is considerable variation in role enactment, the NP role is often acknowledged as a clinical practice role, with the focus being direct patient/client care and less time spent on other role activities, including research (DiCenso & Bryant-Lukosius, 2010). Barriers to implementation of the NP role stem from many levels, including the health system, organization, and practice setting (Sangster-Gormley, Martin-Misener, Downe-Wambolt, & DiCenso, 2011). Such barriers can affect the ability of the NP to fully enact and engage in research competency–related activities. Specific barriers to the research competencies include lack of dedicated time/role expectations, lack of confidence in research skills, and lack of access to current literature and practice guidelines.

Lack of Dedicated Time/Role Expectations

With the emphasis on direct clinical care associated with the role, NPs have little or no dedicated time for research-related activities, even at the level of having time to access and appraise new research and guidelines. In their synthesis report on advanced nursing practice, DiCenso and Bryant-Lukosius (2010) reported that NPs spent between 60 and 90% of their time focused on direct clinical care. A study of hospital-based NPs in Ontario reported that the research domain was where the least amount of the NP's time (7%) was focused (van Soeren, Hurlock-Chorostecki, & Reeves, 2011), while another study of acute care NPs reported an average of 9.1% spent on research activities; again, the lowest of all domains including clinical practice, management, education, and research (Sidani et al., 2000). Recently, Kilpatrick et al. (2012) reported on two cases of NP practice in acute care at different hospitals. Their findings suggested variability in the amount of time spent in the research role component, with the NPs in the first case spending 10.2% of time on research and the NPs in the second case only 0.9%. Some of these studies included NPs in teaching hospitals, which usually have an increased prevalence of research activity. Little is known about the time spent in research activities by Canadian NPs outside of academic hospital settings, such as those in primary care, where time for research-related activities may be even scarcer.

The NP, managers, and physicians may have differing views of how the NP should focus their time. Managers may have more support for the non-clinical components of the role than physicians, who may feel the need for the NP to be focused full-time on provision of clinical care (Kilpatrick et al., 2010). The study by Kilpatrick et al. (2012) illustrates differences that can exist between practice settings with regards to the NPs' ability to enact the research competencies, and the influence of nursing and medical leadership for this activity.

Strategies

Implementation of the NP role in a way that includes the other domains of advanced practice, including research-related activities, must involve the stakeholders, physicians, and managers who potentially influence role enactment (Kilpatrick et al., 2010; Murray, Reidy, & Carnevale, 2010; Sangster-Gormley et al., 2011). Inclusion of stakeholders in implementation of the role facilitates coming to a common understanding, as well as shared vision of the NP role (Sangster-Gormley et al., 2011). Furthermore, delineating the intention of what the role is meant to accomplish (role definition) and acceptance of the role by the team are important aspects of NP role implementation (Sangster-Gormley et al., 2011).

Lack of Confidence in Research Knowledge and Skills

It has been suggested that some NPs may not feel prepared or confident with their research skills (DiCenso & Bryant-Lukosius, 2010; Sidani et al., 2000). This could be due in part to educational preparation. While current education standards support graduate education for NPs with graduate-level coursework in research (CASN, 2012) and most NPs in acute care have master's degrees (Kilpatrick et al., 2010), there remain some primary care NPs who are graduates of baccalaureate or diploma programs (Donald et al., 2010). As graduate education prepares the NP to take on advanced practice activities, such as critiquing and evaluating research (Donald et al., 2010), this variability in educational preparation could potentially affect the confidence and ability of NPs to meet the research competencies.

Another influence on research skills is experience. Lack of confidence in research skills may be more acutely felt by the novice NP, who is often focused on consolidating new and expanded clinical skills and less focused on the other domains of practice. Even with graduate coursework in research, the research experience of novice NPs in may be limited and affect confidence as many master's-level nursing programs now offer a choice of thesis or course-based programs. Graduates of course-based programs would certainly have preparation in research critique and evaluation, but may not have experience in formal research. Whether there is a difference in NPs who have completed course-based versus thesis master's programs in terms of enacting the NP research competencies has not been studied.

Strategies

As NPs develop in their role, mentoring in research skills and having the opportunity to participate in both quality improvement and research studies is essential to the growth of skill and confidence. Other strategies may include continuing education related to development of skills and knowledge in research-related areas included in the competencies. Bryant-Lukosius et al. (2007) reported that NPs and other APNs identified the need for further education in research.

Lack of Access to Current Literature and Best Practice Guidelines

In some settings, NPs may lack access to library services, other information sources, current research, and best practice guidelines that limit the ability to address the research competencies. This may be more pronounced in rural settings (Hunter, Murphy, & Babb, 2015), although a rigorous comparison of urban versus rural NP access to research in Canada has not been published. Although discussed anecdotally, NP access to current literature and practice guidelines as a barrier to addressing the research competencies requires further investigation.

Strategies

NPs and their managers need to ensure that the NP has access to current, evidence-informed literature. The provincial professional association and regulatory body may also have a role to play in facilitating access.

Conclusion

The research competencies for NPs are fundamental in providing and evaluating the outcomes of evidence-based care. There is variation in how these are enacted, and the ability of the NP to meet the competencies is based on experience and education, as well as system and organizational influences such as the nursing and medical leadership understanding of the NP role within the practice setting. Barriers to enacting the competencies are only partially understood and further research on these, including access to current literature, is needed. Different expectations for the novice NP compared to the more experienced NP need to be established. In the future, the increase in the number of NPs with doctoral preparation will support mentorship as well as a growth in research activity.

Critical Thinking Questions

1. Novice NPs often focus on their clinical practice competencies as they gain confidence and experience. How can the novice NP be supported in developing research competencies? Why is this critical to patient outcomes?
2. Nursing and medical leadership often influence enactment of the NP role. What other influences (system, organizational, and practice settings) might facilitate or impede the NP from enacting the research competencies?

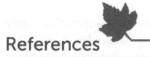

References

Bryant-Lukosius, D., Green, E., Fitch, M., Macartney, G., Robb-Blenderman, L., McFarlane, S., … Milne, H. (2007). A survey of oncology advanced practice nurses in Ontario: Profile and predictors of job satisfaction. *Nursing Leadership, 20*(2), 50–68.

Brykczynski, K.A. (2014). Role development of the advanced practice nurse. In A.B. Hamric, C.M Hanson, M.R. Tracy, & E.T. O'Grady (Eds.), *Advanced practice nursing: An integrative approach* (5th ed.), (pp. 86–111). St. Louis, MO: Saunders Elsevier.

Canadian Association of Schools of Nursing (CASN). (2012). *Nurse practitioner education in Canada: National framework of guiding principles and essential components.* Ottawa, ON: CASN. Retrieved from www.casn.ca/2014/12/nurse-practitioner-education-canada-national-framework-guiding-principles-essential-components/

Canadian Nurses Association (CNA). (2007). *Position statement: Advanced nursing practice.* Ottawa, ON: CNA. Retrieved from http://www.cna-aiic.ca/~/media/cna/page-content/pdf-en/ps60_advanced_nursing_practice_2007_e.pdf?la=en

CNA. (2009). *Position statement: The nurse practitioner.* Ottawa, ON: CNA. Retrieved from http://www.cna-aiic.ca/~/media/cna/page-content/pdf-en/ps_nurse_practitioner_e.pdf?la=en

CNA. (2010). *Canadian nurse practitioner core competency framework.* Ottawa, ON: CNA. Retrieved from www.cna-aiic.ca/~/media/cna/files/en/competency_framework_2010_e.pdf

DiCenso, A., & Bryant-Lukosius, D. (2010). *Clinical nurse specialist and nurse practitioners in Canada: A decision support synthesis.* Ottawa, ON: CHSRF. Retrieved from www.cfhi-fcass.ca/sf-docs/default-source/commissioned-research-reports/Dicenso_EN_Final.pdf?sfvrsn=0

Donald, F., Martin-Misener, R., Bryant-Lukosius, D., Kilpatrick, K., Kaasalainen, S., Carter, N., … DiCenso, A. (2010). The primary healthcare nurse practitioner role in Canada. *Nursing Leadership, 23*(Special Issue December), 88–113. doi: 10.12927/cjnl.2013.22271

Hunter, K.F., Murphy, S., & Babb, M. (2015, September 23). *Benefits and challenges faced by a nurse practitioner working in an interprofessional setting in rural Alberta.* Presentation at the 2015 Canadian Association of Advanced Practice Nurses (CAAPN) Biennial Conference, Winnipeg, MB.

Hunter, K.F., Voaklander, D., Hsu, Z.Y., & Moore, K.N. (2013). Lower urinary tract symptoms and falls risk among older women receiving home support: A prospective cohort study. *BioMed Central Geriatrics, 13*(46). doi: 10.1186/1471-2318-13-46

Kilpatrick, K., Harbman, P., Carter, N., Martin-Misener, R., Bryant-Lukosius, D., Donald, F., … DiCenso, A. (2010). The acute care nurse practitioner role in Canada. *Nursing Leadership, 23*(Special Issue December), 114–139.

Kilpatrick, K., Lavoie-Tremblay, M., Ritchie, J.A., Lamothe, L., Doran, D., & Rochefort, C. (2012). How are acute care nurse practitioners enacting their roles in healthcare teams? A descriptive multiple-case study. *International Journal of Nursing Studies, 49*(7), 850–862. doi: 10.1016/j.ijnurstu.2012.01.011

Leipert, B.D., Delaney, J.W., Forbes, D., & Forchuk, C. (2011). Canadian rural women's experiences with rural primary health care nurse practitioners. *Online Journal of Rural Nursing and Health Care, 11*(1), 37–53.

Murray, L., Reidy, M., & Carnevale, F.A. (2010). Stakeholders' conceptualizations of the nurse practitioner role in the pediatric emergency department. *Nursing Leadership, 22,* 88–100.

Panel on Prevention of Falls in Older Persons, American Geriatrics Society, & British Geriatrics Society. (2011). Summary of the updated American Geriatrics Society/British Geriatrics Society clinical practice guideline for prevention of falls in older persons. *Journal of the American Geriatrics Society, 59*(1), 148–157. doi: 10.1111/j.1532-5415.2010.03234.x

Sangster-Gormley, E., Carter, N., Donald, F., Martin-Misener, R., Ploeg, J., Kaasalainen, S., ... Wickson-Griffiths, A. (2013). A value-added benefit of nurse practitioners in long-term care settings: Increased nursing staff's ability to care for residents. *Nursing Leadership, 26*(3), 24–37.

Sangster-Gormley, E., Martin-Misener, R., Downe-Wamboldt, B., & DiCenso, A. (2011). Factors affecting nurse practitioner role implementation in Canadian practice settings: An integrative review. *Journal of Advanced Nursing, 67*(6), 1178–1190. doi: 10.1111/j.1365-2648.2010.05571.x

Sidani, S., Irvine, D., Porter, H., O'Brien-Pallas, L., Simpson, B., McGillis Hall, L., ... Redelmeir, D. (2000). Practice patterns of acute care nurse practitioners. *Canadian Journal of Nursing Leadership, 13*(3), 6–12.

Tetroe, J. (2007). Knowledge translation at the Canadian Institutes of Health Research: A primer. *Focus: Technical Brief, 18.* Retrieved from http://www.ktdrr.org/ktlibrary/articles_pubs/ncddrwork/focus/focus18/Focus18.pdf

van Soeren, M., Hurlock-Chorstecki, C., & Reeves, S. (2011). The role of nurse practitioners in hospital settings: Implications for interprofessional practice. *Journal of Interprofessional Care, 25*(4), 245–251. doi: 10.3109/13561820.2010.539305

Chapter 8

Leadership Competency

Part A: Leadership Competency by the Clinical Nurse Specialist

Mary-Lou Martin

Mary-Lou Martin is a CNS–Mental Health in the Forensic Program at St. Joseph's Healthcare in Hamilton, Ontario. She also holds an appointment as an Associate Clinical Professor at McMaster University, School of Nursing.

KEY TERMS

change agent
leaders
leadership
multiple system levels

OBJECTIVES

1. Explore the development of the clinical nurse specialist (CNS) leadership competency.
2. Describe the leadership competencies for the CNS role.
3. Describe the evidences related to CNS leadership in Canada.

Introduction

Leadership is a process of influencing the movement of an individual or a group toward goal setting and goal achievement (Bernhard & Walsh, 1995). CNSs are nursing **leaders** who implement innovative, evidence-informed approaches to care (CNA, 2014). They are part of the leadership team and provide guidance for nurses and other interprofessional health care providers. CNSs provide leadership in managing change and influencing clinical practice and the political process at all systems levels to achieve accessibility to care and to advance nursing services (CNA, 2008). Systems leadership competencies are identified in the *Pan-Canadian Core Competencies for the Clinical Nurse Specialist* by the CNA (2014). This chapter will demonstrate the leadership competency of the CNS and the role that CNSs play as nursing leaders who advance nursing practice and make a difference to the health outcomes of Canadians (CNA, 2013).

Leadership Competency

In Canada, the CNS role emerged to address the changing complexity of nursing practice, to provide leadership with care at the bedside, and to promote continuity of care across the different levels of the health care system (CNA, 2006). Later, CNA (2008) described the CNS role as providing guidance and leadership to nurses who manage complex care, to enhance the quality of care and to promote evidence-based care. In the same year, the CNA published *Advanced Nursing Practice: A National Framework*, which was inclusive of both CNS and nurse practitioner (NP) roles in Canada. The four domains of advanced nursing practice were identified as: clinician, researcher, leader, and consultant/collaborator. In 2009, the CNA published a position statement on the CNS role to include five domains of practice: clinician, educator, researcher, consultant, and leader. Although some differences are apparent in the two CNA documents, the identification of the leader/leadership competency is clearly defined in both descriptions.

Leadership by the CNS is reflected in the advancement of evidence-informed specialty nursing practice and the promotion of quality client care at local and national levels. Leadership is also enacted through acting as a change agent and as a resource, facilitator, coordinator, role model, and advocate. The CNA also recognizes that CNSs demonstrate leadership by developing clinical guidelines and protocols, utilizing and promoting the use of evidence, and providing consultation and clinical expertise. Characteristics identified by the CNA (2013) as important to the CNS role include spheres of influence at multiple system levels, such as the individual, aggregate, community, organization, and health care.

Leadership is an important aspect of the CNS role. There are dynamic relationships between the CNS domains of practice, and leadership works in synergy with the other domains. CNSs can move across health sectors and between different clinical settings, and thus they work at both micro and macro system levels to influence clients, staff, and organizational systems (Thompson & Lutham, 2007). CNSs are significant influencers in the transformation of the Canadian health care system by contributing to better care for individuals, better health for populations, and lowering health care costs through their capacity for initiating, implementing, and supporting innovation to enhance the delivery of nursing and health care services (Canadian Centre for Advanced Practice Nursing Research [CCAPNR], 2012).

Evidence of Clinical Nurse Specialist Leadership

CNSs are involved in the development, implementation, and evaluation of new practices and policies related to complex health care issues, quality assurance, and change (CNA, 2009). The changing health care system demands that CNSs reflect and re-examine how they practice and engage in leadership. There is limited literature about the leadership competency of CNSs in Canada; however, some relevant Canadian studies will be reviewed.

In order to be a change agent, CNSs use their knowledge and skills related to practice, education, research, and administration to improve patient care and influence change at the individual, unit, and organizational levels (Pauly et al., 2004; Schreiber et al., 2005). CNSs improve outcomes related to quality of care, nursing knowledge and skills, patient satisfaction, and patient confidence in self-care abilities (Fulton & Baldwin, 2004).

In a Canadian study, Canam (2005) conducted a qualitative study to understand advanced practice with CNSs ($n = 16$) who were working with children with complex health needs and their families. The findings suggested that CNSs play an important role in program development, consultation, educational outreach, clinical guidelines, and policies, with a focus on the system level of health care and population health needs. CNSs indicated they were aware of their influence on the system level, which included efficient use of resources, as well as policy and guideline development. CNSs indicated they interacted with many patients and families, which led to their awareness of the needs at the population level. This level was seen by CNSs as having the most potential for influencing the cost and quality of health care.

A Canadian Health Services Research Foundation (CHSRF) report explored the roles of advanced practice nurses (APNs), their contexts of work, and health care system factors that impact advanced practice nursing. The findings indicated inconsistencies in perceptions and practices regarding the roles of APNs (DiCenso et al., 2010). In the report, administrators indicated that the strength of CNSs was their capacity to integrate clinical expertise with leadership and research skills to support decision-making at the administrative level, as well as with academic goals in teaching hospitals. Administrators also recommended APNs should have multi-dimensional roles that include clinical practice, education, research, and leadership, along with project management and quality improvement.

The leadership role of the CNS is important to the nursing profession and the health care system (Bryant-Lukosius et al., 2010). Administrators and physician informants reported CNSs to be more involved in the support of other health care providers, leading education and evidenced-based practice in addition to quality assurance and program development activities. Informants reported that CNSs can improve the health of Canadians and address policy issues related to accessibility of care for patients, patient safety, cost and quality of care, evidence-based practice, and advancing nursing practice.

Axen (2011) conducted an integrative literature review of 12 studies with a focus on CNS leadership competency from the viewpoint of others. The review revealed that the perceptions of CNSs reflected the view that CNSs are contributing to positive change at the systems level, including policy and guideline development and effective use of resources.

Rourke (2012) conducted a qualitative research study related to policy to explore the practice of CNSs ($n = 11$) working in British Columbia. The findings were similar to past studies in that they revealed that CNSs were involved in policy development at clinical, institutional, and systems levels of the health care system.

One study suggests that CNSs are positioned to take a major leadership role in guiding staff and the health care system to improve care at both micro and macro levels. Finkelman (2013) highlighted that this would mean integrating quality improvement content and experiences into Canadian graduate education curricula, as well as placing greater emphasis on the leadership competency in CNS preparation.

CNSs engage in policy development at the clinical, institutional, and system levels (CNA, 2008; Canam, 2005; Seenandan-Sookdeo, 2012). Policy development at different levels of health care is important. CNSs are strategically positioned to develop policy that can advance nursing and improve patient outcomes (CNA, 2008; Fulton, 2010, Seenandan-Sookdeo, 2012). Bryant-Lukosius et al. (2010) suggests that CNS survival in the next decade is dependent on CNSs having a national voice and being prominent clinical leaders in the health care system. This means that CNSs must use intersectoral approaches and demonstrate stronger national leadership through the Canadian Association of Advanced Practice Nurses (CAAPN) to facilitate building relationships with key stakeholders and gain access to relevant policy tables. The appointment of CNSs as leaders at strategic planning and policy-making levels will ensure quality nursing practice and quality patient care.

CNSs have contributed to quality improvement and patient safety by participating at multiple levels of the health care system; however, this type of work has made it more challenging to associate specific patient outcomes to the work of the CNS or any specific member of the health care team (MacNeil & MacKinnon, 2011).

The current evidence related to the leadership role of CNSs in Canada is sparse and limited by sample size, design, and methodology. More research is required on the leadership outcomes of CNS practice. As well, CNSs need to support, coach, and mentor novice CNSs in the development of their leadership competencies. It is important for CNSs to disseminate through presentations and publications some exemplars of CNS leadership that have demonstrated quality and safety improvements in nursing practice and patient care.

CASE STUDY

The Story of Markaela

Markaela is a clinical nurse specialist (CNS) with 10 years' experience who is employed by an urban academic health care organization. She has a high level of expertise in the clinical specialty of mental health and addiction, and has a clinical appointment with a university's school of nursing. Markaela's clinical practice time is allocated into four domains: clinical care (30%), advancement of nursing practice (25%), evaluation and research (20%), and leadership (25%).

Markaela was requested, by the nursing staff on an acute care mental health unit, to consult on Dorsey, a female patient with a complex mental health condition who had been in seclusion for two days due to threatening behaviour towards patients and staff. While in seclusion, Dorsey had attempted self-harm by banging her head against the wall and biting herself. The staff had attempted to take Dorsey out of seclusion when she seemed settled but were met with no success. Dorsey reported to staff that she did not feel safe leaving seclusion. The staff were anxious about supporting the patient once she had left seclusion because of their concerns about safety, and also identified concerns about the demands on staffing.

Discussion

A process of change began when the CNS, Markaela, met with the nurses to learn about the patient Dorsey. Together, they assessed Dorsey's risks, strengths, overall health status, and mental status to start planning her care. Dorsey had a learning disability, multiple trauma experiences, past violence towards self and others, hypertension, no social support, and was homeless. Dorsey indicated she was a lesbian and that she would like to have a sexual relationship with a female staff member. The nurses reported Dorsey had touched the breasts of two nurses and that she often masturbated and would not cover up when asked.

Markaela asked Dorsey if she could talk with her about her experiences and the patient agreed. In this way, Dorsey participated in the development of her care plan. Evidence-informed therapeutic interventions were identified and outcomes were evaluated. Markaela and the primary nurse met together with Dorsey to provide trauma counselling and dialectical behavioural therapy. When Dorsey was discharged to the community, Markaela continued to meet with her regularly to support her transition to the new community care providers.

Another process of change occurred when there was a hospital review of Code White incidents and restraint utilization. Markaela co-chaired the Code White Committee, which noted an increase in Code White calls and restraint events. She recommended a literature search and survey of other hospitals to determine the evidence regarding the use of restraints. It was found that many hospitals were currently engaged in projects to reduce and/or eliminate restraints. Of note was the number of deaths identified, directly associated with the use of restraints. Many individuals with mental health and addiction issues were found to have had experiences with violence and trauma. An evaluation of restraint use in the mental health and addiction program (MHAP) revealed that many patients experienced greater frequency and duration in restraints when compared to other settings. The committee agreed that work was needed to reduce restraint use and introduce trauma-informed care.

Markaela and her co-chair carried out a SWOT analysis to identify strengths, weaknesses, opportunities, and threats, before developing a business plan. The business plan was then submitted to the senior leadership team for approval and sponsorship. The leadership team endorsed the plan, and the restraint reduction initiative subsequently became part of the strategic plan for the MHAP.

In accordance with the business plan, Markaela facilitated with other colleagues a two-day workshop for all staff on the prevention of restraint use. After attending the workshop, senior leaders acknowledged that an organizational culture shift was required. A problem-solving and strategic-planning process for changing the culture began.

The MHAPs leadership group decided that working groups would take on the task of creating organizational culture change. Markaela co-chaired the Workforce Development Group, and she was a member of both the Leadership Group and the Prevention Group. She also had opportunities to contribute to the Data Evaluation Group that designed the quality improvement project using a plan-do-study-act (PDSA) cycle. Using the PDSA cycle, Markaela and other members from the Leadership Group revised the Code White and restraint policies.

As the co-chair of the Workforce Group, Markaela collaborated with team members and proposed a plan to support the restraint reduction initiative. A restraint philosophy and related competencies were developed and introduced to all clinical staff, as well as integrated into all clinical job descriptions, job postings, interview questions, and performance appraisals. Crisis prevention training programs were reviewed and recommendations made, including integrating education about restraint and best practices into both the general and unit-based orientations.

As a member of the Prevention Group, Markaela participated in conducting an environmental scan focusing on prevention, early intervention, and a decrease in the potential for conflict. A patient comfort plan was developed and introduced to staff and patients, and a comfort room was developed for each of the units. Markaela and the nurse educator then developed the curriculum for a two-hour mandatory session on prevention of restraint use and trauma-informed care for all clinical staff. In the first year of the initiative, restraint use was reduced by 24%.

Nurses on the acute care unit communicated with Markaela that they had concerns about patients' risks for violence to self and others. Markaela was able to identify that patients' risks were not being assessed using a structured, professional judgment approach. No appropriate tools were available, so she developed a risk assessment guide that would also look at strengths. The risk assessment guide was tested through research and subsequently published. Other international clinicians and researchers have continued to use and test this guide.

Markaela offered to participate in developing a new best practice guideline related to restraint use with the province's professional nursing association. She spent two years working with others to create a Best Practice Guideline on Alternatives to Restraint, and disseminated and assisted in integrating this best practice guideline into the MHAP.

Markaela influenced others beyond her own organization by contributing knowledge at national and international conferences, as well as through publications about restraint and trauma-informed care. She also brought back knowledge from these experiences and translated it into patient care and the restraint reduction initiative. The utilization of research findings into practice proved a powerful influence.

Upon reflection, Markaela learned that successful planning for a restraint reduction initiative was dependent upon planned change, assertive leadership, committed stakeholders, a significant organizational cultural shift, and work at multiple system levels. In reflecting on her own learning, Markaela determined that she needed further knowledge and skills in quality improvement. She asked the chair of the Quality Improvement and Safety Council to act as a mentor so that she could successfully lead a quality improvement activity the following year. Markaela's journey of leadership was successful because she had the capacity to be a change agent and influence nursing practice and best practice guidelines. Her work also influenced the education of others, quality improvement, and research, and improved outcomes at the patient, unit, and system level.

Conclusion

CNA (2013) asserts that in the future, CNSs will lead change that includes measurable outcomes, system efficiencies, quality improvement, evaluation, and patient sensitive indicators. CNSs make a difference because of their dynamic interaction with other domains of practice. In Canada, the evolution of leadership by CNSs has been driven by goals to meet the needs of both clients and nurses, use evidenced-based care, control costs, use resources efficiently, and improve patient care and outcomes. To move forward, CNSs need enhanced leadership training in their graduate preparation, along with mentoring in their work experience. CNSs also need to educate others about the impact of their role on outcomes related to nursing practice, patient care, and the health care system. Research and communication about the leadership role of CNSs is also crucial to marketing their speciality expertise, so that their contributions to the multi-level health care system are visible within the Canadian context.

Critical Thinking Questions

1. How is the leadership competency of the CNS relevant to APN scope of practice?
2. What are the dynamic and interacting components of CNS leadership?
3. What can CNSs do to increase the visibility of CNS leadership?

References

Axen, L. (2011). *Does graduate education grant greater visibility to the work of the nurse? A literature review of perceptions of the CNS role.* Unpublished MSN thesis. University of Victoria, Victoria, BC. Retrieved from https://dspace.library.uvic.ca:8443/bitstream/handle/1828/4014/Axen_Linda_MN_2011.pdf?sequence=1&isAllowed=y

Bernhard, L.A., & Walsh, M. (1995). *Leadership: The key to the professionalization of nursing* (3rd ed.). St. Louis, MO: Mosby.

Bryant-Lukosius, D., Carter, N., Kilpatrick, K., Martin-Misener, R., Donald, F., Kaasalainen, S., ... DiCenso, A. (2010). The clinical nurse specialist role in Canada. *Nursing Leadership, 23*(Special Issue December), 140–166.

Canadian Centre for Advanced Practice Nursing Research (CCAPNR). (2012). *The clinical nurse specialist: Getting a good return on healthcare investment.* Hamilton, ON: CCAPNR. Retrieved from http://international.aanp.org/Content/docs/CNS_EN.pdf

Canadian Nurses Association (CNA). (2006). *Report of 2005 dialogue on advanced nursing practice.* Ottawa, ON: CNA.

CNA. (2008). *Advanced nursing practice: A national framework.* Ottawa, ON: CNA. Retrieved from: https://www.cna-aiic.ca/~/media/cna/page-content/pdf-en/anp_national_framework_e.pdf

CNA. (2009). *Position statement: Clinical nurse specialist.* Ottawa, ON: CNA. Retrieved from https://www.cna-aiic.ca/~/media/cna/page-content/pdf-en/clinical-nurse-specialist_position-statement.pdf?la=en

CNA. (2013). *Strengthening the role of the clinical nurse specialist in Canada: Pan-Canadian roundtable discussion summary report.* Ottawa, ON: CNA. Retrieved from https://www.cna-aiic.ca/~/media/cna/page-content/pdf-fr/clinical_nurse_specialist_role_roundtable_summary_e.pdf?la=en

CNA. (2014). *Pan-Canadian core competencies for the clinical nurse specialist.* Ottawa, ON: CNA. Retrieved from http://cna-aiic.ca/~/media/cna/files/en/clinical_nurse_specialists_convention_handout_e.pdf

Canam, C., (2005). Illuminating the clinical nurse specialist role of advanced practice nursing: A qualitative study. *Nursing Leadership, 18*(4), 70–89.

DiCenso, A., Bryant-Lukosius, D., Bourgeault, I., Martin-Misener, R., Abelson, J., Kaasalainen, S., ... Harbman, P. (2010). *Clinical nurse specialists and nurse practitioners in Canada: A decision support synthesis.* Ottawa, ON: Canadian Health Research Foundation. Retrieved from http://www.chsrf.ca/Libraries/Commissioned_Research_Reports/Dicenso_EN_Final.sflb.ashx

Finkelman, A. (2013). The clinical nurse specialist: Leadership in quality improvement. *Clinical Nurse Specialist, 27*(1), 31–35. doi: 10.1097/NUR.0b013e3182776d8f

Fulton, J.S., (2010). Evolution of clinical nurse specialist's role: Practice in the United States. In J.S. Fulton, B.L. Lyon, & K.A. Goureau (Eds.). *Foundations of Clinical Nurse Specialist Practice,* (pp. 3–13). New York, NY: Springer.

Fulton, J., & Baldwin, K. (2004). An annotated bibliography reflecting CNS practice and outcomes. *Clinical Nurse Specialist, 18*(1), 21–39.

MacNeil, J., & MacKinnon, K. (2011). Making visible the contributions of the clinical nurse specialist. *Nursing Leadership, 24*(4), 88–98.

Pauly, B., Schreiber, R., MacDonald, M., Davidson, H., Crickmore, J., Moss, L., ... Hammond, C. (2004). Dancing to our own tune: Understanding of advanced nursing practice in British Columbia. *Nursing Leadership, 17*(2), 47–57.

Rourke, S.N. (2012). *Canadian clinical nurse specialists: Understanding their role in policy within a British Columbian context.* Unpublished MSN thesis. University of Victoria, Victoria, BC. Retrieved from https://circle.ubc.ca/bitstream/handle/2429/43268/ubc_2012_fall_rourke_sarah.pdf?sequence=3

Schreiber, R., MacDonald, M., Pauly, B., Davidson, H., Crickmore, J., Moss, L., ... Hammond, C. (2005). Singing in different keys: Enactment of advanced nursing practice in British Columbia. *Nursing Leadership, 18*(2), 1–17. Retrieved from http://www.longwoods.com/product.php?productid=19026

Seenandan-Sookdeo, K.A. (2012). The influence of power in the Canadian healthcare system. *Clinical Nurse Specialist, 26*(2), 107–112.

Thompson, P., & Lulham, K. (2007). Clinical nurse leader and clinical nurse specialist role delineation in the acute care setting. *Journal of Nursing Administration, 37*(10), 429–431.

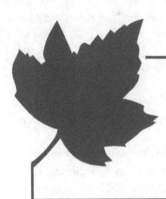

Leadership Competency

Part B: Leadership Competency by the Nurse Practitioner

Tammy O'Rourke

Tammy O'Rourke is an Assistant Professor at the University of Alberta, School of Nursing in Edmonton. She is an NP–Family/All Ages and led the development of one of the initial NP-led clinics in Belleville, Ontario, as well as serving as the clinic's Chief NP/Clinic Director. Tammy has also held an appointment as a Professor in the nursing program at Loyalist College in Belleville, Ontario.

KEY TERMS

clinical leadership
leaders
leadership

OBJECTIVES

1. Discuss the importance of the nurse practitioner's (NP) role as a leader in today's complex health care environment.
2. Explore the Canadian Nurses Association (CNA) NP leadership competency.
3. Discuss the outcomes associated with NP leadership.

Introduction

Canada faces multiple challenges in its efforts to redesign health care services. Most importantly, Canada lacks a shared vision to support long-term health reform and there are not enough **leaders** in Canada to support large system redesign. Several factors can complicate the ability to increase leadership capacity and engage health care providers in leadership activities to support widespread system transformation. In Canada, these factors include the fact that relationships between leadership activities and system outcomes, and between leadership programs and initiatives, are not well established, and current Canadian health care system arrangements confound the situation. Finally, progress is being made, but it is slow (Lavis, Moat, & Rizvi, 2014).

Leadership is a critical contributing factor in the success of health-system redesign (Ham et al., 2011). As Canada moves towards delivering new and improved services that are patient-centred and integrate relevant social determinants of health, we need NPs to demonstrate leadership in clinical practice environments. NPs are well poised to provide leadership and there are several recent examples of NPs leading change to better care, better value, and better health within in Canada's health care system. This chapter describes the role that NPs play as leaders in Canada's health care system and provides recommendations pertaining to the activities important to enacting the Canadian Nurses Association (CNA) core leadership competencies for all NPs.

Leadership Competency

The leadership competency is defined by the CNA (2009) and states that **leadership** is "about the competent and engaged practice of nurses, who provide exemplary care, think critically and independently, inform their practice with evidence, delegate and take charge appropriately, advocate for patients and communities, insist on practicing to their full and legal scope, and push the boundaries of practice to innovative new levels" (p. 1). However, **clinical leadership** is hard to define and often difficult to measure in regards to NP practice (Watson, 2008). In practice, NPs can find it difficult to enact these competencies due to organizational constraints and/or limited resources to support leadership activities. Enacting the CNA leadership competencies in today's complex health care system can be a challenging yet rewarding experience for NPs. Leadership requires perseverance and NPs must engage in activities aimed at influencing others. This influence is exerted as a means of developing collective groups to ensure that visions become realities.

Leaders frequently face opposition as they challenge the status quo and seek to improve health care systems through activities aimed at shaping, sharing, and protecting visions for change in their organization, community, and/or province. The development of leadership potential is widely recognized as an essential component of the educational preparation and practice expectations for NPs. However, a well-accepted theory for nursing leadership has yet to emerge in the literature. Despite increasing knowledge in the area of outcomes associated with leadership in nursing practice, the strength of the evidence is limited to mostly correlational studies (Cummings, 2013; Wong, Cummings, & Ducharme, 2013). Leadership is recognized by the CNA as one of six core competencies for NPs (CNA, 2010); box 8.1 provides a description of the leadership competency.

BOX 8.1

Canadian Nurses Association Leadership Competencies
The nurse practitioner:

1.25 Provides leadership in the management of clinical care and is a resource person, educator, and role model.

1.26 Acts as a preceptor, mentor, and coach to nursing colleagues, other members of the health care team, and students.

1.27 Articulates and promotes the role of the nurse practitioner to clients, other health care providers, social and public service sectors, the public, legislators, and policy-makers.

1.28 Provides leadership in the development and integration of the nurse practitioner role within the health care system.

1.29 Advocates for and participates in creating an organizational environment that supports safe client care, collaborative practice, and professional growth.

1.30 Guides, initiates, and provides leadership in the development and implementation of standards, practice guidelines, quality assurance, and education and research initiatives.

1.31 Guides, initiates, and provides leadership in policy-related activities to influence practice, health services, and public policy.

Source: Canadian Nurses Association (CNA), 2010.

The story of Kristy demonstrates how NP leadership can have an impact on health care system change.

CASE STUDY

The Story of Kristy

Kristy is an NP living in a city of approximately 40,000 people. The city provides central services to a larger rural population of approximately 100,000 people. Currently, over 40,000 people in this area do not have access to primary health care services. The city was having issues attracting high-quality primary health care providers and grassroot efforts to successfully obtain government funding for team-based primary health care had been unsuccessful. As a result, Kristy was unable to find employment. There were no funded positions in the city for NPs. At the same time, local decision-makers had set up a physician recruitment committee. This committee was supporting physician relocation at the cost of $150,000 per physician. The committee was using funds awarded to them from city council for this purpose.

To keep her clinical practice skills up-to-date and follow her passion of being an NP, Kristy was forced to travel 90 minutes to provide primary health care services in a different community. Patients in her community were forced to seek access to primary health care services through the emergency room and urgent care clinics. These patients required care that would be better provided by an interprofessional primary health care team and Kristy wanted to provide the leadership to make this happen. Kristy set out to make the vision for an NP-led clinic in her community a reality. The anticipated outcome for the introduction of this new service was improved access to team-based primary health care and decreased utilization of high cost urgent care and emergency medical services. After months of hard work, the proposal for the community's clinic received funding and today it serves almost 3,000 patients through the support of an interprofessional primary health care team.

Discussion

Kristy's story demonstrates how NP leadership can have an impact on health care system change to achieve positive outcomes for their community and profession, and for patients who lack access to primary health care services. Kristy was successful in introducing and implementing an innovation: an NP-led clinic. Successful leaders transform systems through these types of initiatives. Her leadership activities were aimed at generating strategic change and these activities required a certain level of sophistication. Kristy took several steps to gain in-depth knowledge of the change process and develop skills used to engage several key stakeholders in the decision-making process relevant to the change.

The type of leadership required to make change similar to that involved in this case requires a strong spirit of commitment and the courage to face strong opposition. Kristy demonstrated critical thinking, encouraged and supported the introduction of innovation, positioned herself to be successful in the future, and championed change. She saw a brighter, different future for her community's health care system and was optimistic that change could occur in her community. She anticipated issues and identified tools and strategies to encourage stakeholders to think positively about the change. Canada's health care system needs leaders who are enthusiastic about change and possess the drive and credibility to get things done.

Throughout the process, Kristy learned several lessons about stakeholder engagement. One of the key lessons was that physicians need to be engaged early in the process and that it is important to support recognition for the importance of teamwork in health care environments. Early in the development phase of the project, Kristy spoke to multiple physicians in the community in an effort to educate them about the model and garner support for the project. Unfortunately, many local physicians were supportive of a different model of care, namely family health teams (FHT). FHTs are similar to NP-led clinics; however, these teams are led and managed by physicians. Kristy worked diligently to identify physician champions both locally and provincially who would assist in developing the clinic. She was successful in her efforts and two physicians came forward to support the work of the clinic.

Once the clinic was funded, Kristy was required to engage in activities, such as human resource recruitment and management, policy development, and team building for the purpose of improving clinical services to change patient outcomes. At times, this was more challenging than the activities required to get funding for the clinic. These leadership skills were essential to ensuring that patient outcomes would be better through the use of this type of care model. Key drivers to the development of clinical leadership in practice settings include highlighting the importance of the NP role, evidence-based practice, clinical outcome measurement, empowering clinicians, and supporting NP participation in clinical decision-making (Davidson, Elliott, & Daly, 2006). In the case study, the NP-led clinic was in the spotlight for several reasons; it was the second clinic of its kind in the province and it had received funding despite competition from a physician-led model proposal for the same community. Kristy was now faced with the challenge of developing an interprofessional team while everyone watched.

NPs play important leadership roles in the development of interprofessional teams. Their purpose as leaders within these teams is to design strategies to support colleagues' efforts to achieve higher levels of functioning that contribute to health care system efficiency (Rigolosi, 2005). Clinical leadership contributes to the development of effective teams, and NP clinical leaders lead their teams into the future, which is often an unknown entity (Davidson, Elliott, & Daly, 2006). However, most NPs are clinical leaders who are eager to enact their obligation of advocacy for patients at all system levels (Carryer, Gardner, Dunn, & Gardner, 2007).

In the case study, Kristy had to set the direction for a group of health care providers and build an integrated system of patient-centred care out of fragmented parts. She was self-motivated and goal-oriented. Kristy worked to create a work environment where everyone wanted to come to work and where they felt supported to do their best work. It was the biggest challenge in her career to date and although she made mistakes (as many do when setting out for the first time), she continued to learn throughout the process and she used her authority to make decisions that were in the best interest of the providers and patients she served. Kristy decided to engage the assistance of experts in human resource management. These experts supported the team's development and each member grew from their increasing knowledge of self and others. These management experts assisted Kristy in her recruitment efforts through the use of strength-based assessments and team-building sessions.

During the same time that Kristy was developing and supporting the newly formed interprofessional team, she was focused on crossing boundaries into national and international arenas. She was able to influence others who had the decision-making capacity to enact change at the macro system level and contribute to the development of the profession. Kristy took the time to engage with her professional organizations. She attended several teleconferences and meetings for both the RN and NP associations in her province, as well as becoming a board member for the Registered Nurses' Association of Ontario (RNAO).

This position provided her with the opportunity to engage with multiple provincial decision-makers. These decision-makers included the executive director of the Association of Family Health Teams in Ontario (AFHTO), the provincial chief nursing officer, the provincial minister of health, and others. Professional NP leaders should hold memberships in their professional organizations and volunteer on local, provincial, and national committees because, as a professional NP leader, this allows for ongoing contributions on a macro systems level (Elliott et al., 2012). Kristy demonstrated strong professional leadership skills as she led the way to professional recognition and increased autonomy using her socio-political savvy. This type of savvy requires NPs to possess an increased level of confidence in the value of their profession and the ability to recognize opportunities for both silence and the use of voice.

Kristy's enactment of the CNA leadership competencies was crucial to the introduction and sustainability of the NP-led clinic in her community. She led the way to the development of an interprofessional team that now provides primary health care services for almost 3,000 patients. The clinic she developed is well known for adopting innovation and for high-functioning team-based performance, and has been recognized provincially and nationally for its work.

Conclusion

NPs require strong leadership skills as they lead the way to the development and introduction of NP-led service models that will provide cost-effective, high-quality alternatives to outdated models of care for Canadian citizens. As the NP profession moves forward with the next phase of its development, more NP leaders will be required to enact the leadership competencies defined by the CNA. Activities associated with leadership include addressing sustainability of the NP role, leading team-based care in a variety of health care environments, and demonstrating the importance NPs have to exhibit "better health, better care and better value" for the Canadian population (Health Council of Canada, 2013).

Critical Thinking Questions

1. What type of leaders do you believe Canada's health care system needs to develop a shared vision for long-term health care reform?
2. What are the next steps in increasing leadership capacity within the current NP workforce and future generations of NPs?
3. Is there an opportunity within your organization, community, and/or province for the introduction of an NP-led innovation? How would this impact on "better value, better care, and better health" for the Canadian population?

References

Canadian Nurses Association (CNA). (2009). *Position statement: Nursing leadership*. Ottawa, ON: CNA. Retrieved from http://www.cna-aiic.ca/~/media/cna/page-content/pdf-en/nursing-leadership_position-statement.pdf?la=en

CNA. (2010). *Canadian nurse practitioner core competency framework*. Ottawa, ON: CNA. Retrieved from http://www.cno.org/Global/for/rnec/pdf/CompetencyFramework_en.pdf

Carryer, J., Gardner, G., Dunn, S., & Gardner, A. (2007). The core role of the nurse practitioner: Practice, professionalism and clinical leadership. *Journal of Clinical Nursing, 16*(10), 1818–1825. doi: 10.1111/j.1365-2702.2007.01823.x.

Cummings, G. (2013). Nursing leadership and patient outcomes. *Journal of Nursing Management, 21*(5), 707–708.

Davidson, P., Elliott, D., & Daly, J. (2006). Clinical leadership in contemporary clinical practice: Implications for nursing in Australia. *Journal of Nursing Management, 14*(3), 180–187. doi: 10.1111/j.1365-2934.2006.00555.x

Elliott, N., Higgins, A., Begley, C., Lalor, J., Sheerin, F., Coyne, I., & Murphy, K. (2012). The identification of clinical and professional leadership activities of advanced practitioners: Findings from the specialist clinical and advanced practitioner evaluation study in Ireland. *Journal of Advanced Nursing, 69*(5), 1037–1050. doi: 10.1111/j.1365-2648.2012.06090.x

Ham, C., Baker, R., Docherty, J., Hockey, P., Lobley, K., Tugendhat, L., & Walshe, K. (2011). *The future of leadership and management in the NHS: No more heroes*. Retrieved from http://www.kingsfund.org.uk/sites/files/kf/future-of-leadership-and-management-nhs-may-2011-kings-fund.pdf

Health Council of Canada. (2013). *Better health, better care, better value for all: Refocusing health care reform in Canada*. Toronto, ON: Health Council of Canada. Retrieved from https://www.cahspr.ca/web/uploads/conference/2014-02-14_Better_Health_Better_Care_Better_Value_For_All.pdf

Lavis, J., Moat, K., & Rizvi, Z. (2014). *Issue brief: Fostering leadership for health-system redesign in Canada*. Hamilton, ON: McMaster Health Forum. Retrieved from http://

www.mcmasterhealthforum.org/docs/default-source/Product-Documents/issue-briefs/fostering-leadership-health-system-redesign-canada-ib.pdf?sfvrsn=2

Rigolosi, E. (2005). *Management and leadership in nursing and health care: An experiential approach* (2nd ed.) New York, NY: Springer.

Watson, C. (2008). Assessing leadership in nurse practitioner candidates. *Australian Journal of Advanced Nursing, 26*(1), 67–76.

Wong, C., Cummings, G., & Ducharme, L. (2013). The relationship between nursing leadership and patient outcomes: A systematic review update. *Journal of Nursing Management, 21*(5), 709–724. doi: 10.1111/jonm.12116

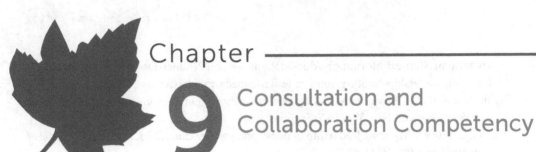

Chapter

9

Consultation and Collaboration Competency

Part A: Consultation and Collaboration Competency by the Clinical Nurse Specialist

Marcia Carr

Marcia Carr is a CNS–Medicine Clinical Service Network at Fraser Health Authority in Delta, British Columbia. She has adjunct faculty appointments in the schools of nursing at the University of British Columbia, University of Victoria, Simon Fraser University Gerontology Research Centre, and McMaster University. Marcia has also served as President of the Clinical Nurse Specialist Association of British Columbia (CNSABC).

KEY TERMS

collaboration
collaborator
consultant
consultation

OBJECTIVES

1. Explore the Clinical Nurse Specialist (CNS) role of consultant.
2. Explore the CNS role of collaborator.
3. Apply CNS consultant and collaborator role competencies for complex patient, health care system, and specialized population issues.

Introduction

A fundamental part of clinical nurse specialist (CNS) practice is the **consultant** competency, which is enacted using a collaborative practice approach. The *Pan-Canadian Core Competencies* for the CNS articulates four overarching competencies that include clinical care, systems leadership, advancement of nursing practice, and evaluation and research (CNA, 2014). These competencies further validate the importance of the consultant role to influence and impact care for individuals, direct-care health care providers, and organization system levels (Schreiber et al., 2005). Furthermore, the scope of practice for the CNS also incorporates these levels when assessing, planning, implementing, and evaluating strategies to construct micro and macro processes that are aimed at facilitating safe, quality care and positive health outcomes (Schreiber et al., 2005). The CNS utilizes the **collaborator** role to facilitate inclusiveness in the building of respectful and trusting partnerships that will improve care and practice changes among all care stakeholders.

Consultation

Consultation as it applies to the CNS enactment of the competencies is defined as the meeting with key informants and/or care providers to discuss the complex care and practice issues requiring advanced practice nursing expertise in order to achieve measurable care improvement outcomes.

The CNS Role and Function as a Consultant

The CNS applies expert advanced practice competencies, based on Benner's levels of clinical competence (1982), when completing the advanced assessment, critical analysis, and synthesis of root causes and system care gap processes. Additionally, through a systematic process, the CNS in the consultant role provides evidence-informed, fiscally accountable strategies that have measurable outcomes to improve the system and care gaps.

Why and When Is the CNS Asked to Consult?

The CNS is asked to consult when a patient presents with complex problems requiring specialized advanced practice nursing (APN) expertise; when the health care system requires a clinical lens that scopes broadly at the direct care, system-wide, and external stakeholder levels for resolution of care gaps; and when specialized population needs are at risk for negative impacts and outcomes. The CNS is able to facilitate a systematic review that includes a root cause analysis, and provides best practice strategies to improve and/or resolve the presenting problem. Additionally, the CNS role is positioned to influence changes and improvements at the patient/family, direct care provider, and internal/external system level.

Who Approaches the CNS to Consult?

Any member of the health care team and/or health care system may call upon the CNS to discuss a presenting patient/population/system or clinical care problem, concern, or issue. However, the CNS may independently determine the need to provide consultation beyond the original request because of discoveries made during the consultation process.

The CNS Consultation Process

One method that is often utilized in the consultation process is to initiate the Appreciative Inquiry (AI) (Bushe, 2011) in order to clarify and establish desired outcomes from the consultation. From this process, the CNS is able to analyze, assist with decision-making, and create strategic change among the targeted stakeholders. This strength-based approach facilitates the building of change strategies that are received more positively by those who will be affected. Therefore, the people that are directly impacted (e.g., patients, families, communities) are needed to gather their subjective perceptions along with the objective facts. A systematic gap analysis reveals actual and potential root causes and helps synthesize out data that can be used to evaluate outcomes (Gomez-Mejia, Balkin, & Cardy, 2008).

Collaboration

Collaboration as it applies to the CNS enactment of the competencies is a process through which the CNS methodically builds relational partnerships with key informants and stakeholders to achieve measurable outcomes. It means more than gathering participants and talking. It is building a foundation of mutual trust among the partners from which respectful, realistic improvements and change can grow. The way that the CNS applies the collaborative process ultimately can determine outcomes for individuals, population groups, and systems affected. Furthermore, each one of the collaborations has the potential to build a resource network that the CNS may call upon to influence and impact other desired improvements.

The following case study demonstrates how a CNS role was instrumental in targeting specific strategies by collaborating with others in the health care team to improve the health outcomes for other patients.

CASE STUDY

The Story of Esther

Esther was a vital, bright, and articulate 77-year-old retired schoolteacher living in British Columbia. She was planning to go on a European trip with her husband following elective hip arthroplasty at her community hospital. During her pre-operative workup with anesthesiology, she stated that she did not react well to general anesthesia. From previous experiences, she stated that she became very confused post-operatively on opioids, and that codeine had caused her significant constipation. She also stated that although she had some heart problems, she was normally quite well despite having part of her lung removed due to cancer.

During the pre-operative workup, the anesthesiologist reassured Esther that she would receive local anesthesia, not a general anesthetic. Additionally, he noted that the analgesic ordered post-operatively be hydromorphone. On the day of surgery, a different anesthesiologist administered her anesthesia, resulting in Esther receiving a general anesthetic and post-operatively being written an order for meperidine rather than hydromorphone. Since she was experiencing low oxygen saturations and hypotension in the post-anesthesia care unit (PACU), Esther was transferred to the intensive care unit (ICU) for stabilization. She experienced episodes of confusion and agitation while in the ICU. On day four, Esther was transferred to a medical unit for a few days and then transferred to the activation unit where her restlessness and confusion continued. Staff put Esther's bedside rails up while she was in bed, and she had restraints on while in a chair. Her family tried to be with her as much as possible to reassure and calm her, and to advocate for her care. Esther kept stating that she had terrible abdominal pain, for which she received additional analgesia. Subsequently, Esther was found on the floor beside her bed. The on-call physician gave a telephone order for lorazepam 1 mg po to sedate her. A few hours later, Esther was again found on the floor. Initially, she was unresponsive and though later responsive, Esther was considerably more restless and agitated. There was bruising on the side of her face and around her eye. The family hated seeing Esther like this and asked that a physician evaluate her as soon as possible. Diagnostic tests were ordered, however Esther's condition continued to decline rapidly. The physician spoke with the family about a do-not-resuscitate (DNR) order, which the family agreed to. Esther had sporadically received stool softeners and laxatives throughout her hospitalization, but there had not been a consistent tracking of whether she was having any bowel movements. Esther continued to complain about abdominal pain and an abdominal X-ray was ordered. Despite medical intervention, Esther passed away the next day.

As this was classified as an unexpected death, the case was referred to the provincial coroner. Two years later, the coroner's inquest concluded that death was attributed to ischemic infarction of the bowel due to profound fecal impaction and cerebral ischemia due to prolonged post-operative oxygen desaturation and hypotension. All of these findings contributed to Esther's cognitive and functional changes and decline. The coroner directed that the College of Registered Nurses of BC (CRNBC) and the College of Physicians and Surgeons of BC (CPSBC) address the clinical care issues that contributed to Esther's death.

Family, nursing, and allied health staff were all devastated by Esther's death. She had been well known in her small community and a number of staff knew her because she had been a local teacher. The morale at the hospital was affected, as there was a feeling of shame and blame being perceived due to the directive for a coroner's inquest. The family considered litigation, but decided, in accordance with what they believed would be Esther's wish, to actively participate in preventing the same thing from happening to anyone else.

Discussion

Esther's story is an example of a patient's hospitalization journey that should have been straightforward. However, due to a number of clinical care and system issues, Esther tragically died within two weeks of her admission.

The BC provincial nursing regulator consulted with the practicing CNS in geriatric psychiatry/geriatric medicine where Esther was hospitalized to review Esther's case and initiate the necessary steps to improve the hospital's care of acutely ill older adults. At the same time, the provincial regulatory body for physicians and surgeons was also directed to address these concerns in relation to communication and transition of care between physicians. The CNS worked in collaboration with the nursing regulator, the nursing unit managers, and the interprofessional health care team to identify the possible root causes and care gaps contributing to this adverse patient outcome.

Prior to proceeding with any plans, the CNS formed a collaborative working group composed of unit managers, hospital directors, and direct care nursing staff to establish mutual respect and trust with those affected. The CNS purposefully built the working group's agenda and acted primarily in the consultant role to aide them in their development of the strategic plan. The CNS used the AI process (Bushe, 2011) with the working group to enable open and respectful group formation, as well as acquire vital information on their wants and desired outcomes.

In order to have a concrete kick-off point from which the group was able to develop the strategic plan, the CNS developed an environmental scan tool derived from the least restraint and fall/injury prevention literature. This included identifying characteristics (e.g., no clutter, non-glare accessible lighting, low-rise beds, half-height bed railings, and fall prevention equipment) of what the hospital environment should look like in order to be an older adult–friendly hospital unit. The CNS additionally assessed the staff's knowledge, abilities, and attitudes about delirium, dementia, depression, fall prevention strategies, and de-conditioning effects on mobility, pain, and bowel management. The CNS was highly mindful in ensuring a non-blame approach to support the already "hurting" staff, including senior administration who decided that the approaches and plans needed to be hospital-wide and not just for the units that participated in Esther's care. The working group decided not to use surveys or questionnaires to determine staff's knowledge of, ability in relation to, and attitudes toward caring for older adults, as they believed it did not reflect how they currently worked together. They also decided that one of them would act as the guide/host for the CNS so that introductions and observations could be facilitated in an unobtrusive fashion. This approach provided the CNS opportunities to not only meet, but also open up informal "in the moment" conversations, with the staff about their thoughts and feelings related to caring for older adults in order to set the foundation upon which relational trust could be built.

As part of the plan, the CNS completed a full chart review including timelines of cardinal events during Esther's hospitalization. Having knowledge of the findings of the coroner's inquest, the CNS paid particular attention to documentation and current nursing forms in place. From a macro-level lens, the CNS reviewed hospital policies related to post-operative care pathways, pain management, restraints, bowel management, and fall prevention.

An analysis of the data gathered from the various sources informed the identification of areas of strengths and areas for improvement. The CNS presented the findings to the working group. The major strength revolved around staff expressing their desire to contribute to improving their ability to care for acutely ill older adults. They were seeking pragmatic and feasible actions that they could implement immediately, as well as ones that they could work on. While the assumption was that care for any adult was the same as caring for older adults, this became the dominant root cause of the overall care issues that arose with Esther's hospitalization. Staff readily admitted that there were knowledge gaps in caring for acutely ill older adults. This resulted in not knowing whether a problem even existed, let alone how to articulate or address the problem. Additionally, the need to prioritize revisions to policies and clinical practice guidelines on post-operative care, pain management, bowel management, least restraint, and fall prevention, in addition to improvements needed related to clear and consistent communication and documentation, was required. The working group decided that staff education was essential, and this was to be the first part of the remediation plan.

Concurrently, communication with staff required a plan that was purposefully designed by the CNS to focus on what they were doing well, what they would suggest may need improving, and what they would like to start working on first. Building trust and credibility among the staff was mindfully evaluated throughout all interactions, as it was essential that the CNS be perceived as a positive partner in helping them achieve their desired outcomes. By continually using the AI process, this assisted the facilitation process and in reinforcing the consultation role and how the CNS could assist with advanced clinical assessments, care planning, and evaluation of outcomes. Additionally, this provided the CNS with opportunities to demonstrate timely support and education that further built credibility and trust among the staff.

To address the identified, targeted knowledge gaps, the CNS developed a hospital-wide, interprofessional education program. The hospital's management team committed to supporting quality and safety improvements including staff attendance at education seminars, equipment changes and purchases, and environmental revisions (e.g., de-cluttering, cleaning over-the-bed lights). Working in close cooperation with a network of CNS colleagues in surgery and critical care ensured consistency of care and practices across the hospital. In addition to nursing competencies specifically focusing on the care of acutely ill older adults, interprofessional competencies were developed to ensure alignment of all providers' scopes of practice to achieve the quality improvement goals.

The CNS provided four, three-and-a-half hour education sessions that were repeated several times to capture the majority of staff and management. The clinical nurse educators (CNE) were integral partners in the education process, as they provided direct education support to the various units on an ongoing basis. This supported sustainment of practice changes on the units and provided the CNE material to use during new staff orientation. As the CNS was regionally positioned rather than single hospital or unit-based, there was a requirement to ensure the new structure could be sustained at this hospital and be replicated at other hospitals where other acutely ill older adults were cared for. The opportunity to build and pilot the strategic plan that was developed at this hospital provided the CNS with valuable information and lessons to apply to the whole health authority. The CNS consultant role expanded the sphere of influence and impacted the care of other complex patients.

Reviewing, revising, and, in some cases, streamlining communication and documentation practices can help prevent care gaps (e.g., one location to record bowel movements rather than several different places, pre-hospital cognitive and functional status to prevent assumption of dementia rather than delirium). Clearly, CNEs and CNSs have a synergetic relationship complementing each other's practice. With the CNEs primary focus on staff education, the CNSs were able to support their abilities through ensuring currency for knowledge translation with their staff related to best practice clinical guidelines, protocols, policies, and procedures. The hospital's commitment to a "never again" attitude helped to facilitate everyone's abilities, allowed strengths to improve, and sustained best practice care for acutely ill older adults.

Outcome measurement is vital to sustainability. Random audits of direct care were observed and chart reviews were completed based upon the working group's strategic plan to review areas for improvement, and to assist with future care planning and reinforcement of best practices for acutely ill older adult care.

Esther's family was an integral part of the improvement process that took place in the hospital. It was very important to engage and communicate with the family throughout all processes and activities. Their support in joining in the "never again" attitude provided a stronger message because of their learning and insights of how families' voices can be better heard. The family developed, and currently maintains, a website telling Esther's story to support other families (www.esthersvoice.com.) In this way, they continue to honour both Esther and other older adults. Esther's daughter personally responds to any members of the public who want to know how their voices as family members can be heard. Esther's daughter states, "Esther was always a teacher to her core and she would want her legacy to be about learning not blaming." The CNS continues to work with Esther's daughter to ensure the family voice remains heard.

The CNS also continues to engage with expert partners in geriatric medicine, geriatric psychiatry, and interactive media development from two universities. Together, they collaborate and consult with the daughter's computer software development company to create programs that will help patients, families, and staff. The "Mindful Garden," which is actively in development, is a computer program that aims at utilizing visual, olfactory, and auditory cues to facilitate an environment that is reassuring and calming. The structure and concept for the computer program is related to delirium, dementia, and depression. Collaboration produces networks that enable CNSs' ability to innovatively intersect with different networks to create more opportunities and greater impact. If Esther could have seen the "Mindful Garden," showing her in the prairie wheat fields, hearing the swishing of the wind through each stalk, and smelling the clean air, the research development team believes that Esther's agitation and restlessness might have been calmed and would have had a greater potential for recovery.

Esther is but one example of the need for health care systems to improve the quality and safety of care for acutely ill older adults. At this pivotal time, the BC Ministry of Health and the Nursing Directorate enabled the engagement and collaboration of all British Columbia health authorities to improve care of acutely ill older adults throughout the province. Their provision of grants for five years, to a group of five CNSs from three different health authorities, provided funds for the collaborative development of the Acute Care Geriatric Nurse Network (ACGNN) in years one through four, and the Geriatric Emergency Nurse Initiative (GENI) in year five. The ACGNN and GENI work continues to support care of acutely ill older adults through the www.acgnn.ca website. During the grant funding years, the group travelled throughout BC—especially to rural and remote areas—to educate and disseminate best practices for acutely ill older adults, as CNS expertise is not available in every area. All disciplines and administration are included in learning sessions and their attendance adds greater understanding of the need for collaboration. The yearly evaluations that include participants' "wish list," enabled the CNSs to advocate with and inform the health authorities' Chief Nursing Officers, as well as the Ministry of Health, about required system changes. Additionally, the *Geriatric Giants Quick Reference* continues to help sustain the knowledge translation fostered by the CNSs (ACGNN, 2013). The ACGNN CNSs have a viable and robust network, sustained through volunteering of their own time to ensure availability of information and resources to influence and impact improvements in the care of acutely ill older adults both provincially and nationally. The resources and information have spread to Japan, Ireland, and the United States, to name but a few.

Conclusion

The CNS role and functions, which are now clearly articulated in the *Pan-Canadian Core Competencies for the CNS* (CNA, 2014), are illustrated in Esther's story. By applying consultant and collaborator approaches, CNSs demonstrate how they can influence and impact direct patient care, the health care system, and policy decisions. CNSs continually strive to ensure and facilitate safe, best practice care for individuals, populations, and health care delivery services.

Critical Thinking Questions

1. Why would a regulatory nursing body choose to consult with a CNS in responding to a coroner's recommendation?
2. What impact can the CNS competency of consultant and collaborator have in improving best practices at the individual, population, and health care system levels?
3. What key characteristics differentiate the CNS role and function from the CNE and manager's roles and functions to enable best practices?

References

Acute Care Geriatric Nurse Network (ACGNN). (2013). *Geriatric giants quick reference* (3rd ed.). Burnaby, BC: ACGNN. Retrieved from http://www.acgnn.ca/

Benner, P. (1982). From novice to expert. *American Journal of Nursing. 82*(3), 402–407.

Bushe, G.R. (2011). Appreciative inquiry: Theory and critique. In D. Boje, B. Burnes, & J. Hassard (Eds.). *The Routledge companion to organizational change* (pp. 87–103). Oxford, UK: Routledge.

Canadian Nurses Association (CNA). (2014). *Pan-Canadian core competencies for the clinical nurse specialist.* Ottawa, ON: CNA. Retrieved from http://cna-aiic.ca/en/news-room/news-releases/2014/canadian-nurses-association-launches-core-competencies-for-clinical-nurse-specialists

Gomez-Mejia, L.R., Balkin, D.B., & Cardy, R.L. (2008). *Management: People, performance, change* (3rd ed.). New York, New York: McGraw-Hill.

Schreiber, R., MacDonald, M., Pauly, B., Davidson, H., Crickmore, J., & Moss, L., ... Hammond, C. (2005). Singing in different keys: Enactment of advanced nursing practice in British Columbia. *Nursing Leadership, 18*(2), 1–17. Retrieved from http://www.longwoods.com/content/19026

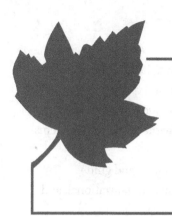

Consultation and Collaboration Competency

Part B: Consultation and Collaboration Competency by the Nurse Practitioner

Monica Parry

Monica Parry is an Assistant Professor and Director of the Nurse Practitioner Programs at the Lawrence S. Bloomberg Faculty of Nursing, University of Toronto. She is an NP–Adult specializing in cardiac surgery, and assisted in developing the innovative Primary Health Care/Global Health area of emphasis in the NP program.

KEY TERMS

collaboration
consultation
referral
transfer-of-care

OBJECTIVES

1. Discuss the difference between a consultation and a referral.
2. Explain the essential components of a consultation.
3. Recognize when a consultation results in a transfer-of-care.
4. Identify the antecedents, attributes, and consequences of collaborative practices.

Introduction

Nurse Practitioners (NPs) consult and collaborate in both familiar and unfamiliar clinical situations in order to practice at advanced and extended levels. The purpose of this chapter is to describe the six core NP consultation, collaboration, and referral competencies as described by the Canadian Nurses Association (CNA), which are as follows:

1. Consults with and/or refers clients to other health care providers at any point in the care continuum when a client's condition is not within the nurse practitioner scope of practice or the individual nurse practitioner's competence.
2. Acts as a consultant to and/or refers and accepts referrals from health care providers, community agencies, and non-allied health care professionals.

3. Advocates for clients in relation to therapeutic intervention, health care access, the health care system, and policy decisions that affect health and quality of life.
4. Collaborates with members of the health care team to provide and promote interprofessional client-centred care at the individual, organizational, and systems levels.
5. Collaborates with members of the health care team to promote and guide continuous quality improvement initiatives at the individual, organizational, and systems levels.
6. Applies advanced knowledge and skills in communication, negotiation, coalition building, change management, and conflict resolution, including the ability to analyze, manage, and negotiate conflict. (CNA, 2010, p. 9)

These competencies apply to all NP roles, including NP–Adult, NP–Pediatrics, and NP–Family/All Ages, and are grounded in the five World Health Organization (WHO) principles of primary health care: accessibility, public participation, health promotion, appropriate technology, and intersectoral collaboration.

Consultation

Consultation is an explicit request from one health care professional to another to provide guidance or advice in the care of a client. NPs consult other health care professionals when client care extends beyond their legal scope of practice, beyond their individual competence, if a diagnosis or treatment plan is unclear, or when the client would benefit from the expertise of another health care professional (Association of Registered Nurses of Prince Edward Island [ARNPEI], 2012; College of Nurses of Ontario [CNO], 2011). NPs also provide consultations to other health care professionals when their expertise will improve quality of care or reduce risk for clients.

Consultations can be informal (patient care rounds) or formal (written request for an opinion or recommendation), and can occur during the assessment, diagnosis, or therapeutic management of a client. During any consultative process the NP must describe their level of involvement, as well as the reason for and the level of urgency of the consultation (College of Registered Nurses of British Columbia [CRNBC], 2012). Formal consultations with other health care providers require client information that describes demographics, medications, allergies, past health history, pertinent family or social history, diagnostic test results, other relevant consultations, and a summary of the current problem. It is the responsibility of the NP to follow-up on the consultation findings to ensure resolution, or advocate for any outstanding issues impacting the client's health. It is also expected that the NP clearly document the consultative process within the client's medical record.

When the consultation results in the need to transfer care, the decision for this transfer is jointly made between the NP, the receiving health care professional, and (if appropriate) the client. Transfer-of-care is a process whereby an NP transfers management for some or all of a client's care to another health care provider who explicitly agrees to accept this responsibility. With a transfer-of-care there is a clear transfer of accountability, and clear communication with the client about this process. The NP must ensure that the accepting health care provider has the necessary clinical information to assume care, which would include a summary of any active medical problems and the treatment plan for the client. A transfer-of-care usually occurs when the primary care responsibilities required for appropriate patient care fall outside the NP's scope of practice. This transfer-of-care may be temporary or permanent.

Collaboration

The word *collaborate*, derived from the Latin *collaborare*, means "to labour together" (Henneman, Lee, & Cohen, 1995). The WHO suggests that collaborative practice occurs when multiple health workers from different professional backgrounds provide comprehensive quality services across settings to patients, families, caregivers, and communities (2010). The CNA believes that interprofessional collaborative models for health service delivery are critical for improving access to client-centred care (2011). The six principles of interprofessional collaboration include client engagement, access, trust and respect, effective communication, a population-health approach, and provision of the best possible care and services (Enhancing Interdisciplinary Collaboration in Primary Care [EICP], 2006). Clients are the priority focus; the services NPs provide must be responsive to their needs and clients must be actively engaged in decisions about the management of their health. When interprofessional collaboration is present, clients have access to the "right care in the right place at the right time," and by the "right health professional" (Government of Ontario, 2014).

Collaboration implies that people are able to view themselves as members of a team and feel that they contribute to a common goal (Henneman et al., 1995). Collaborative practice is common among physicians and NPs. It is unique to each practice setting and optimizes the skills of each participant to provide care within their scope of practice (Resnick & Bonner, 2003). Collaboration implies a non-hierarchical relationship where power is shared, and is not synonymous with supervision of an NP's practice. Henneman et al. (1995) define the antecedents, attributes, and consequences of collaborative practice. NPs must understand their role and level of expertise, be confident in their competence, and recognize their scope of practice within federal, provincial, and jurisdictional boundaries. They must also have good communication skills and trust and respect for their collaborating partners. In some jurisdictions in Canada, NPs are required by legislation to form a collaborative practice relationship with a physician (or a group of physicians), as well as their employing organization (College of Registered Nurses of Nova Scotia [CRNNS], 2011). This collaborative practice arrangement enables the NP and physician(s) to work together, using their separate and shared knowledge and skills to provide optimal client-centred care (CRNNS, 2011). Both sides must willingly participate in order to share planning, decision-making, and responsibility of care. Members can then engage in respectful, open communication and decision-making, practice to their full scope based on best evidence, strive to achieve optimal client outcomes, and support the continued competence and professional development of each team member. NPs who are involved in collaborative practice models experience increased confidence in their skills, as well as an enhanced sense of self-worth. Effective collaboration promotes interprofessional cohesiveness, increased job satisfaction, and better patient outcomes.

In Ontario, NP-led clinics are part of the primary health care system. NPs manage clinics to provide primary health care services that focus on preventive, curative, rehabilitative, and supportive/palliative care. These services aim to improve accessibility, public participation, health promotion, appropriate technology, and intersectoral collaboration (CNA, 2000). They consult physicians when circumstances extend beyond their scope of practice (DiCenso & Bryant-Lukosius, 2010). NPs and other health professionals collaborate on government policy to build capacity for the design and delivery of intersectoral health care services. Most recently, amendments to Ontario's Regulation 965 of the Public Hospital Act enabled NPs to admit, treat, and discharge hospital in-patients. There has been a shift toward more collaborative practice for the delivery of health services in Canada, necessitating a critical importance for NPs to understand effective role utilization across all health care settings.

Referral

A referral is an explicit request from one health care professional to another to provide time-limited, client-specific health services (CNO, 2011). A referral is a form of consultation that is episodic or concurrent; it is distinctly different from a consultation because it implies time-limited treatment (Goolsby, 2002). In Canada, different professions and organizations have different referral processes. All physician/specialist referrals, however, require a letter of consultation that outlines the reason for the referral, the client's history, and pertinent physical and diagnostic findings. In Ontario, the *Schedule of Benefits for Physician Services* presented a barrier for efficient access to specialist services (Nurse Practitioners' Association of Ontario [NPAO], 2012). For example, when a written request was made by a family physician for a referral to a specialist, the specialist could claim a medical assessment fee as well as a consultation fee. However, when an NP generated the referral, the specialist could only claim the medical assessment fee. The specialist was also under no obligation to write a consultative note when an NP generated the referral. Even though it was within the NP scope of practice to refer a client to a specialist provider in Ontario, obstacles still exist related to provincial remuneration practices. Restrictions to NP-generated referrals to private health service providers (such as physiotherapists, registered massage therapists, and occupational therapists) or provincial programs and services (such as diabetes education) in Canada are dependent on provincial funding models and extended health insurance plans.

CASE STUDY

The Story of Franko

Franko is a 61-year-old male who lives with his wife in a low-income rental apartment in Southeastern Ontario.

Chief Complaint: Presented with increasing shortness of breath on exertion (SOBOE), which had worsened in the past three months.

Present Illness: History of bicuspid aortic valve disease, an ejection fraction of 53%, and moderate concentric left ventricular hypertrophy. Franko underwent elective aortic valve replacement surgery (tissue) and had an uneventful post-operative recovery. His vital signs were stable, heart sounds normal, had a grade II/VI systolic ejection murmur, normal breath sounds, no nausea/vomiting, no urinary symptoms, and post-operative blood sugar levels were 12–14 mmol/L. Current medications included ECASA 81 mg po daily, Clopidogrel 75 mg po daily, Enalapril 20 mg po daily, HCTZ 25 mg po daily, Rosuvastatin 40 mg po daily, Hydromorphone 2 mg po q3h prn, Metformin 1500 po mg qam and 1000 po mg qpm, and Glyburide 2.5 mg po bid.

Past History: Past health history included T2DM x 14 years (HbA1c 8.1%), osteoarthritis, morbid obesity, peripheral vascular disease, TIA two years ago, previous stent to his left anterior descending coronary artery, permanent pacemaker for complete heart block six years ago, and hypertension x 14 years.

Family History: Father, aged 78, with chronic back pain. Mother, aged 77, with T2DM. Franko has no children.

Personal and Social History: His wife underwent urgent cardiac surgery three months ago and now experiences persistent post-operative sternal pain with costochondral mobility. Neither Franko nor his wife has extended health benefits; they receive Canada Pension Plan (CPP) disability with CPP retirement benefits and do not qualify for Ontario Disability Support Program (ODSP) benefits. Franko is not active, does not take regular walks, and likes to watch television most of the day.

Discussion

This case illustrates how in-hospital consultations with pharmacy and social work optimize discharge planning. The Canadian Diabetes Association's *Clinical Practice Guidelines* (2016) emphasize an aggressive approach to the prevention and management of diabetes. However, affordability and access to diabetes medications, devices, and supplies vary depending on where one lives in Canada (not unlike prescription medication, device, or supply costs associated with other chronic illness conditions). Approximately 57% of Canadians with diabetes do not comply with their prescribed management plan because of affordability issues. Out-of-pocket expenses for Franko's medications, for example, depend on costs related to pharmacy mark-ups, dispensing fees, and public and private insurance coverage. In this case, consultations with pharmacy and social work helped to ensure Franko's individual needs were met. These collaborations assisted in determining the least expensive medication to prescribe, as well as to determine if Franko would qualify for a lower deductible from a drug benefit program.

Post-operatively, Franko's hyperglycemia warranted the addition of a second antihyperglycemic agent. With the assistance of the pharmacist, the NP coordinating Franko's care was able to add a relatively inexpensive second agent. The pharmacist also assisted in choosing this agent based on Health Canada–approved medications available across formularies. They knew that "listed" medications were available and would be of full benefit to Franko; those marked "restricted" (available only to those who are eligible under the public drug plan and who meet specific eligibility criteria) and "not listed" (unavailable on the public drug plan) were not ideal. If Franko had been eligible for Ontario's Trillium Drug Program, he would have received coverage for selected blood glucose strips, as well as oral medications, but would still have been required to pay a deductible based on his income. In Ontario, if Franko required insulin to manage his hyperglycemia post-operatively, he would not have received financial assistance to cover the costs of lancets or a glucose meter. In consultation with the pharmacist and social worker, the NP coordinating Franko's care was able to estimate the daily cost of his medication to be $16.81, or approximately $525/month. The NP was able to make recommendations to manage costs and improve adherence to his recommended diabetes management regime.

In consultation with the collaborating cardiac surgeon, it was decided that Franko would be referred to an endocrinologist. Although the ongoing management of his care coordination would remain with his primary care provider, the endocrinologist would assist in the ongoing evaluation and management of his diabetes and related complications. Diabetes is one of the most prevalent and costliest diseases in Canada, with much of the cost and suffering attributed to complications such as retinopathy, nephropathy, neuropathy, and cardiovascular disease.

This integration and coordination of services ensured Franko received specialist services to maximize his health outcomes. This case illustrates the importance of interprofessional collaboration with medicine, pharmacy, social work, and the client/family. It reinforces the "right care in the right place at the right time" strategy (Government of Ontario, 2014) embraced by many Canadian provinces.

Conclusion

Consultation, collaboration, and referral are essential components to NP practice. Clients are the priority focus; the services provided must be responsive to their needs, and clients must be actively engaged in decisions about the management of their health. When NPs focus on client engagement, access, trust and respect, effective communication, provision of the best possible care and services, and a population health approach, clients will have access to the "right care in the right place at the right time" by the "right health professional" (Government of Ontario, 2014). Collaboration is a complex process that requires confidence, competence, trust, and respect from all individuals. A lack of collaboration contributes to fragmentation of care, client dissatisfaction, and poor client outcomes.

Critical Thinking Questions

1. Compare and contrast the concepts of collaboration and teamwork.
2. Describe the organizational and systems level policies that would facilitate collaborative practice environments in your province.
3. Discuss possible strategies for negotiation and conflict resolution in managing restrictions to the NP scope of practice in your province or territory. Compare and contrast how other jurisdictions are dealing with these issues.
4. What elements would you incorporate into your toolkit to integrate the NP role into a collaborative practice environment?

References

Association of Registered Nurses of Prince Edward Island (ARNPEI). (2012). *Nurse practitioner standards for practice*. Charlottetown, PEI: ARNPEI. Retrieved from http://www.arnpei.ca/images/pdf/Nurse%20Practitioner%20Standards%20for%20Practice.pdf

Canadian Diabetes Association (CDA). (2016). *Clinical practice guidelines*. Retrieved from http://guidelines.diabetes.ca/

Canadian Nurses Association (CNA). (2000). *The primary health care approach.* Ottawa, ON: CNA. Retrieved from http://cna-aiic.ca/~/media/cna/page-content/pdf-en/fs02_primary_health_care_approach_june_2000_e.pdf?la=en

CNA. (2010). *Canadian nurse practitioner core competency framework.* Ottawa, ON: CNA. Retrieved from https://www.cna-aiic.ca/~/media/cna/files/en/competency_frame-work_2010_e.pdf

CNA. (2011). *Position statement: Interprofessional collaboration.* Ottawa, ON: CNA. Retrieved from http://www.cna-aiic.ca/~/media/cna/page-content/pdf-en/interproffessional-collaboration_position-statement.pdf?la=en

College of Nurses of Ontario (CNO). (2011). *Practice standard: Nurse practitioner.* Toronto, ON: CNO. Retrieved from http://www.cno.org/Global/docs/prac/41038_StrdRnec.pdf

College of Registered Nurses of British Columbia (CRNBC). (2012). *Scope of practice for nurse practitioners: Standards, limits and conditions.* Vancouver, BC: CRNBC. Retrieved from https://www.crnbc.ca/Standards/Lists/StandardResources/688ScopeforNPs.pdf

College of Registered Nurses of Nova Scotia (CRNNS). (2011). *Guidelines for collaborative practice teams and employers of nurse practitioners: Strategies for integrating nurse practitioners in healthcare teams.* Halifax, NS: CRNSS. Retrieved from http://www.crnns.ca/wp-content/uploads/2015/02/GuidelinesforCollaborativePracticeTeams.pdf

DiCenso, A., & Bryant-Lukosius, D. (2010). *Clinical nurse specialists and nurse practitioners in Canada: A decision support synthesis.* Ottawa, ON: Canadian Health Services Research Foundation (CHSRF). Retrieved from http://www.cfhi-fcass.ca/sf-docs/default-source/commissioned-research-reports/Dicenso_EN_Final.pdf?sfvrsn=0

Enhancing Interdisciplinary Collaboration in Primary Health Care (EICP). (2006). *The principles and framework for interdisciplinary collaboration in primary health care.* Ottawa, ON: EICP. Retrieved from http://www.eicp.ca/en/principles/march/eicp-principles-and-framework-march.pdf

Goolsby, M.J. (2002). *Nurse practitioner secrets: Questions and answers to reveal the secrets to successful NP practice.* Philadelphia, PA: Hanley & Belfus.

Government of Ontario. (2014). *2014 mandate letter: Health and long-term care. Putting patients at the centre—the right care, right place, right time.* Toronto, ON: Gov.ON.

Henneman, E.A., Lee, J.L., & Cohen, J. (1995). Collaboration: A concept analysis. *Journal of Advanced Nursing, 21*(1), 103–109. doi: 10.1046/j.1365-2648.1995.21010103.x

Nurse Practitioners' Association of Ontario (NPAO). (2012). *Briefing note on NP referral to specialists.* Toronto, ON: RNAO. Retrieved from http://npao.org/wp-content/uploads/2012/07/Briefing-Note-on-NP-Referral-to-Specialists-February-22-2012-to-ADM-McGurn.pdf

Resnick, B., & Bonner, A. (2003). Collaboration: Foundation for a successful practice. *Journal of the American Medical Directors Association, November/December,* 344–349. Retrieved from https://www.gapna.org/sites/default/files/download/RegulatoryEnvironment/resnick.pdf

World Health Organization (WHO). (2010). *Framework for action on interprofessional education & collaborative practice.* Geneva, CH: WHO. Retrieved from http://whqlibdoc.who.int/hq/2010/WHO_HRH_HPN_10.3_eng.pdf?ua=1

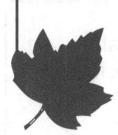

SECTION III

Advanced Practice Nursing Specialty Roles in Canada

This section provides the reader with depictions of advanced practice nursing (APN) roles that are enacted across Canada. The clinical nurse specialist's (CNS) roles of geropsychiatry, mental health, and ambulatory care are discussed but are not exhaustive of the roles that CNSs contribute to the Canadian health care system. The discussion of nurse practitioner (NP) roles is organized around primary health care, as well as the acute and chronic roles that have developed across practice settings. At the core, based on the foundational background as a registered nurse, all APNs build and expand their roles with an overall goal of facilitating timely and accessible care within fiscally challenging environments to provide optimal health services for Canadians.

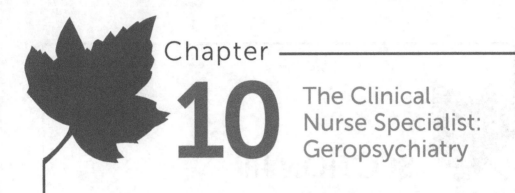

Chapter 10

The Clinical Nurse Specialist: Geropsychiatry

Gloria McInnis-Perry

Gloria McInnis-Perry is an Associate Professor at the University of Prince Edward Island in Charlottetown. She is a specialist in seniors' mental health in acute and long-term care, in community and hospital-based settings, in both Canada and the United States.

KEY TERMS

clinical nurse specialist (CNS)
geropsychiatric clinical nurse specialist (GPCNS)
mental illness
older adults

OBJECTIVES

1. Describe the role of the geropsychiatric clinical nurse specialist (GPCNS).
2. Explore the role functions of the GPCNS.
3. Identify the unique challenges in providing mental health care to older adults.

Introduction

In Canada, persons aged 65 years and older comprise approximately 15.6% of our population; by 2030, this number is anticipated to increase to 23% (Statistics Canada, 2010). Concurrently, Canadian men and women are living longer, with a life expectancy of 80 and 84.2 years respectively (Decady & Greenberg, 2014). Approximately 75% of Canadians aged 65 and over report having at least one of the seven most common health problems (arthritis, cancer, chronic obstructive lung disease, diabetes, heart disease, high blood pressure, and mood disorders), with many reporting the coexistence of two or more of these conditions (Health Council of Canada, 2010). **Older adults** with high comorbidity who have three or more chronic conditions report poorer health, take more prescriptions, have an increased risk of functional dependency, and have a higher number of health care visits (Canadian Institute Health Information [CIHI], 2011).

Living a long and healthy life is a desire for many older adults. For others, coping with changes, such as retirement, relocation, social losses, and normal decline in physical health, poses risks to mental health at a time when strengths and resources may be reduced. The most common **mental illnesses** after age 65 are mood and anxiety disorders, cognitive and mental disorders due to a medical condition (including dementia and delirium), substance misuse (including prescription drugs and alcohol), and psychotic disorders (Public Health Agency of Canada [PHAC], 2006). Depressive episodes, agoraphobia, and panic disorder can present as first episode disorders for the 60 years and over age group (Kessler, Amminger, Aguilar-Gaxiola, Lee, & Üstün, 2007). The prevalence of mental illness increases after the age of 69 and, by 90 years of age, there is a 42% chance one will develop such a condition (Mental Health Commission of Canada [MHCC], 2014).

In Canada, seniors' specialized mental health treatment programs, support services, research, and knowledge are lacking (MacCourt, Wilson, & Tourigney-Rivard, 2011). Nonetheless, many older adults' mental health problems can be managed with adequate preventive strategies, timely recognition and diagnosis, and delivery of person-centred interventions. This chapter examines the role of the **geropsychiatric clinical nurse specialist** (GPCNS), and includes discussion of the educational preparation for the role, consideration of aging issues, and advanced mental health nursing care of mentally ill older adults and their families. A case study will demonstrate how the advanced practice nursing (APN) role competencies are integrated into the daily practice of the GPCNS.

Geropsychiatric Clinical Nurse Specialist

The geropsychiatric clinical nurse specialist (GPCNS) is a **clinical nurse specialist** (CNS) with a professional specialty in the mental health of older adults, and has expert knowledge in normal age-related changes and common psychiatric, cognitive, and comorbid medical disorders occurring in later life. The GPCNS has a high level of expertise in assessing patients, making diagnoses, and treating the complex health responses of individuals, groups, and communities. Role functions of the GPCNS include educating and coaching patients, families, and nurses; performing in-depth physical, social, and psychological assessments; providing direct physical and psychological interventions; consulting and collaborating with family caregivers, nursing staff, physicians, and other disciplines to plan and evaluate individualized care based on assessments; managing interprofessional care over a defined period of time; serving as leaders by changing practices or directing interprofessional teams; and conducting or participating in research activities (Bourbonniere & Evans, 2002).

Issues Related to Aging in Canada

GPCNSs are aware of the current issues facing the older adult. Understanding the bio-logical changes related to normal aging and aging well, as well as the social/ethno-cultural/spiritual/religious context of the mentally ill older adult and their families, are central to person-centred and recovery-focused care. The aging process is universal, highly com-plex, diverse, and influenced by changes in the biological/psychological/social/ethno-cul-tural/spiritual aspects of the individual. Grouping older adults based on chronological age remains the most common means of assessing the elderly and determining their suitability for a wide variety of programs. However, the GPCNS must consider cohort effects that take into account the influence of historical time and the attributes of a particular generation, as well as how events may be experienced differently between and within various cohorts.

Agism, Stigma, and Discrimination

Older adults face issues of agism, stigma, and discrimination. Agism is the existence of negative attitudes towards a person on the basis of their chronological age. Older adults with mental health problems face overlapping stigma: the stigma of mental illness, as well as the stigma of being elderly (MHCC, 2012). Moreover, these older adults most likely experience extrapyramidal symptoms due to the use of conventional antipsychotics whose side effects can be quite disabling for the older adult and may lead to further social stigma-tization. Many older adults with serious and persistent mental illness have greater difficulty accessing age-related services, such as nursing homes. Conversely, an older adults' age may limit access to certain health care services. Addressing issues of agism, stigma, and/or dis-crimination is part of the recovery philosophy, and a part of the GPCNS's ethical practice.

Aging Well

Aging well is "a lifelong process optimizing opportunities for improving and preserving health and physical, social, and mental wellness; independence; quality of life; and enhancing successful life-course transitions" (Peel, Bartlett, & MacClure, 2005, p. 298). Emphasizing a wellness perspective of aging encourages consideration of the person's strengths, resilience, resources, and capabilities (Touhy, Jett, Boscart, & McCleary, 2012). The social determinants of health, including income and social status, social support networks, physical health and social environments, personal health practices, coping skills, and health services, are all factors that impact older adults' well-being.

Social, Cultural, and Spiritual/Religious Context

Consideration of the social/cultural/spiritual context in which older adults live and how these shape their world view are essential to ensure a holistic approach when providing psychiatric care. These fundamental areas, along with the physical aspects, determine how mental health and mental illness is understood. Many older adults prefer to "age in place" (in their own home), supported by family and friends, and with the necessary professional health care. Social support is important to human health (Gottlieb & Bergen, 2010), is interactional (O'Reilly & Thomas, 1989), and is derived from various social networks. Older adults who have strong social networks are often happier and perceive themselves as healthy (Gilmour, 2012). Nonetheless, many older adults live alone. The majority of these are women, who are lonely and without the social support of their immediate family, friends, and community (Aday, Kehoe, & Farney, 2006; Newall et al., 2009; Victor, Scambler, Bowling, & Bond, 2005). Age and gender differences in social support needs must be considered, especially with factors such as social assessments, strengthening relationships, addressing social isolation, and providing opportunities for older adults to participate in meaningful activities (McInnis-Perry, Weeks, & Styrn, 2013).

Among older Canadians, there is great cultural and ethnic diversity, which presents challenges in the provision of a comprehensive, recovery-focused mental health care system. Culture and ethnicity are often linked; however, culture is a way of life (behaviours, values, attitudes, and geographic and political factors) that is attributed to a group of people, while ethnicity refers to race, origin or ancestry, identity, language, and religion (Phinney, 1996). The expression, interpretations, and care of mental illness vary within and among culture groups.

Spirituality is expressed and understood in a cultural context. The GPCNS's understanding of the older adult's beliefs, values, and spirituality are essential aspects in providing holistic nursing care. The term *religion* is often used interchangeably with *spirituality*, yet the two are distinct. Religion is "the organized set of beliefs, traditions, and behaviours that relate to some greater entity outside the self," and spirituality is "the inner life of personal development, the search for meaning that may or may not be a part of any religion or a relationship to a higher power" (Chandler, 2012, pp. 578–579). The importance of religion and spirituality as a source of protection is well documented, as it affects older adults' mental health and positive health outcomes such as higher quality of life; lower rates of depression, anxiety, and suicide; mental health status; and treatment effects (Baetz & Bowen, 2011; Weber & Pargament, 2014). However, the expression of one's religion/spirituality may pose challenges in mental health care, as these experiences may be seen as a "normal cultural experience," "sacred," or a "blessing" versus a delusional symptom. Often, negative psychological outcomes are related to adverse religious coping, spiritual struggle, misunderstanding, miscommunication, or negative beliefs (Weber & Pargament, 2014).

The GPCNS needs to understand how older adults define and describe their religious/spiritual beliefs and experiences, and how these may differ from the GPCNS's personal beliefs. As well, it is important to understand the role that religion and spirituality play in the older adult's life and how they influence their day-to-day functioning. If the older adult's preoccupation with religion and religious rituals becomes so destructive that they cannot function with daily life, then the consideration of an underlying psychopathology must be assessed.

Recovery-Focused Care

A mental health system that addresses the complex interaction between the individual and social dimensions that influence mental health outcomes must be both person-centred and comprehensive in its approach to recovery and well-being. Much effort is needed to promote the mental health of older adults, as good physical health, meaningful activities, and secure and supportive relationships all contribute to good mental health and quality of life for older adults. In a recovery-oriented system, people who experience mental health problems and illnesses are treated with dignity and respect. The concept of recovery is person-centred and built on the principles of choice, respect, hope, empowerment, self-determination, and responsibility (MHCC, 2009). Older adults living with mental illness who participate as fully as possible in their own care and well-being make informed choices with the support of health care professionals, family, and friends. Essential to recovery is the removal of all barriers in order for the person to have access to the right mix of evidence-informed service at the right time (MHCC, 2009). Early intervention at the first indication of mental illness and/or addiction symptoms is important as it can shorten the recovery journey.

BOX 10.1

Applying Recovery Principles to the Assessment of the Older Adult

Listed below are some considerations when assessing older adults:

1. Always assess and consider the older adult's strength and ability to function.
2. Distinguish between normal and abnormal aging. Older adults are more likely to have somatic complaints, and attribute these to physical problems rather than mental health problems. To the older adult, these symptoms are real and the GPCNS needs to acknowledge these feelings. Exploring the temporal context of the symptoms will provide the GPCNS with a better understanding of the history, possible triggers, and whether or not the symptoms are part of normal worry versus a mental health disorder.
3. Consider the effect that medical illnesses and medications have on the presentation of mental illness.

4. Some older adults exhibit sub-syndromal symptoms of an illness, in which severity and symptoms are not high enough to be diagnosed with a formal psychiatric diagnosis; however, therapeutic interventions may relieve symptoms, improve functional status, prevent a more serious illness, and improve overall quality of life.
5. The loss of a loved one, social status, pet, or object may be quite a significant loss to the older adult, as the ability to replace these losses may be more difficult than for a younger person.
6. Always complete a risk assessment and consider the personal context of the older adult.
7. If suicidal ideation is assessed, implement safety measures and inform appropriate personnel.

Geropsychiatric Clinical Nurse Specialist Competencies

Clinical

Caring for the older adult who exhibits signs and symptoms of a mental health disorder can present some unique challenges. The GPCNS must consider the biological/psychological/social/cultural/spiritual influences on the older adult, and integrate this knowledge with individualized treatment of various mental disorders. The GPCNS must also take into account the most common mental illnesses in the older adult, the clinical considerations of providing evidence-informed holistic care, and keep abreast of relevant and ongoing research in this area. Growing older, for some, means living longer with a recurrent serious and persistent mental illness, experiencing late onset mental illnesses, living with behavioural and psychological symptoms associated with dementia, and living with chronic medical problems with known correlations with mental illnesses such as Parkinson's disease, cerebral vascular disease, and chronic obstructive lung disease (Horgan et al., 2009).

Assessment

The GPCNS assesses clients, develops and contributes to the plan of care, and intervenes in complex health care situations within the specialty of geropsychiatry. The process begins with a comprehensive mental health assessment based on the GPCNS's underlying philosophy, theoretical framework, experience, access to electronic charting, assessment databases, and workplace policy. The GPCNS collects, documents, and analyzes client information and draws conclusions supported by this information. Since many older adults being cared for by the GPCNS present with complex mental health issues, a high level of clinical reasoning skills supported by evidence guide the care.

The GPCNS considers both the process and the content of the assessment. This includes engaging the client in a therapeutic relationship, maintaining appropriate boundaries, and utilizing recovery principles and techniques. The GPCNS must be alert to inconsistencies during the interview and consider the ongoing nature of the assessment process. It is important for the older adult to feel valued, listened to, and safe. The assessment should consider the interview environment: whether the interview is formal or informal; structured, semi-structured, or unstructured; and whether the older adult has communication deficits or barriers requiring modifications.

The GPCNS completes an assessment that targets various aspects of functioning such as cognitive, psychological, affective, and physical performance, as well as social and psychosocial abilities. The GPCNS reviews already existing medical (diagnostic and laboratory tests, medications) and general nursing data (activities of daily living, nutrition, sleep hygiene, etc.) in addition to collecting new information from the older adult, family, and formal caregivers over the course of care.

Screening tools may be used to assist in the assessment and monitoring of mental illness; however, one must consider the selection and use of tools on factors such as the characteristics of the situation, the presenting problem, and the older adult's abilities to self-report. Many diagnostic criteria and instruments used for defining and identifying mental illnesses have been developed and validated in younger adults, which may not adequately capture the older adults' experience, subclinical symptoms, and influence of race, culture, and educational level. It is recommended that, where possible, the GPCNS purposely select screening and assessment tools that have been validated for older adults.

Nursing Diagnoses

Assessment skills are used to identify nursing diagnoses and to develop nursing interventions that reduce symptoms, risks, or functional decline. The use of nursing diagnoses with consideration of medical diagnoses, including those related to the *Diagnostic Statistical Manual of Mental Disorders-5* (DSM-5) (American Psychological Association [APA], 2013) will assist in the identification of specific interventions.

Interventions and Outcomes

Nursing interventions should be based on a comprehensive assessment and be evidence-informed, while patient/client outcomes should be nurse-sensitive, desirable, achievable, and measurable. There are many interventions available to the GPCNS in the care of the older adult living with a mental illness. The use of evidence-informed nursing protocols and guidelines should be considered. Often, the GPCNS provides formal and informal education to the client, family, nursing, and staff, or provides advocacy. There are many educational opportunities for the GPCNS while fulfilling the competencies inherent in the role. As a clinician, the GPCNS educates the client and family about mental illness, mental health issues, and care practices. As part of an interprofessional team, the GPCNS can develop continuing education, orientation, and mentor programs to support the team process. As a mentor/coach/trainer, the GPCNS supervises and educates other nurses as a way to strengthen psychiatric mental health nursing, gerontological competencies, and promoting the standards of practice.

A step-by-step approach to care is individualized to the older adult's present needs, mental health disorder, symptoms, functional level, existence of comorbidities, present and past medication usage, and access to available resources and a collaborative team. Depending on these factors, the GPCNS will begin with the least intrusive approach to care. Non-pharmacological interventions are suggested as the first step, such as individual and group activity (music, art, exercise, relaxation, reminiscent, dietary, sleep hygiene, reality orientation), environmental situation (therapeutic and safe, sensory-sensitive, and orienting), and addressing caregiver issues (communication, care practices, stress, and grieving) through education and supportive therapy (self-help groups or formal therapy).

After prompt identification and assessment provision of education about the mental health issue or illness is provided, advice on self-medication use and risk of over-the-counter medications is given. Active monitoring of symptoms and functioning is of prime importance to the GPCNS. If no improvement is evident, then individual or group counselling and/or self-help groups are suggested before moving on to more formalized psychotherapeutic interventions. The use of medications may come into play if the prior interventions do not work, or if the older adult's functioning level declines and/or the risk of self-harm increases. More intense and multiagency services, such as community mental health or in-patient care, may be necessary. Psychopharmacotherapy, used in conjunction with psychotherapy, is a common practice in treating the older adult.

Researcher

As a researcher, the GPCNS disseminates research findings and educates patients/clients, families, students, health care providers, and policy-makers. The GPCNS generates and synthesizes, and are experts in leading evidence-based practice, evidence-informed practice, and professional practice at all levels based on multiple sources of knowledge (CNA, 2013). The research competencies are integral components of the role of the GPCNS, as every aspect of the advance practitioner's role is influenced by research.

Leadership

Leadership is a hallmark of the GPCNS's practice (Lyon, 2014). The GPCNS is a transformational leader, one who appeals to others' values, helps them see a higher vision, and encourages them to exert themselves in helping to achieve that vision. The GPCNS possesses leadership skills necessary to transform the mental health system, specifically older adults' mental health care. They participate in professional organizations and act as role models, which impacts on geropsychiatric mental health care (Tringali, Murphy, & Osevala, 2008). The GPCNS leads, coaches, and mentors direct care nurses in providing evidence-informed care to older adults living with mental health issues. In addition, they design and provide mental health promotion and risk reduction programs and initiatives. The GPCNS works collaboratively within the interprofessional team to provide older adults' mental health care. Many GPCNSs lead, or become part of, initiatives such as strategic planning, the development and/or revision of policies and procedures, and the education of patients, staff, and families.

Consultation and Collaboration

Consultation and collaboration are integral parts of the GPCNS's role (CNA, 2009). Consultation is the indirect provision of care through helping others implement change (Pearson, 2014). The GPCNS provides expertise (and may be consulted on a complex patient case) that is group-specific to staff or patients or to organizational-specific issues for the purpose of improving health care. The GPCNS "collaborates with other health care providers and other interested parties to maximize health benefits to persons receiving, while recognizing and respecting the knowledge, skills and perspectives of all" (CNA, 2008, p.10). Collaborative practice is envisioned as an interprofessional process of communication and decision-making that enables the separate and shared knowledge and skills of health care providers to synergistically influence the client/patient care provided (Way, Jones, & Busing, 2000).

Depending on where the GPCNS practices and whether the CNS has a practice base versus an independent external consultant role (Doody, 2014), consultation and collaboration may be a more common or a more selective role (for example, being a CNS as part of an older adult's mental health community team versus the director of the team). Whether based in the community, long-term care centre (LTC), or hospital setting, the role of the consultant will depend on the reason for the consult, the patient, available resources, and level of expertise of the CNS. The GPCNS completes a thorough assessment, identifies problems, suggests interventions, and evaluates outcomes. Interventions usually involve the client, family, and health care providers. Important in a recovery-focused philosophy is the client/provider collaborative care, in which clients are engaged in and participate fully in treatment decisions. Collaborative care can take many forms and can include setting goals for treatment, preparing a treatment or action plan, and having patients participate in treatment decisions.

The GPCNS is often a facilitator of interprofessional teams, which requires strong team-building and communication skills. Communicating the plan of care to all involved is essential. If further medical or diagnostic testing is required, referral or consultation to medicine may be required. The GPCNS may make specific recommendations to nursing staff, such as medication monitoring, completion of behavioural checklists, and implementation of behavioural management strategies. Other interventions may require referral to other health care professionals such as social work, occupational therapist, and nutritionist.

CASE STUDY

The Story of Bea

Bea, an 85-year-old widow who moved to a nursing home three months ago, is recently referred to the GPCNS by her general practitioner (GP) for assessment of changes in her behaviour (restlessness, agitation, argumentative, yelling, verbal abuse towards nursing staff, social withdrawal, crying, insomnia, and refusal to attend group activities). Bea has a diagnosis of dementia (vascular and probable Alzheimer's disease), herpes zoster, hypertension, hyperlipidemia, hip fracture, and osteoarthritis in both hips. She is on Aricept, Zocor, Lopressor, Neurontin, and Aspirin.

The GPCNS visits the nursing home and begins a comprehensive nursing assessment, which includes a review of Bea's health status as documented in her health file. The GPCNS notes Bea's pre-admission cognitive screening on the Mini Mental State Exam (MMSE) was 20/30, and the Geriatric Depression Scale (GDS) was 3/10. The GPCNS completes the geropsychiatric mental health assessment tools (repeated MMSE and GDS) and a social/environment assessment. They coordinate a meeting with Bea, her family, GP, and nursing and other care providers. The GPCNS findings are: MMSE 19 (moderate CI); GDS 9/15 (moderate depression); no SI nor HI. Laboratory tests were also normal. Bea has an unsteady gait and uses a walker. She has a hearing deficit, and pain in her hips and upper torso. She has had a reported weight loss of 2.2 kg over the last two weeks. Bea scored positive on the behavioural checklist.

Bea's room is located at the end of a long, dimly lit, poorly oriented corridor. She has infrequent visits from her family and friends. Bea expresses anger towards her family for sending her to LTC, and for not visiting. She misses working in the garden and attending daily mass. Bea seems frustrated with the inconsistency in staff care and not receiving adequate pain relief during the night, which makes it difficult to sleep comfortably.

Bea's nursing diagnoses are: chronic confusion, alteration in mood, grief, pain, disturbed sensory perception (auditory), self-care deficit, imbalanced nutrition (less), impaired physical mobility, disturbed sleep pattern, ineffective individual coping, insomnia, risk for loneliness, and family alteration.

Subsequent to these findings, the GPCNS requests a behavioural monitoring checklist and more laboratory tests. Working collaboratively with the interprofessional team, it is determined the geropsychiatrist is to see Bea to rule out major depression/dysfunctional grieving. The GP is to assess pain management and make referrals for a hearing test, nutritionist, and physiotherapist to assess gait. The GPCNS will provide education to the staff on person-centred care, depression, relocation issues, pain management and comfort measures, effective communication issues, self-care, and diversional activities. As well, the GPCNS will provide individual supportive therapy to Bea to help with the transitional stress to LTC, coping with the responses to her depression, monitoring her response to antidepressant and pain medication, and will repeat the GDS. The GPCNS will involve Bea's family and caregivers, as well as attend Bea's case conferences for six months.

Conclusion

The GPCNS provides expert advanced nursing care for older adults living with complex mental health issues across the health care continuum. Education and support of older persons, their family, nurses, interprofessional staff, and the facilitation of change are all components of GPCNS practice. The GPCNS is an evolving specialty in an ever-evolving health care system, which requires the development and use of evidence-informed knowledge and skills in order to keep abreast of changing holistic care practices when caring for the mentally ill older adult and their families.

Critical Thinking Questions

1. What are the roles of the geropsychiatric clinical nurse specialist (GCNS)?
2. What unique factors must the GPCNS consider when working with older adults?
3. What modifications of the comprehensive mental health assessment are necessary in caring for the older adult mentally ill?

References

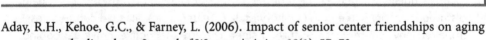

Aday, R.H., Kehoe, G.C., & Farney, L. (2006). Impact of senior center friendships on aging women who live alone. *Journal of Women & Aging, 18*(1), 57–73.

American Psychological Association (APA). (2013). *Diagnostic and statistical manual of mental disorders* (5th ed.). Arlington, VA: APA.

Baetz, M., & Bowen, R. (2011). Suicidal ideation, affective lability, and religion in depressed adults. *Mental Health, Religion & Culture, 14*(7), 633–641.

Bourbonniere, M., & Evans, L. (2002). Advanced practice nursing in the care of frail older adults. *Journal of the American Geriatrics Society, 50*(12), 2062–2076.

Canadian Institute for Health Information (CIHI). (2011). *Health care cost drivers: The facts.* Ottawa, ON: CIHI. Retrieved from https://secure.cihi.ca/free_products/health_care_cost_drivers_the_facts_en.pdf

Canadian Nurses Association (CNA). (2008). *Code of ethics for registered nurses.* Ottawa, ON: CNA. Retrieved from http://www.cna-aiic.ca/~/media/cna/files/en/codeofethics.pdf

CNA. (2009). *Position statement: Clinical nurse specialist.* Ottawa, ON: CNA. Retrieved from www2.cna-aiic.ca/CNA/documents/pdf/publications/PS104_Clinical_ Nurse_Specialist _e.pdf

CNA. (2013). *Strengthening the role of the clinical nurse specialist: Pan-Canadian roundtable discussion summary report.* Ottawa, ON: CNA. Retrieved from www.cna-aiic.ca/en/professional-development/nurse-practitioner-and-clinical-specialists/clinical-nurse-specialists

Chandler, E. (2012). Religious and spiritual issues in DSM-5: Matters of the mind and searching of the soul. *Issues in Mental Health Nursing, 33*(9),577–582.

Decady, Y., & Greenberg, L. (2014). *Health at a glance: Ninety years of change in life expectancy.* Ottawa, ON: Statistics Canada. Retrieved from http://www.statcan.gc.ca/pub/82-624-x/2014001/article/14009-eng.htm

Doody, O. (2014). The role and development of consultancy in nursing practice. *British Journal of Nursing, 23*(1), 32–39.

Gilmour, H. (2012). Social participation and the health and well-being of Canadian seniors. *Statistics Canada Health Reports, 23*(4). Retrieved from http://www.statcan.gc.ca/pub/82-003-x/2012004/article/11720-eng.pdf

Gottlieb, B., & Bergen, A. (2010). Social support concepts and measures. *Journal of Psychosomatic Research, 69*(5), 511–520.

Health Council of Canada. (2010). Helping patients help themselves: Are Canadians with chronic conditions getting the support they need to manage their health? *Canadian Health Care Matters,* January, Bulletin 2, Toronto, ON. Retrieved from http://publications.gc.ca/collections/collection_2011/ccs-hcc/H173-1-2-2010-eng.pdf

Horgan, S., LeClair, K., Donnelly, M., Hinton, G., MacCourt, P., & Krieger-Frost, S. (2009). Developing a national consensus on the accessibility needs of older adults with concurrent and chronic mental and physical health issues: A preliminary framework informing collaborative mental health care planning. *Canadian Journal on Aging. 28*(2), 97–105.

Kessler, R.C., Amminger, G.P., Aguilar-Gaxiola, S., Alonso, J., Lee, S., & Üstün T.B. (2007). Age of onset of mental disorders: A review of recent literature. *Current Opinion in Psychiatry, 20*(4), 359–64.

Lyon, B.L. (2014). Transformational leadership as the clinical nurse specialist's capacity to influence. In J.S. Fulton, B.L. Lyon, & K.A. Goudreau (Eds.). *Foundations of clinical nurse specialist practice,* (2nd ed., pp. 163–172). New York, NY: Springer.

MacCourt, P., Wilson, K., & Tourigny-Rivard, M.F. (2011). *Guidelines for comprehensive mental health services for older adults in Canada.* Calgary, AB: MHCC. Retrieved from http://www.mentalhealthcommission.ca/English/system/files/private/document/mhcc_seniors _guidelines.pdf

McInnis-Perry, G., Weeks, L., & Stryhn, H. (2013). Age and gender differences in emotional and informational social support insufficiency in older adults in Atlantic Canada. *Canadian Journal of Nursing Research, 45*(4), 50–68.

Mental Health Commission of Canada (MHCC). (2009). *Toward recovery and well-being: A framework for a mental health strategy for Canada.* Calgary, AB: MHCC. Retrieved from http://www.mentalhealthcommission.ca/English/system/files/private/FNIM_Toward_Recovery_and_Well_Being_ENG_0.pdf

MHCC. (2012). *Changing directions changing lives: The mental health strategy for Canada.* Calgary, AB: MHCC. Retrieved from http://strategy.mentalhealthcommission.ca/pdf/strategy-images-en.pdf

MHCC. (2014). *Why investing in mental health will contribute to Canada's economic prosperity and to the sustainability of our health care system.* Calgary, AB: MHCC. Retrieved from http://www.mentalhealthcommission.ca/English/system/files/private/document/mhstrategy_case_for_investment_backgrounder_eng_0.pdf

Newall, N.E., Chipperfield, J.G., Clifton, R.A., Perry, R.P., Swift, A.U., & Ruthig, J.C. (2009). Causal beliefs, social participation, and loneliness among older adults: A longitudinal study. *Journal of Social and Personal Relationships, 26*(2–3), 273–290.

O'Reilly, P., & Thomas, H.E. (1989). Role of support networks in maintenance of improved cardiovascular health status. *Social Science & Medicine, 28*(3), 249–260.

Pearson, G.S. (2014). Consultation in the clinical nurse specialist role. In J.S. Fulton, B.L. Lyon, & K.A Goudreau (Eds.). *Foundations of clinical nurse specialist practice* (pp. 269–276). New York: Springer.

Peel, N., Bartlett, H., & McClure, R. (2005). Healthy ageing: How is it defined and measured? *Australasian Journal on Ageing, 23*(3), 115–119.

Phinney, J. (1996). When we talk about American ethnic groups, what do we mean? *American Psychologist, 51*(9), 918–927.

Public Health Agency of Canada (PHAC). (2006). *The human face of mental health and mental illness in Canada 2006.* Ottawa, ON: PHAC. Retrieved from http://www.phac-aspc.gc.ca/publicat/human-humain06/pdf/human_face_e.pdf

Statistics Canada. (2010). *Projected population by age group and sex according to three projection scenarios for 2006, 2011, 2016, 2021, 2026, 2031 and 2036.* Ottawa, ON: Statistic Canada. Retrieved from http://www.statcan.gc.ca/tables-tableaux/sum-som/l01/cst01/demo23a-eng.htm

Touhy, T., Jett, K., Boscart, V., & McCleary, L. (2012). *Ebersole and Hess' gerontological nursing and healthy aging* (1st Cdn. ed.). Toronto, ON: Elsevier.

Tringali, C., Murphy, T., & Osevala, M. (2008). Clinical nurse specialist practice in a care coordination model. *Clinical Nurse Specialist, 22*(5), 231–239.

Victor, C., Scambler, S., Bowling, A., & Bond, J. (2005). The prevalence of, and risk factors for, loneliness in later life: A survey of older people in Great Britain. *Ageing & Society, 25*(6), 357–375.

Way, D., Jones, L., & Busing, N. (2000). *Implementation strategies: Collaboration in primary care—family doctors & nurse practitioners delivering shared care.* Toronto, ON: Ontario College of Family Physicians. Retrieved from http://ocfp.on.ca/docs/public-policy-documents/implementation-strategies-collaboration-in-primary-care---family-doctors-nurse-practitioners-delivering-shared-care.pdf?Status=Master

Weber, S., & Pargament, K. (2014). The role of religion and spirituality in mental health. *Current Opinion in Psychiatry, 27*(5), 358–363.

Chapter 11

The Clinical Nurse Specialist: Mental Health

Josephine Muxlow and Bernadine Wallis

Josephine Muxlow is a CNS–Adult Mental Health with the Atlantic Region (Halifax) First Nations and Inuit Health Branch with Health Canada in Halifax, Nova Scotia. She was a pioneer of the CNS role at Health Canada and holds an appointment as Adjunct Professor at Dalhousie University, School of Nursing.

Bernadine Wallis is an Instructor at the University of Manitoba, Faculty of Nursing. She was previously a CNS–Mental Health with the First Nations and Inuit Health Branch with Health Canada in Winnipeg.

KEY TERMS

advanced practice
clinical nurse specialist (CNS)–Mental Health
direct care
indirect care
system leadership

OBJECTIVES

1. Understand the role of the CNS–Mental Health in the Canadian health care system.
2. Analyze and evaluate how the CNS–Mental Health functions independently and collaboratively within a health care setting.
3. Understand how the Canadian Nurses Association's (CNA) *Pan-Canadian Clinical Nurse Specialist Core Competencies* become the pillars of CNS–Mental Health practice.
4. Identify strategies the CNS–Mental Health uses for advancing nursing, system leadership, and quality management in a mental health setting.

Introduction

In Canada, mental illness is the second leading cause of disability and death (Lim, Jacobs, & Dewa, 2008). It is estimated that one in five Canadians experiences major mental illness, with an annual economic impact of at least $50 billion dollars (Mental Health Commission of Canada [MHCC], 2012: Smetanin et al., 2011). Over the past decade, mental health and mental illnesses have been brought to the forefront in Canada by several reports and initiatives (Government of Canada, 2006; MHCC, 2009, 2012). The following list outlines the evidence that mental health seriously impacts our society:

- The majority of the 4,000 Canadians who die by suicide each year experienced a mental health problem or issue.
- As high as 70% of young adults with mental health problems experienced issues from childhood.
- Absenteeism related to mental health problems or illnesses costs $6 billion in lost productivity annually.
- Projections indicated that the rate of mental illness for adults between the ages of 70 and 89 will be higher than any other age group in Canada. (MHCC, 2012, p. 1)

The **CNS–Mental Health** in an **advanced practice** nursing role has the opportunity, through system and transformational leadership, to contribute to an efficient, effective, patient-centred mental health care system. An equitable and efficient mental health system not only aligns care and services with client needs, but also enhances quality care with positive health outcomes related to wellness and recovery.

This chapter focuses specifically on the role of the CNS–Mental Health. It is important to acknowledge that there are other health care professionals with multiple titles and classifications who practice in various psychiatric and mental health settings supporting the Canadian population (see Chapter 10 for a discussion related to the geropsychiatric CNS role).

The Role of the Clinical Nurse Specialist–Mental Health

The CNS is one of two advanced practice nurse (APN) roles identified by the Canadian Nurses Association (CNA); the nurse practitioner (NP) is the other. The CNS–Mental Health is "a registered nurse who holds a graduate degree in nursing and has a high level of expertise in the clinical speciality of psychiatric mental health nursing" (CNA, 2014, p. 1). The CNS–Mental Health "analyzes, synthesizes and applies nursing knowledge, theory, research evidence to foster system-wide changes" and advances psychiatric mental health nursing care (CNA, 2014, p. 1). Within this context, the CNS–Mental Health plays a pivotal role in the transformation of the mental health system by enhancing care and services, promoting better health, reducing cost, and promoting equity and social justice in mental health care.

Currently, the CNS–Mental Health practices within the provincial or territorial scope of practice for registered nurses because legislation and regulation specific for the advanced CNS role is not available. There is also no national credentialing for the CNS, although the CNA has a national certification examination that is available to all practicing psychiatric and mental health nurses and other nursing specialty groups. The two national professional associations that support the CNS–Mental Health and promote quality improvement are the Canadian Association of Advanced Practice Nurses/L'Association Canadienne des Infirmières et Infirmiers en Pratique Avancée (CAAPN-ACIIPA) and the Canadian Federation for Mental Health Nurses.

Fulton, Lyon, and Goudreau (2014) described developmental differences between an experienced registered nurse and a CNS pertaining to the "breadth and depth of the specialty area, clinical practice, system leadership, the understanding of inner self, emotions and inner leadership, ethical practice, and professional practice and affiliation" (p. 19). One key difference is the CNS consultation role and system leadership skills related to coaching, mentoring, and analysis of ethical issues.

The APN role competencies are clinical, research, leadership, and consultation and collaboration (CNA, 2008). The CNS-specific core competencies were adopted in June 2014, and their domains of competencies are clinical care, system leadership, advancement of nursing practice, evaluation, and research (CNA, 2014). The CNS–Mental Health embeds the *Pan-Canadian Core Competencies* in the advanced practice role regardless of the area of specialty and practice setting. In addition, the CNS–Mental Health provides both **direct care** and **indirect care**, and uses a variety of approaches and strategies in providing client-centred care, advanced nursing practice, system leadership, and evaluating and critically appraising nurse-sensitive outcomes (see Figure 11.1).

Clinical Care

In order to provide client-centred care the CNS integrates trauma-informed practice in conjunction with holistic and public health nursing approaches, as well as psychotherapeutic care, the nursing process, and broad theoretical approaches. The integration of trauma-informed practice enables the CNS to apply the advanced knowledge of pathophysiology within the context of the ripple effect of a traumatic event on the physical, emotional, mental, spiritual, and relationship aspects of the client's life. The CNS's knowledge of the impact of a traumatic event on regulating emotions, manifestation of trauma through feelings of shame, guilt, powerlessness, helplessness, self-esteem, and loss of identity become an integral part of the therapeutic intervention. An essential component of developing a care plan with the client is the identification of the client's strengths, resilience, meaning, and goals.

FIGURE 11.1: The Clinical Nurse Specialist: Domains, Role, and Functions

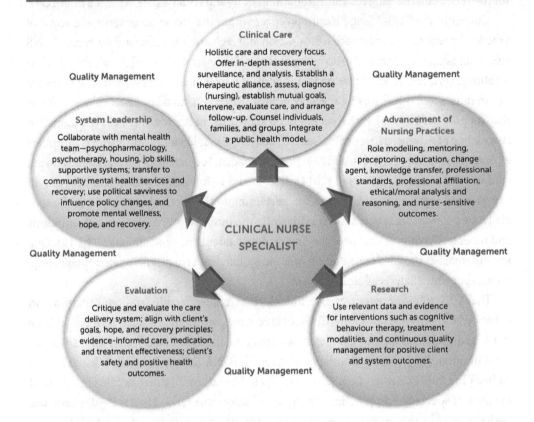

This figure describes the domains of clinical care, advancement of nursing practice, research, evaluation, and system leadership as they pertain to the roles and functions of the clinical nurse specialist with the focus of a quality management perspective.

Source: Created by Josephine Muxlow; adapted from Canadian Nurses Association (CNA), 2014.

The CNS–Mental Health promotes mental health/mental wellness by integrating public health approaches and the social determinants of mental health in clinical practice. The evidence shows that key determinants of mental health are employment, education, housing and income, supportive relationships (peer), involvement in social activities, community engagement, and freedom from discrimination and stigma (Centre for Addiction and Mental Health [CAMH], 2009; World Health Organization [WHO], 2004, 2015). Many Canadians living with mental health problems and mental illness fail to experience these key determinants of health and therefore have difficulties achieving goals to increase resilience and decrease risk factors.

The direct and indirect care provided by the CNS–Mental Health is grounded in cultural competence that integrates the client's ways of knowing and doing, meaning of care, and the reality of the client's life, as well as the ability to engage and interact effectively with the client regardless of the client's mental health status. The CNS incorporates best practices and critical analysis during the holistic assessment, monitoring, and interventions phases of care to achieve positive health outcomes. Likewise, the CNS applies system level and leadership skills when consulting and collaborating with other health professionals to improve the health of the population.

Direct Care

The CNS–Mental Health uses clinical expertise and advanced knowledge and skills in psychiatric mental health when working with clients with complex and persistent mental health and addiction problems and social issues. They apply a holistic model (see Figure 11.2) by demonstrating expert knowledge, skills, and competencies, integrating values and beliefs, building interpersonal relationships and therapeutic alliance (trust, respect, dignity, engagement, and communication skills), and analyzing the social and cultural determinants of health so that they are meaningful to the client. The CNS also demonstrates the political competence required to navigate both the internal and external mental health system for client safety and positive health outcomes. Likewise, the CNS applies system level and leadership skills when consulting and collaborating with other health professionals to improve the health of the population.

The percentage of the CNS–Mental Health's practice activities related to direct care varies with the organization and practice setting. Components of direct care provided by the CNS include comprehensive holistic assessment (i.e., validation, implementation, and evaluation) with a systematic approach using problem-solving skills and techniques to manage a wide range of clients with compounding mental, physical, social, and economic issues. Direct care also includes monitoring the effect of medication(s), counselling (individual, families, and group), co-therapy with other health professionals, crisis intervention and stabilization, and psycho-educational activities related to promoting mental health, wellness, and recovery. Knowledge and application of public health nursing enhances the CNS's ability to address complex health-related issues, health inequities, and social justice issues while providing direct care. In addition, the CNS–Mental Health incorporates clinical inquiry, system theory, and research to evaluate and critically appraise nurse-sensitive outcomes and continuous quality improvement initiatives under the umbrella of quality management.

Other relevant aspects of the CNS's practice include working with clients to attain goals and promote positive mental health activities to achieve mental wellness, hope, and recovery. The CNS has the opportunity to integrate knowledge and information gained through engagement and communication into policy and clinical guidelines whenever there are identifiable risks for client safety, quality care, continuous quality improvement, and positive health outcomes. The evidence of the increasing need for mental health services discussed earlier in the

FIGURE 11.2:   Holistic Model for the CNS–Mental Health

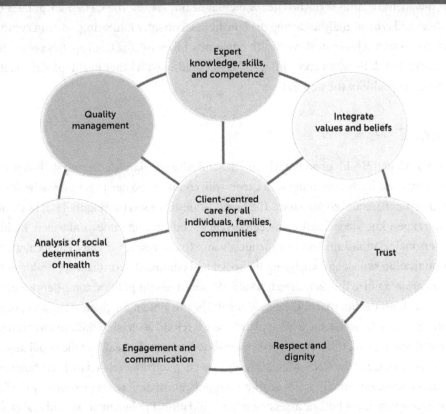

This figure illustrates the components of holistic care used by the CNS–Mental Health to provide client-centred care to individuals, families, and communities.

Source: Created by Josephine Muxlow.

chapter demonstrates the need for the CNS–Mental Health to continue to advocate for a full scope of practice in hospital and community mental health settings. At the forefront of the mental health system, the CNS's practice is improving the health status of clients whose health and well-being are compromised as a result of physical, emotional, and psychosocial problems with or without complex and persistent mental health issues and concurrent disorders.

Indirect Care

Consultation and Collaboration

Consultation and collaboration are two key components of the CNS's indirect practice. It is important to differentiate between the CNS providing direct care to clients with complex health issues and the CNS providing consultation on complex and persistent mental health issues to care providers and decision-makers. Depending on the practice setting, both direct and indirect care falls under the CNS role. It is also important to acknowledge that the CNS becomes a consultee with the psychiatrist, pharmacist, and other health care team members when addressing risk management and psychopharmacology issues. At this time, prescribing rights are not available to the CNS working in the Canadian health care system, although they are generally available to the larger community of CNSs practicing in the United States, and mental health nurses in the United Kingdom (Hemingway & Ely, 2009; Mangle, Phillips, Pitts, & Laver-Bradbury, 2014). Consultation is interwoven in all aspects of the CNS role. Keltner, Schwecke, and Bostrom (1991) defined consultation as "an interactive process between two professionals to discuss a work-related problem at the individual, family, group, program, or system level" (p. 151). This core competency is widely acknowledged in the CNS community (CNA, 2008; National Association of Clinical Nurse Specialists [NACNS], 2010).

The CNS functions as an expert consultant in psychiatric mental health nursing, and is instrumental in assisting nurses and mental health practitioners in addressing complex and persistent mental health issues within or outside their own full scope of practice. For example, in an institutional setting, the expert consultation may include health professionals working on non-psychiatric mental health units or clinics. Inherent in the consultation process is having a clear understanding of the issues, knowledge, skills, and competence in teaching and learning techniques, issues management and resolution, and individual, group, and system dynamics. The CNS provides advanced knowledge when consultation is requested by a health care provider for an issue or a problem that is outside the health provider's scope of practice or level of competence. In 2009, Erchul and the American Board of Professional Psychology (ABPP) described Caplan's four types of mental health consultation (see Figure 11.3).

Keltner, Schwecke, and Bostrom (1991) state that the psychiatric consultant nurse uses their expertise to provide three types of consultation: patient-focused, consultee-focused, and system- or organization-focused. They listed the following as key factors in the consultation process:

- Consultant should be in a staff position rather than a supervisor/management position to promote open communication.
- Consultees freely accept the consultant's recommendations with free will.
- Issues addressed are work-related and remain professional not personal.
- Consultee remains responsible for the client.
- Consultant and consultee develop a professional peer relationship for problem solving, rather than one of staff supervisor/manager. (p. 152)

In the Canadian health care system, the CNS–Mental Health provides consultation mainly on an informal basis without the formal contractual agreement advocated by Caplan, Caplan, and Erchul (1995). In a publicly funded in-patient mental health setting, the CNS

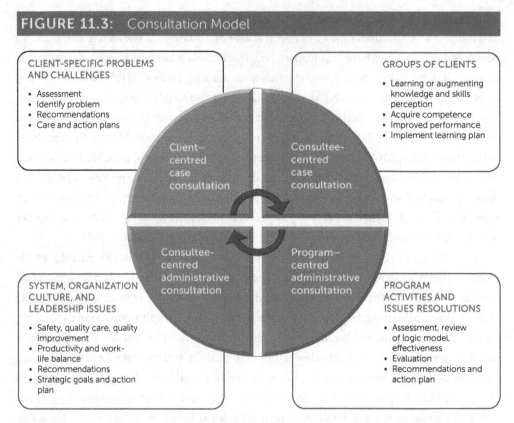

FIGURE 11.3:   Consultation Model

CLIENT-SPECIFIC PROBLEMS AND CHALLENGES

- Assessment
- Identify problem
- Recommendations
- Care and action plans

GROUPS OF CLIENTS

- Learning or augmenting knowledge and skills perception
- Acquire competence
- Improved performance
- Implement learning plan

Client–centred case consultation

Consultee–centred case consultation

Consultee–centred administrative consultation

Program–centred administrative consultation

SYSTEM, ORGANIZATION CULTURE, AND LEADERSHIP ISSUES

- Safety, quality care, quality improvement
- Productivity and work-life balance
- Recommendations
- Strategic goals and action plan

PROGRAM ACTIVITIES AND ISSUES RESOLUTIONS

- Assessment, review of logic model, effectiveness
- Evaluation
- Recommendations and action plan

This figure uses Caplan's (1970) four categories of consultation, with additional clarifications of CNS activities related to client-specific problems, system, organization culture, and leadership issues, as well as groups of clients, programs activity, and issues resolutions.

Source: Created by Josephine Muxlow; adapted from Caplan, Caplan, & Erchul, 1995.

provides consultation services as a member of the mental health team in the organization. There may be variation from province to province based on provincial mandates, outreach services affiliated with the organization, service delivery contracts, and memorandum of understanding for clinical mental health services between the health authority and specific community health agencies. The CNS affiliated with a community-based mental health setting may extend consultation services to include interprovincial organizations such as correctional services and community health centres within the catchment or zone area.

Regardless of the type of consultation and principles adhered to during the consultation process, Keltner, Schwecke, and Bostrum (1991) describe six phases of the consultation process (which are similar to the nursing process) as

1. opening and contracting: clarification of roles, expectations, anticipated outcomes, and contractual agreement;
2. assessment and diagnosis: perceptions of the issue, previous interventions, and current expectations;
3. setting of specific, realistic, and time-sensitive mutually agreed goals with recommended actions and anticipated outcomes;
4. implementation of the recommended actions, performed by the consultee;
5. evaluation of outcomes: assess for goal attainment and anticipated outcomes; and
6. closing, disconnecting, and documentation. (p. 158)

The CNS–Mental Health has the unique opportunity to facilitate formal and informal consultations of all types for both health care and non-health care staff, policy-makers, and administrators whose portfolios have an indirect effect on clients with mental health problems and illness. The CNS uses evidence to augment knowledge to influence policy development and changes at the local and political level, and contribute to mental wellness initiatives to improve client health outcomes. The areas of consultation include, but are not limited to, suicide prevention, crisis intervention and stabilization, safety and use of restraints, capacity building in communities, staff professional development, and promoting community wellness across the lifespan.

CASE STUDY

The Story of Jay

Jay, a 38-year-old male who lives in a Community Living residential home, was admitted to a psychiatric in-patient unit two weeks ago with symptoms of an acute psychotic episode.

Jay has a history of type 1 diabetes and has been non-adherent with self-care management. He has been on antidepressants for a year and has been treated for substance misuse in the past. Jay has a known history of hepatitis C and is visited weekly at his residential home by the home- and community-care nurse.

Management of psychotic episodes includes insight-oriented therapy and investigation, as well as laboratory testing. Jay will be returning to the residential home in two weeks. Case management and discharge planning processes commenced for follow-up and continuity of care. A plan for his return home was developed and implemented with the client, home and community care, addiction services, the diabetes day clinic coordinator, and the nurse practitioner at the hepatology clinic.

Collaboration is also a function of the CNS's indirect care practice. The CNS works collaboratively with members of the interprofessional team to meet the client's desired goals and is a part of the mental health team. Through case management, the CNS facilitates collaboration among health sectors and community agencies in advocating for care, services, and support to meet the client's identified biopsychosocial and cultural needs. The CNS also focuses on the client's strengths and holistic approaches in the collaborative relationship with the client, families, and mental health team. An integral component of the CNS's collaboration role is the coordination of care and services on a continuum for client safety (personal and environmental), and the promotion of mental wellness and recovery. Open communication with colleagues, other health sectors, and community agencies, and the ability to appreciate each team member's contribution, is essential in a collaborative relationship.

System Leadership

The CNS–Mental Health requires knowledge on addiction and the interrelationship between mental health, addiction, and chronic physical diseases. The evidence on mental health, mental illness, and addiction published by the Mental Health Commission of Canada (2012) strengthens the call for changes to and transformation of the current mental health system. The mental health system is a complex, open system with competing inputs and outputs that feed back into the environment. The system provides services and/or programs for clients across the lifespan, although the level of service or program varies from province to province. Programs and/or services are provided in an acute care unit, general psychiatric unit, assessment and short stay units, specialized units for clients with serious and persistent mental illness, forensic units, and community-based clinics/health centres with or without assertive and intensive community and mobile crisis teams.

The current emphasis and initiatives on mental health, mental illness, and mental health strategies provincially, nationally, and globally target mental health promotion and prevention, and the reduction of health inequities. The CNS, as a transformational leader and change agent, leads and influences changes within the system for continuous quality improvement, promoting mental wellness, and fostering recovery.

The CNS influences and leads change at the clinical, program, and system levels. Interpersonal and communication skills are central to motivate, inspire, and influence system changes. At the clinical level, the CNS facilitates collaboration with the interprofessional team across services and sectors in promoting teaching and learning for safe quality care and positive health outcomes. In addition, the CNS creates an environment for the professional growth of the health team through role modelling, mentoring, and team building.

At the program level, the CNS analyzes and synthesizes evidence and leads the development and implementation of clinical guidelines and policies for continuous quality improvement. Similar processes are used with the addition of program management skills to develop and implement programs and activities such as mental wellness, managing symptoms and behaviour, suicide prevention, and stress management.

At the system level, the CNS may conduct environmental scans and use other evaluation tools to evaluate gaps in the system that affect client and staff safety, present findings to senior management, and develop strategies to reduce risk and enhance quality management. **System leadership**, within a mental health setting, includes the promotion of a safe environment and maintaining a supportive and healthy work environment. The CNS intervenes by creating a safe space (physical and emotional) through open communication, shared power, activities that foster hope and peer support, and provision of required tools and resources, as well as therapeutic milieu, psycho-education, negotiation, and policy.

Advancing Nursing Practice

The CNS, as a member of the interprofessional mental health team, advances nursing practice through role modelling, mentoring, and coaching. The CNS demonstrates the importance of professional development through continuous learning, professionalism, ethical and moral conduct in keeping with nursing standards of practice and code of ethics, reflective practice, and professional and academic affiliations. The CNS uses knowledge and evidence to facilitate learning with clients and families, mentoring members of the interprofessional team, and as a preceptor for undergraduate and graduate students.

It is important to recognize different learning styles and teaching principles, and to be aware of and employ various techniques to accommodate learners' needs. The CNS as an educator assesses the learner's readiness and motivating factors, and is flexible in their approaches in engaging the client or staff member. Two key success factors include understanding the learner's readiness for change and applying adult learning principles when working with adults.

The CNS mentors staff members using formal or informal processes on an ongoing basis to acquire knowledge, skills, and competencies. Mentoring occurs in assessment and evaluation of anticipated outcomes, and the provision of treatment modalities and liaising with other health care disciplines internally or externally across the continuum of care.

Evaluation and Research

The CNS–Mental Health researches, retrieves, critically appraises, and synthesizes systematic reviews and other research literature relevant to mental health and addiction as part of their competencies. Evidence is integrated into clinical practice for assessments, interventions, developing strategies, quality management, and evaluation of positive health outcomes. Interventions include strategies the CNS uses in case management and building therapeutic relationships.

In addition, the CNS–Mental Health utilizes evidence from a variety of key data sources such as Statistics Canada's Community Health Survey, the Canadian Institute for Health Information (CIHI), best practice guidelines, the Centre for Addiction and Mental Health (CAMH), and the Mental Health Commission of Canada (MHCC) to shape interventions, outcome evaluation, policy revisions, and program redesign. It is essential that the CNS demonstrates competence to measure and evaluate health outcomes.

The CNS as a system leader uses research and evaluation to demonstrate cost analysis and cost containment related to safe quality care and positive health outcomes. The CNS also leads and/or participates in research at the organization level and/or an academic level. In the organization, the CNS engages and disseminates evidence as a knowledge translator to members of the interprofessional team through face-to-face presentation, journal club, video conference, and publication in organizational newsletters and nursing journals.

Conclusion

The focus of the CNS–Mental Health practice is creating a safe environment for the client and staff through the creation of therapeutic relationships and the promotion of positive mental health and recovery. Promoting positive mental health requires that the CNS appraise, synthesize, and apply evidence that informs practice utilizing a client-centred and a holistic strengths-based model of care, and develops and implements initiatives and strategies that would increase protective factors, reduce risk factors, and foster resilience.

The CNS–Mental Health demonstrates specialized knowledge, skills, and competence at the expert level as a role model, mentor, and a consultant to members of the interprofessional team for complex mental, physical, and addiction issues. The CNS–Mental Health also utilizes advanced and specialized knowledge and skills for problem solving, ethical dilemmas, and issues resolution.

The pillars of the CNS–Mental Health practice are the CNS core competencies, whereby quality management is interwoven through every aspect of care and service delivery. The CNS–Mental Health is required to demonstrate in-depth knowledge, skills, and competencies in pathophysiology, psychotherapeutic approaches, and psychopharmacology in addressing the stigma, system inefficiencies, and complex and persistent issues within a health care setting.

Finally, the CNS–Mental Health leads and influences change in the health care system that supports the client in achieving their goals and desired health outcomes through transformational leadership. The CNS promotes best practices, evidence-informed care, and client safety to advance the nursing profession by developing clinical guidelines, policies and protocols, and measurement tools for continuous quality improvement. As a transformational leader, the CNS develops and implements initiatives that align with the organization's strategic goals for positive health outcomes.

Critical Thinking Questions

1. Analyze and evaluate the impact of the role of the CNS–Mental Health in a health care setting. What are the linkages to a holistic model of care, client safety, advancing nursing care, and quality improvement?
2. A client living with mental illness and co-occurring addiction issues is admitted to a mental health unit. What theoretical framework would determine the practice of a CNS with this client? Why?
3. A mental health nurse is working with Jay, the client identified in the case study. Describe how you would implement the consultant role of the CNS.

References

Canadian Institute for Health Information (CIHI). (2009). *Improving the health of Canadians: Exploring positive mental health.* Ottawa, ON: CIHI. Retrieved from http://www.cihi.ca/cihi-ext-portal/pdf/internet/improving_health_canadians_en

Canadian Nurses Association (CNA). (2008). *Advanced nursing practice: A national framework.* Ottawa, ON: CNA. Retrieved from http://www.cna-aiic.ca/~/media/cna/page-content/pdf-en/anp_national_framework_e.pdf

CNA. (2014). *Pan-Canadian core competencies for the clinical nurse specialist.* Ottawa, ON: CNA. Retrieved from http://cna-aiic.ca/~/media/cna/files/en/clinical_nurse_specialists_convention_handout_e.pdf

Caplan, G. (1970). *The theory and practice of mental health consultation.* New York, NY: Basic Books.

Caplan, G., Caplan, R.B., & Erchul, W.P. (1995). A contemporary view of mental health consultation: Comments on "types of mental health consultation" by Gerald Caplan (1963). *Journal of Education and Psychological Consultation, 6*(1), 23–30. doi: 10.1207/s1532768xjepc0601_2

Centre for Addiction and Mental Health (CAMH). (2009). *Knowledge exchange: Social aetiology of mental illness.* Toronto, ON: CAMH. Retrieved from http://www.camh.ca/en/research/research_areas/knowledge_exchange_and_training/Pages/Social-Aetiology-of-Mental-Illness-Training-Program.aspx

Erchul, W.P., & American Board of Professional Psychology (ABPP). (2009). Gerald Caplan: A tribute to the originator of mental health consultation. *Journal of Educational and Psychological Consultation, 19*(2), 95–105. doi: 10.1080/10474410902888418

Fulton, J.S., Lyon. B.L., & Goudreau, K. (Eds.) (2014). *Foundations of clinical nurse specialist practice* (2nd ed.). New York, NY: Springer.

Government of Canada. (2006). *Out of the shadows at last: Transforming mental health, mental illness and addiction services in Canada*. Ottawa, ON: Parliament of Canada. Retrieved from http://www.parl.gc.ca/Content/SEN/Committee/391/soci/rep/rep02may06-e.htm

Hemingway, S., & Ely, V. (2009). Prescribing by mental health nurses: The UK perspective. *Perspectives in Psychiatric Care, 45*(1), 24–35. Retrieved from http://onlinelibrary.wiley.com/doi/10.1111/j.1744-6163.2009.00197.x/pdf

Keltner, N.L., Schwecke, L.H., & Bostrom, C.E. (1991). *Psychiatric nursing: A psychotherapeutic management approach* (1st ed.). St. Louis, MO: Mosby-Year Book.

Lim, K.L., Jacobs, P., & Dewa, C. (2008). *How much should we spend on mental health?* Institute of Health Economics/Alberta Health Services. Retrieved from http://www.ihe.ca/documents/Spending%20on%20Mental%20Health%20Final.pdf

Mangle, L. Phillips, P., Pitts, M., & Laver-Bradbury, C. (2014). Implementation of independent nurse prescribing in UK mental health settings: Focus on attention deficit/hyperactivity disorder. *Attention Deficit and Hyperactivity Disorders 6*(4), 269–279. Retrieved from http://link.springer.com/article/10.1007%2Fs12402-014-0138-x#page-1

Mental Health Commission of Canada (MHCC). (2009). *Toward recovery & well-being: A framework for a mental health strategy for Canada*. Calgary, Alberta: Mental Health Commission of Canada. Retrieved from http://www.mentalhealthcommission.ca/English/system/files/private/FNIM_Toward_Recovery_and_Well_Being_ENG_0.pdf

MHCC. (2012). *Changing directions changing lives: The mental health strategy for Canada*. Calgary, Alberta: Mental Health Commission of Canada. Retrieved from http://strategy.mentalhealthcommission.ca/pdf/strategy-images-en.pdf

National Association of Clinical Nurse Specialist (NACNS). (2010). *Clinical nurse specialist core competencies: Executive summary 2006–2008*. Philadelphia, PA: NACNS. Retrieved from http://www.nacns.org/docs/CNSCoreCompetenciesBroch.pdf

Smetanin, P., Stiff, D., Briante, C., Adair, C.E., Ahmad, S., & Khan, M. (2011). *The life and economic impact of major mental illnesses in Canada*. Ottawa, ON: Mental Health Commission of Canada. Retrieved from https://www.mentalhealthcommission.ca/English/system/files/private/document/MHCC_Report_Base_Case_FINAL_ENG_0.pdf

World Health Organization (WHO). (2004). *Promoting mental health: Concepts, emerging evidence, practice: Summary report*. Geneva, CH: WHO. Retrieved from http://www.who.int/mental_health/evidence/en/promoting_mhh.pdf

WHO (2015). *Mental health: Strengthening our response. Media Fact Sheet, No 220*. Geneva, CH: WHO. Retrieved from http://www.who.int/mediacentre/factsheets/fs220/en/

Chapter

12

The Clinical Nurse Specialist: Ambulatory Care

Jennifer Price

Jennifer Price is an APN, and has held both CNS and ACNP roles at the Women's College Hospital's Women's Cardiovascular Health Initiative in Toronto, Ontario.

KEY TERMS

ambulatory care
ambulatory care nursing
    (ACN)
chronic disease
    management
self-management
self-management
    support

OBJECTIVES

1. Define ambulatory care nursing (ACN).
2. Explore the rationale for ambulatory care.
3. Explore the role of the clinical nurse specialist (CNS) in ambulatory care.

Introduction

To understand the role of the advanced practice nurse (APN) in **ambulatory care**, we need to look to the roots of ambulatory care. This chapter will explore the shift from in-patient care to ambulatory care, and highlight the importance of the clinical nurse specialist (CNS) as a key provider in the ambulatory setting.

The Shift to Ambulatory Care

Shifting health care services to the community has been a long-standing political priority in Canada (Royal College of Nursing [RCN], 2014; van Soeren, Hurlock-Chorostecki, Pogue, & Sanders, 2008). With the population living longer, more people are living with comorbidities and requiring ongoing complex interventions, which they prefer to receive within their own community (Rich, Lipson, Libersky, & Parchman, 2012; Vlasses & Smeltzer,

2007). Moving care out of acute care facilities into the ambulatory setting not only delivers positive health outcomes, but also frees up hospital beds and resources to provide the most acute and specialized care to individuals with high acuity levels.

The shift to increasing ambulatory volumes occurred over time, but the early 1990s saw a definite movement of care from the hospital setting into the community. Several factors have contributed to the expansion of ambulatory care services. Financial policies during the late 1980s and early 1990s dictated the closing of acute care hospital beds, causing patients to be discharged to the community earlier (Canadian Institute for Health Information [CIHI], 2005; Hastings, 1986; Katz, Martens, Chateau, Bogdanovic, & Koseva, 2014). These patients had higher acuities and required more intensive care in the community. Fortunately, as fiscal caps for hospital care moved patients into the ambulatory care setting, advances in technology enabled more care and diagnostics to be delivered through minimally invasive or non-invasive procedures (Vlasses & Smeltzer, 2007). Pharmacotherapy evolved as a treatment easily managed in the ambulatory setting allowing, for example, the management of post-operative pain at home or the infusion of intravenous antibiotics (Nevius & D'Arcy, 2008). Improved technology has also allowed the management of care to become seamless and portable through use of electronic patient records (Vlasses & Smeltzer, 2007). The vast majority of health care in Canada occurs outside the hospital walls. This applies to both physician services and services provided by other health care practitioners, including nurses. While this seems obvious, as the Canadian health care system is widely acknowledged for having a strong focus on primary care, what is not as well understood is the increasing volume of specialty care including surgery, interventional procedures, and diagnostics delivered in the community (Katz et al., 2014). The Canadian Institute for Health Information (CIHI) reports on hospital stays and ambulatory care visits within the hospital sector. Ambulatory care in this context includes visits to the emergency department (ED), outpatient surgery, and visits to an ambulatory clinic. Between 1986 and 2002 the average in-patient admissions per day decreased 15.9%, while the number of visits to ambulatory care departments doubled in those years and is now over 50 million visits per year. These statistics demonstrate the transfer of care from in-patient settings to ambulatory care (CIHI, 2005). Further demonstration of care transfer is the emergence of ambulatory hospitals in the province of Ontario with several in Toronto, Ottawa, and Kingston.

Ambulatory Care Nursing

Mastal (2010) describes the ambulatory setting as historically belonging to physicians. The majority of outpatients were seen in physician offices and referred on for other specialties or different levels of service, such as hospitalization. In the past, numbers of registered nurses (RN) were few in the ambulatory setting as patients were primarily cared for by the physician. As health care has shifted to the ambulatory setting from the acute care sector the need for professional **ambulatory care nursing (ACN)** has exponentially increased with a resultant growth in numbers of professional nurses in an ambulatory setting. Over the last three decades these nurses have also grown in their ability to distinguish themselves as a specialty with a unique realm of practice, as evidenced by the two associations founded by professional ambulatory nurses (Mastal, 2010).

ACN has been recognized as a specialty in the United States (US) for several decades with their professional group, The American Academy of Ambulatory Care Nursing (AAACN), being founded in 1978 as an educational forum for administrators. Membership is now open to all nurses, as well as other health professionals who are interested in ambulatory care and telehealth nursing (AAACN, 2014).

The Canadian Association of Ambulatory Care (CAAC) was founded more recently, in 2012, to highlight the groundbreaking work in ambulatory care in Canada. The CAAC provides a forum for all professionals working in any area of ambulatory care to share their knowledge and skills through networking and education (CAAC, 2012).

Both organizations define ACN in similar ways, stating that these professionals care for individuals, families, groups, communities, and populations. The setting for ambulatory nursing is distinctively different from other nurses as they practice in the home, primary and specialty outpatient venues, and non-acute surgical and diagnostic outpatient settings in the community.

The patient flow in ambulatory care is vastly different from the hospital setting. ACN is characterized by RNs caring for high volumes of patients in a relatively short period of time (always less than 24 hours), dealing with issues that can be both unknown and unpredictable. Assessments are rapid and focused and the nurse/patient/family relationships are typically long term. Unlike the hospital, the ambulatory care nurse frequently works in isolation. While they may provide direct patient care the ACN is more likely to be an organizer or manager of care, directing patients in self-care or helping them make behavioural changes. The ambulatory care nurse addresses a patient's wellness, acute illness, chronic issues, and end-of-life requirements. These nurses are patient advocates, navigators, and coordinators of all health care (AAACN, 2011, 2014; CAAC, 2012). This type of working environment requires a strong clinical background, leadership skills, and autonomous critical thinking ability. Nurses work with fewer resources in the community setting, making it more difficult to get a second opinion from a nursing colleague. In addition, ambulatory care nurses interact with patients face to face and via telephone or Internet. Lack of direct contact with patients demands different assessment and communication skills, as the direct non-verbal sensory input of facial expressions and body language is lost.

With the increasing complexity of the care required, the AAACN recognizes the requirement for all levels of nursing in the ambulatory setting, including the APN roles of the nurse practitioner (NP), CNS, and nurse researcher (AAACN, 2014).

The Role of the APN in Ambulatory Care

Throughout the history of nursing, nurses have developed, refocused, and expanded their roles to meet patient and population requirements. The emergence of the APN, which includes both the CNS and the NP, is an excellent example of this. A more recent example is the emergence of the APN in the ambulatory setting. Specifically, there has been widespread adoption of the CNS in chronic disease management. With their advanced preparation and clinical expertise they are perfectly positioned to provide education, clinical care, guidance, and support to families and other providers.

At the heart of chronic disease management is self-management, a term used widely in the health care literature with no gold-standard definition (Barlow, Wright, Sheasby, Turner, & Hainsworth, 2002). Self-management includes the work individuals assume to live well with their ongoing medical conditions. This includes physical tasks, as well as role management and the confidence to carry out this work (Adams, Greiner, Corrigan, & Institute of Medicine (US), 2004).

Self-management support is critical to the development of self-management and emphasizes patients' central role in managing and being responsible for their health because the locus of responsibility rests with them. In addition, self-management support involves collaborative relationships with patients and their families and goes beyond the provision of education and support. Patients and providers work together to define problems/barriers, develop priorities, and set goals while the provider offers problem-solving support and strategies to build confidence. While self-management support can be provided by a variety of health care professionals, the APN in ambulatory care is ideally positioned to provide self-management support to their patients and families.

Self-management approaches have been shown to have positive impacts on the well-being of individuals with chronic illness (Barlow, Turner, & Wright, 2000; Warsi, Wang, LaValley, Avorn, & Solomon, 2004). In addition, Lorig's work suggests improved health behaviour, health status, and decreased health care utilization in patients participating in a chronic disease self-management program (CDSMP) (Lorig & Visser, 1994; Lorig & Holman, 2003; Lorig, Ritter, Laurent, & Fries, 2004; Lorig, Ritter, Laurent, & Plant, 2008).

Several studies have specifically examined the role of the APN in ambulatory care, as they provide self-management support or assist patients' transition to the home setting. A randomized, controlled trial in patients with rheumatoid arthritis compared a CNS ambulatory intervention with in-patient care and a multidisciplinary day care team. No significant differences were found between the groups during the two-year follow-up except visits to the CNS were more frequent and home help was less frequent. The authors concluded that the CNS intervention was effective in this patient population, and a useful alternative to other multidisciplinary strategies in the setting of the complex care requirements of individuals with rheumatoid arthritis (Tijhuis, Zwinderman, Hazes, Breedveld, & Vlieland, 2003).

Brooten et al. (2001) examined prenatal, infant, and maternal outcomes over a one year period post-delivery where half the prenatal care was delivered in the home by CNSs. Results showed that the group cared for in the home by the CNS had fewer fetal/infant deaths, fewer preterm infants, and fewer re-hospitalizations. The researchers also found that the CNS prenatal homecare saved hospital days, which translated to a cost savings of $2.5 million dollars.

Brooten, Yougblut, Deatrik, Naylor, and York (2003) published further work that examined five clinical trials of APN interventions with the intent to describe the patient problems and time and type of intervention. All the trials were examining APN transitional care, that is, comprehensive discharge planning and home follow-up. Groups with greater mean APN time and contacts per patient had better health outcomes and greater health care cost savings. Of all the APN interventions, surveillance was the most predominant in all patient populations, accounting for over 50% of the 150,131 interventions. Health teaching, guidance, and counselling was the second-most frequent category of APN intervention in four of the five trials. Treatments and procedures accounted for less than 1% of the interventions across all groups. The final category of interventions, case management, accounted for 12 to 25% of the interventions, depending on the trial. The authors conclude that to provide this type of transitional care APNs had to have advanced skills in assessment, collaboration, teaching, counselling, communications, and health behaviour management. These trials support the value of the APN role in ambulatory care, demonstrating improved health care outcomes in the setting of improved cost savings.

CASE STUDY

The Story of Rebecca

Rebecca is an 81-year-old woman with a primary diagnosis of atrial fibrillation whose cardiologist referred to cardiac rehabilitation (CR). Six weeks into the program the clinical nurse specialist (CNS) was asked to see Rebecca regarding her swollen legs and fatigue.

A review of Rebecca's history revealed that she had been diagnosed with atrial fibrillation one year ago while being investigated for sleep apnea. She does not describe any chest pain or discomfort, but finds herself increasingly fatigued and reports a reduction in physical activity. Her previous medical history includes osteoarthritis in her right hip and left knee, sleep apnea treated with CPAP, and self-declared feelings of depression for which she has never sought help.

Today, Rebecca is alert and oriented but appears short of breath at rest. She complains that her legs are feeling tight and uncomfortable. Initial vital signs are BP right arm sitting 125/80, AR 110, RR16; weight 62.2 kg, height 1.55 m, BMI 26, and waist circumference 86 cm. On physical examination, her air entry is equal to the bases and clear. Rebecca has normal heart sounds with no murmurs, but JVP is elevated, liver is palpable, and has 3+ pitting edema to above the knees. She is anxious and appears scared. A Beck Depression Inventory screening reveals a score of 20, and it is noted that Rebecca self-scores as pessimistic. A review of her medications reveals she is not taking any prescription medications, preferring supplements as prescribed by her naturopathic doctor.

An initial problem list for Rebecca included tachycardia, hepatomegaly, anxiousness/frightfulness, and depression. In the past, this is a patient who would have been sent to an emergency department (ED) for diagnosis and workup. Today, in ambulatory care, these patients with complex medical and psychosocial issues are routinely assessed and treated. Rebecca is referred to the medical day unit (MDU) for physician assessment and diagnostic testing. Referrals to social work, pharmacy, and the dietitian are also made.

The CNS focuses on assisting Rebecca both to understand and come to terms with her diagnosis of atrial fibrillation. The CNS often has to have difficult conversations with patients and families. This includes open discussions concerning medications to control her heart rate and prevent stroke, and provides an opportunity to assist the front-line staff in understanding why patients choose not to take medications and which strategies may or may not be successful in promoting medication adherence. Rebecca will benefit from ongoing follow-up to assist with self-management support. Learning how to recognize symptoms is an important surveillance skill patients with chronic diseases require to help them manage their chronic condition. Developing healthy behaviours around exercise and nutrition will also be part of the long-term plan for Rebecca.

In the above case study, the CNS utilizes many of the advanced skills described by Brooten et al. (2003). Assessment must be timely and focused, as the individual is usually scheduled for a short appointment. Collaborating with the interprofessional health care team was critical to managing Rebecca's acute exacerbation in the outpatient setting, as well as the diagnosis and treatment of medical issues. In Rebecca's story, health education and counselling were key to helping her understand her condition and work towards caring for herself to ensure the best quality of life.

While the CNS in ambulatory care can provide excellent self-management support, an important component of the role is teaching and coaching nursing colleagues. This part of the practice is an excellent way to disseminate evidence-based practice. CNSs often act as role models for other nursing staff, as well as conducting formal and informal education sessions.

Conclusion

In Canada, health care is shifting from in-patient acute care to a variety of outpatient ambulatory and community care centres. This movement and shifting of resources has been a political priority in Canada since the 1980s.

This shift has been enabled by advancements in minimally invasive surgery, improved diagnostics, pharmaceutical therapies, and technology enhancing the transfer of patient information. These advancements in medical and health technology have also enabled the population to live longer. As a result, many more individuals are living longer with multiple complex comorbidities requiring ongoing complex care interventions.

The increasing complexity of patients being cared for in the ambulatory setting has resulted in the increased need for professional nursing care. These nurses have been able to articulate a unique realm of practice, and, indeed, have founded two national ambulatory care organizations.

The role of the APN (including the CNS role in ambulatory care) advances with ongoing research evidence to support improved health outcomes and health care cost savings in the setting up of APN interventions. As health care continues to move out of the hospital, opportunities for the APN in ambulatory care will grow as they provide their expert skills in assessment, education, counselling, and research within this diverse and multi-faceted setting.

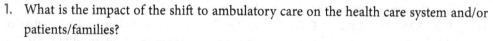

Critical Thinking Questions

1. What is the impact of the shift to ambulatory care on the health care system and/or patients/families?
2. What is the impact of the APN role in ambulatory care now, and what might you anticipate in the future?

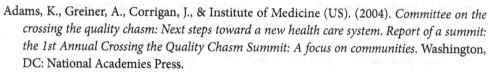

References

Adams, K., Greiner, A., Corrigan, J., & Institute of Medicine (US). (2004). *Committee on the crossing the quality chasm: Next steps toward a new health care system. Report of a summit: the 1st Annual Crossing the Quality Chasm Summit: A focus on communities*. Washington, DC: National Academies Press.

American Academy of Ambulatory Care Nursing (AAACN). (2011). American Academy of Ambulatory Care Nurisng position statement: The role of the registered nurse in ambulatory care. *Nursing Economics, 29*(2), 96.

AAACN. (2014). About American Academy of Ambulatory Care Nursing. Pitman, NJ: AAACN. Retrieved from https://aaacn.org

Barlow, J., Wright, C., Sheasby, J., Turner, A., & Hainsworth, J. (2002). Self management approaches for people with chronic conditions: A review. *Patient Education and Counseling, 48*(2), 177–187.

Barlow, J.H., Turner, A.P., & Wright, C.C. (2000). A randomized controlled study of the Arthritis Self-Management Programme in the UK. *Health Education Research, 15*(6), 665–680.

Brooten, D., Youngblut, J.M., Brown, L., Finkler, S.A., Neff, D.F., & Madigan, E. (2001). A randomized trial of nurse specialist home care for women with high-risk pregnancies: Outcomes and costs. *American Journal of Managed Care, 7*(8), 793–803.

Brooten, D., Youngblut, J.M., Deatrick, J., Naylor, M., & York, R. (2003). Patient problems, advanced practice nurse (APN) interventions, time and contacts among five patient groups. *Journal of Nursing Scholarship, 35*(1), 73–79.

Canadian Association of Ambulatory Care (CAAC). (2012). *About CAAC*. Toronto, ON: CAAC. Retrieved from http://www.canadianambulatorycare.com/about-us.html

Canadian Institute for Health Information (CIHI). (2005). *Hospital trends in Canada: Results of a project to create a historical series of statistical and financial data for Canadian hospitals over twenty-seven years*. Ottawa, ON: CIHI.

Hastings, J.E. (1986). Organized ambulatory care in Canada: Health service organizations and community health centers. *Journal of Public Health Policy, 7*(2), 239–247.

Katz, A., Martens, P., Chateau, D., Bogdanovic, B., & Koseva, I. (2014). Do primary care physicians coordinate ambulatory care for chronic disease patients in Canada? *BMC Family Practice, 15*, 148. doi: 10.1186/1471-2296-15-148

Lorig, K., & Visser, A. (1994). Arthritis patient education standards: A model for the future. *Patient Education and Counseling, 24*(1), 3–7.

Lorig, K.R., & Holman, H. (2003). Self-management education: History, definition, outcomes, and mechanisms. *Annals of Behavioral Medicine, 26*(1), 1–7.

Lorig, K.R., Ritter, P.L., Laurent, D.D., & Fries, J.F. (2004). Long-term randomised controlled trials of tailored-print and small-group arthritis self-management interventions. *Medical Care, 42*(4), 346–354.

Lorig, K.R., Ritter, P.L., Laurent, D.D., & Plant, K. (2008). The internet-based arthritis self-management program: A one-year randomized trial for patients with arthritis or fibromyalgia. *Arthritis and Rheumatism, 59*(7), 1009–1017. doi: 10.1002/art.23817

Mastal, M.F. (2010). Ambulatory care nursing: Growth as a professional specialty. *Nursing Economics, 28*(4), 267–269.

Nevius, K.S., & D'Arcy, Y. (2008). Decrease recovery time with proper pain management. *Nursing Management, 39*(11), 26–32. doi:10.1097/01.NUMA.0000340815.21271.a2

Rich, E., Lipson, D., Libersky, J., & Parchman, M. (2012). *Coordinating care for adults with complex care needs in the patient-centered medical home: Challenges and solutions. White paper*. Rockville, MD: Agency for Healthcare Research and Quality.

Royal College of Nursing (RCN). (2014). *Moving care to the community: An international perspective*. London, UK: RCN Retrieved from http://www.rcn.org.uk/__data/assets/pdf_file/0006/523068/12.13_Moving_care_to_the_community_an_international_perspective.pdf

Tijhuis, G.J., Zwinderman, A.H., Hazes, J.M., Breedveld, F.C., & Vlieland, P.M. (2003). Two-year follow-up of a randomized controlled trial of a clinical nurse specialist intervention, inpatient, and day patient team care in rheumatoid arthritis. *Journal of Advanced Nursing, 41*(1), 34–43.

van Soeren, M., Hurlock-Chorostecki, C., Pogue, P., & Sanders, J. (2008). Primary healthcare renewal in Canada: A glass half empty? *Healthcare Papers, 8*(2), 39–44.

Vlasses, F.R., & Smeltzer, C.H. (2007). Toward a new future for healthcare and nursing practice. *Journal of Nursing Adminstration, 37*(9), 375–380. doi:10.1097/01.NNA.0000285140.19000.f5

Warsi, A., Wang, P.S., LaValley, M.P., Avorn, J., & Solomon, D.H. (2004). Self-management education programs in chronic disease: A systematic review and methodological critique of the literature. *Archives of Internal Medicine, 164*(15), 1641–1649.

Chapter

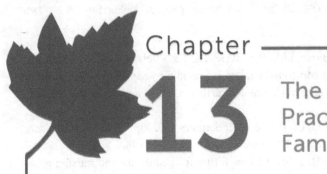

13 The Nurse Practitioner: Family/All Ages

Jane MacDonald and Laura Johnson

Jane MacDonald has worked as an NP since 2001. She is currently employed at a primary care clinic in Winnipeg, with the Winnipeg Regional Health Authority. Jane's urban-based practice includes patients across the age spectrum, with an emphasis on the elderly and chronic disease management. While the majority of her work involves clinical care of patients, she is also engaged in clinic-based quality improvement projects and preceptoring of NP students.

Laura Johnson is a Professor in the BScN Program at Vancouver Island University in Victoria, British Columbia. Prior to this new role, Laura was an NP–Adult in the adult emergency department of Winnipeg's Health Sciences Centre and was an Instructor in the College of Nursing at the University of Manitoba in Winnipeg, Manitoba, where she taught in the NP Program. Laura is the past president of the Nurse Practitioner Association of Manitoba (NPAM).

KEY TERMS

advanced practice
  nursing (APN)
core competencies
direct clinical care
primary health care
  nurse practitioner
  (PHCNP)

OBJECTIVES

1. Understand the role of the primary health care nurse practitioner (PHCNP).
2. Synthesize key competencies fundamental to the NP role.
3. Evaluate critical trends in the health care system and their implications for the PHCNP.
4. Explore the barriers and facilitators to PHCNP practice.
5. Engage in dialogue regarding the role of the PHCNP in the primary health care setting.

Introduction

The fastest growing APN role in Canada is the **primary health care nurse practitioner (PHCNP)** (Donald et al., 2010). The role is also known as Family/All Ages, reflecting the population-based focus of the Canadian Nurse Practitioner Examination (CNPE). To be consistent with current nomenclature from the Canadian APN literature, the chapter will refer to the role as PHCNP.

PHCNPs apply advanced nursing and medical theory acquired at the graduate level in the provision of clinical care for all age groups and a wide variety of medical conditions. While the foundation of the PHCNP role is **direct clinical care**, the non-clinical domains of consultation, collaboration, reflective practice, research, and leadership also define the role. Nurse practitioner (NP) core competencies developed by the Canadian Nurses Association (CNA) (2010a) provide guidance and structure for PHCNPs in the operationalization of the role. Federal and provincial governments, regulatory bodies, and grassroots initiatives also contribute to role actualization.

Primary Health Care Nurse Practitioner Education

The educational preparation of the PHCNP in Canada has fluctuated from post-baccalaureate diploma to a graduate degree (Kaasalainen et al., 2010). Collectively, nursing organizations recommended that the educational standard for all NPs be at the graduate level (Pulcini, Jelic, Gul, & Loke, 2010). Substantial progress toward reaching this goal in Canada has materialized over the last 15 years.

The vast majority of NP educational programs in Canada focus on primary health care, and impart the medical knowledge necessary to competently treat acute episodic illnesses and chronic medical conditions, along with the critical analysis necessary for competency. Further, skills in comprehensive health assessment, diagnostic reasoning, and differential diagnoses are critical to NP educational preparation (Mick & Ackerman, 2000). The development of role autonomy is a hallmark of NP curricula related to diagnostic reasoning and decision-making (Mick & Ackerman, 2000), where the legal authority to order diagnostic tests, treatments, and prescribe medication is within the NP scope of practice (Ackerman, Norsen, Martin, Wiedrich, & Kitzman, 1996; CNA, 2010a; Mick & Ackerman, 2000). Once advanced education has been completed, graduate NPs must write a credentialing examination demonstrating NP competencies in order to gain licensure for the jurisdiction in which they are seeking employment. In most jurisdictions, graduates write the Canadian Nurse Practitioner Exam (CNPE), which is administered by the provincial or territorial regulatory body.

The Canadian Nurse Practitioner Initiative's (CNPI) (2006a) appraisal of the curricula of NP programs across Canada identified shared aims in the types of courses that were included, such as health assessment, pathophysiology, and management of health and disease across the lifespan, including prescribing. Some stakeholders in Canada have appealed for national curriculum standards and a fixed core curriculum for NP programs (Canadian Association of Schools of Nursing [CASN], 2012).

The education of NPs consists of academic as well as extensive clinical experiences. Although NP education readies students for the clinical practice role, there is a lack of standardization in the number of clinical placement hours required, and in the qualifications clinical preceptors should possess (CASN, 2012). Clinical hours provide the opportunity to put into practice the knowledge acquired in the classroom setting. Preceptors are central to clinical education by assisting the student to bridge the gap between clinical practice and theory. Mentoring through preceptorship prepares the NP graduate student to autonomously and independently provide care for conditions within the scope of practice of the NP as a novice. PHCNP clinical practice synthesizes a number of competencies and standards of practice that are acquired through the NP education program and reinforced through clinical practice. The novice PHCNP practice may look vastly different from the practice of a more experienced NP, yet the core standards and competencies are the same (CASN, 2011). The combination of graduate education and direct comprehensive care provides the depth and breadth for NP students to develop competencies of **advanced practice nursing (APN)** for health promotion, treatment, and management of health conditions.

Primary Health Care Nurse Practitioner Role Description

The APN role, such as the NP, is delineated from basic nursing roles (Bryant-Lukosius, DiCenso, Browne, & Pinelli, 2004; Gardner, Hase, Gardner, Dunn, & Carryer, 2007; Ruel & Motyka, 2009) and is defined by educational preparation, direct clinical practice, and in-depth nursing knowledge and expertise allowing one to meet the needs of individuals, families, groups, and/ or populations (CNA, 2008). NPs are advanced practice nurses (DiCenso et al., 2010) and NP competencies are outlined as specific knowledge, skills, and personal attributes required for safe and ethical practice (CNA, 2010a). Nursing practice competencies are essential for NP education and the development of work roles. Role competencies are a means to define work (CNA, 2010a) and commonly confidence is the most frequently mentioned characteristic with respect to facilitating effective work (Jones, 2005). The CNA competencies have applicability across practice settings and are integral to the safe and ethical practice of NPs (CNPI, 2006b; Pohl et al., 2009). Not only do they provide the basis for education programs and guide the regulation and registration of nurse practitioners, they help guide novice and experienced NPs alike in actualizing direct clinical practice and other aspects of the NP role. The *Canadian Nurse Practitioner Core Competency Framework* outlines the following NP competencies:

- professional role, responsibility, and accountability
- health assessment and diagnosis

- therapeutic management
- health promotion and prevention of illness and injury (CNA, 2010a, pp. 8–13)

These core competencies for NPs provide the basis for educational programs and NP registration, and serve to guide the NP in the work setting (CNA, 2010a).

A national definition for PHCNP does not exist but it "is generally accepted that PHCNPs provide services to individuals and families across the lifespan and work in a variety of community-based settings" (Donald et al., 2010, p. 93). PHCNPs focus on health promotion, preventative care, diagnosis, treatment, and management of common acute and chronic conditions through the utilization of evidence-based nursing and medicine.

The introduction of the PHCNP role is linked to countrywide health reform efforts to improve the accessibility and quality of primary health care (Donald et al., 2010). Major health care reform initiatives in the 1990s identified the potential impact nursing and other health care professionals could have on patient care, which led to the reframing of primary health care in Canada. Federal and provincial initiatives aimed to enhance health promotion, support equitable access to service, and increase quality of care. This allowed for the re-introduction of the PHCNP role that was lost in the 1980s. Legislation, regulations, remuneration, and education strategies were developed to aide in role implementation (Donald et al., 2010).

Clinical Practice: The Foundation of Primary Health Care Nurse Practitioner Practice

As direct care providers, NPs synthesize research, education, clinical expertise, leadership, and consultation to provide comprehensive health care. A unique aspect of the work of NPs is the provision of direct patient care in a primary care setting within an advanced scope of practice (title and scope of practice are protected by legislation). The comprehensive activities provided by the NP serve to improve quality of care and facilitate the patients' optimal progression through the health care system.

The PHCNP role allows for the provision of care to individuals across the lifespan in the management of acute episodic illnesses and chronic conditions. The foundation of NP practice is "direct clinical practice ... which unfolds around the premise that individuals seek care for a broad range of health care concerns over time and across the lifespan" (Pohl & Kao, 2014, p. 403). Direct clinical care by a PHCNP requires the critical application of health assessment followed by diagnosis and therapeutic management skills for patients pursuing care. As an autonomous health professional with a graduate education, the PHCNP builds on the registered nurse (RN) foundation of health promotion, illness prevention, and health management by integrating advanced nursing and medical theory in providing comprehensive health services (CNA, 2010a). PHCNPs work collaboratively with patients and other health care professionals to provide care to diverse populations in a variety of settings (CNA, 2010a).

Although there is variation between provincial/territorial jurisdictions, the legislated authority allows for NPs to autonomously order and interpret diagnostic tests, perform minor surgical procedures, and prescribe medications (CNA, 2010a). PHCNPs are accountable to patients regarding their care in terms of clinical findings, diagnoses, and management plans including testing, referrals, pharmaceutical management, and rehabilitation (CNA, 2010a).

PHCNPs work in a variety of settings: government-funded community clinics, private clinics, family health networks, emergency rooms, and outpatient clinics attached to hospitals (DiCenso et al., 2007). The NP role has also been utilized for innovative approaches to health care provision. One such example is Manitoba, where government-created QuickCare clinics operate on the strengths of the NP role: autonomous provision of care for those with acute episodic needs (Dinh, 2012a). Other innovative approaches are also being trialed with such approaches as mobile clinic buses that travel through certain communities on a set rotation. Mobile buses have been implemented in a variety of communities across Canada (Dinh, 2012a) and serve to break down a barrier to health care access and offer a unique and profound opportunity to improve health and expand health care.

The majority of PHCNPs work in community clinics, which is possible through a variety of funding models. The structure, function, governance, and funding vary regionally across Canada but can be broadly categorized into four models: physician-led practices, NP-led practices, community-led practices, and integrated primary care networks (Dinh, 2012a). Community-led clinics (known as community health centres in BC, Manitoba, and Nova Scotia, and family care clinics in Alberta) are the most common setting in which PHCNPs are employed and have a mandate to serve the needs of the community (Dinh, 2012a). They feature multidisciplinary health care teams, in which PHCNPs have patients rostered to them either directly or through a collaborating physician. Physician-led clinics may incorporate a variety of health care disciplines within their structure, of which the PHCNP role may be one. NP-led clinics are relatively new on the primary health care landscape, with models operating in Ontario, Manitoba, and Saskatchewan (Dinh, 2012a). An example of an NP-led clinic is featured in Box 13.1.

BOX 13.1

An Example of an NP-Led Clinic: The Lakehead NPLC

The Lakehead NP-led clinic (NPLC) was first opened in November 2010 and serves the city of Thunder Bay, Ontario, and surrounding area. It provides primary health care to 3,200 patients, with a nurse practitioner (NP) to patient ratio of 1:800. The interprofessional (IP) team includes four NPs, one registered nurse (RN), one registered practical nurse (RPN), one social worker, one registered dietitian (0.8 full-time equivalent), and one pharmacist (0.2 full-time equivalent).

The NPs provide health promotion, disease and injury prevention, treatment, rehabilitation, and other support services. The NPLC's collaborating physician has medical directives in place for the NPs for some controlled acts and is a source for consultation on complex cases. The physician comes to the clinic on a bi-weekly basis to see patients, and a collaborating psychiatrist comes once per month.

The roles of the dietitian, social worker, and pharmacist in the NPLC are similar to other IP collaboration (IPC) team models. The dietitian provides nutrition education to individuals and groups for health promotion and management of chronic diseases. The social worker not only provides counselling support to clinic patients, addressing issues such as depression, anxiety, grief, and chronic pain, but also makes referrals to appropriate community services, helps patients navigate systems, and completes paperwork required to access social supports. The pharmacist conducts individual patient assessments to identify, prevent, and resolve medication-related problems and reviews medical histories, identifies problems, and develops and monitors care plans that are then communicated to the patient and the interprofessional team.

Depending on the type of clinic, new patients may be attached to a PHCNP through a screening process tailored to each clinic's needs. The first point of contact for a patient must be a person who is knowledgeable of both the NP and physician role in order to appropriately match that individual to a provider depending on a patient's medical needs and the strengths, experience, and scope of practice of the NP and physician. An individual not familiar with the NP role may require education about the PHCNP.

Within the community clinic setting, patients seeking care of a PHCNP are usually looking for a regular health care provider whom they can access as necessary for identified health concerns across the lifespan. This could be a parent seeking a provider for a new infant, a teenager no longer needing care under a pediatrician, a patient whose previous provider has retired or moved, a woman requiring prenatal care, or someone who is unhappy with their current provider. There is an identified shortage of providers across Canada, and the integration of the PHCNP into the health care system by a variety of funding mechanisms allows for these types of individuals to become patients of a PHCNP (CNA, 2010b).

For PHCNPs in most community settings, variety and complexity are routine (as is the case for most health care professionals). While the basic structure of the day may be standardized, the patients booked into that day provide the challenge, excitement, and reward of being an NP. A mix of acute episodic, health maintenance, and chronic presentations constitute most days. The ratio varies depending on the day, the community, urban versus rural settings, and community demographics. The ages of the patients booked on a day-to-day basis may range from predominantly elderly/very elderly to an equal mix of young and old to predominantly young. Typically, in NP-led clinics, an NP will have their own practice roster within the clinic, but most clinics work in a team environment therefore supporting each other. This team approach may be actualized by the need for the PHCNP to see other providers' patients for such reasons as medical leave or vacation coverage. A large percentage of the PHCNP's days are spent in clinical practice with a practice roster ranging between 500 to1000 individuals (Dinh, 2012a). There is a paucity of literature regarding NP panel sizes, but what does exist indicates rosters ranging from 330 up to 1000 patients per NP (Dinh, 2012a).

Characteristics of a PHCNP interaction include awareness of scope of practice and operating appropriately within legislation, regulations, and standards. It also requires the integration of applicable cultural elements, awareness of determinants of health while carrying out either a regional exam/history or comprehensive well-person exam. The well-person history and examination for a teenager will look very different than that for an elderly person, and the NP must integrate the developmental and life stages into overall management (CNA, 2010a). PHCNPs must also be able to quickly adapt to change and apply critical thinking to verbal and non-verbal cues of a presentation.

Patient Relationship

The privilege of the PHCNP role is the development of a relationship with a patient as it allows for a deeper, richer understanding of the patient and fosters mutual trust and respect. PHCNP patient visits may be longer than those of their physician counterparts (Venning, Durie, Roland, Roberts, & Leese, 2000) thereby potentially addressing more than one health concern in a visit. Patient satisfaction with NPs is often related to the time element (William & Jones, 2006), which allows for relationship building to occur. The evolution between a patient and PHCNP is an inherent part of the role with mutual trust and respect enhancing relationship development (Pohl & Kao, 2014). A longitudinal study examining NP and patient interactions validated the importance of patient-centred care in the advanced nursing practice (ANP) of PHCNPs. Patient-centred care and the element of time allowed for more concerns identified by either the patient or the PHCNP to be negotiated and managed. The art of embracing and managing issues ultimately resulted in achievement of goals for the patient. There is value to PHCNPs holding on to their nursing roots as a foundation for their approach to patient care while at the same time blending the medical model into practice style (de Leon-Demare, MacDonald, Gregory, Katz, & Halas, 2015).

An understanding of the complexities of a person's personal life, appreciating social, lifestyle, and functional challenges, can allow for a more comprehensive and personalized health care management plan. It is often the long-standing nature of the NP/patient relationship that creates that understanding (Pohl & Kao, 2014).

Commonly Seen Conditions

A typical clinic day will involve a variety of presentations, ranging from acute episodic presentations such as respiratory or genitourinary infections to the management of chronic medical conditions such as diabetes or hypertension. Chronic disease management is a priority and requires an approach that is multi-faceted and interdisciplinary. All presentations require the PHCNP to perform a focused health assessment using assessment tools and techniques based on the individual's needs and relevance to stage of life (CNA, 2010a). Competent NPs will identify limits of their scope of practice. Maturation in the role leads to role evolution and increasing comfort with complexity of care management.

Patient Populations Served

Patient populations vary depending on the community and demographics. Age, gender, and ethnicity are all relevant denominators in providing care and shape the vision of a primary care clinic. Pediatrics may comprise a large percentage of some PHCNPs' practices whereas in other communities the practice may be largely built around a geriatric population. Cultural awareness and sensitivity is also integrated within the PHCNP role and may be more present in some clinic populations than others. In this increasingly global world, the ease of travel requires the NP to be informed of global health and political concerns as well.

Primary and Secondary Prevention

Health promotion and illness/injury prevention is a hallmark of the NP role as it incorporates foundational pieces of undergraduate nursing education with the medical aspect acquired in graduate education. The PHCNP often will incorporate features of both primary and secondary prevention into clinic visits as applicable. This happens more so with a patient's annual physical, which provides the opportunity to touch on well-person topics not normally covered during episodic visits or routine chronic condition visits. The integration of medical knowledge allows for primary and secondary prevention to be tailored by the PHCNP for each individual.

Depending on the type of clinic, PHCNPs may collaborate with the primary care nurses (PCN) in the clinic for health promotion and injury/illness prevention strategies. A strength of primary care clinics is their interdisciplinary nature, which allows other health care professionals such as PCNs to utilize their scope of practice to its fullest by undertaking the primary and secondary prevention aspects of clinical care.

The PHCNP educates patients about primary prevention by counselling about the prevention of the onset of specific diseases via risk reduction. The PHCNP may help a patient alter behaviours that potentially lead to disease, such as smoking cessation or by reducing exposure to a disease through vaccination (Donovan, n.d.). Secondary prevention such as mammography, cervical cytology, and fecal occult blood testing are procedures that detect and treat pre-clinical pathological changes (thereby controlling disease progression) and are essential to a PHCNP's practice. Awareness of changes to primary and secondary prevention recommendations require the PHCNP to keep current on evidence-based literature and recommendations.

Chronic Disease Management

Chronic disease management is another core element of the PHCNP role. Once a patient has developed a chronic disease such as diabetes or hypertension, the PHCNP can lessen the impact of the disease on the patient's function and quality of life through a multi-dimensional approach to care incorporating all the elements of APN. The overall coordination of care is paramount and can be complex for some chronic disease presentations; PCNs, social workers, dietitians, and specialists may all be involved to some degree with chronic disease management and the PHCNP is often the key coordinator.

Collaboration

Collaboration between the NP, the patient and their family, and the community is essential to PHCNP practice. Nurse practitioners must also establish collaborative relationships with all members of the health care team. As the member of the team that provides continuity and stability in the care and management of patients over the long term, PHCNPs often emerge as leaders in primary care teams in health care settings.

Within primary care clinics, foundational staff usually includes support staff, nurses, NPs, physicians, and a clinic manager. Support staff are the first point of contact for the public and require a detailed understanding of roles and responsibilities of all providers, as well as an understanding of clinic process. Other health care professionals associated with a primary clinic will vary depending on community needs and system availability. Mental health specialists (counsellors and/or psychiatrists) are often a part of the primary care team, as is dietitian support. Occupational therapy, physiotherapy, pharmacy, midwifery, social work, and perhaps specialty medicine may be accessible in some form as well. PHCNPs collaborate with a variety of health care professionals within and outside of clinics depending on the community setting and its needs, for example with local church groups or homeless shelters.

Within clinical practice, collaboration may occur multiple times throughout the day. The PHCNP must recognize and balance the needs and expectations of the patient with the boundaries of the system both within the clinic and the larger health care system as a whole. Collaboration between other health care professionals occurs depending on the presentation. Effective collaboration is dependent on team composition, personalities, and requires effort (Pohl & Kao, 2014). Physician collaboration may be formal or informal and is present on some days more than others for a PHCNP. The autonomous nature of the PHCNP's scope of practice does not require physician collaboration to occur at regular intervals, but more so when the PHCNP recognizes a condition or presentation is beyond their scope of practice.

A good portion of the PHCNP's clinical encounters may involve collaboration with the PCNs in the clinic. The PCN role is relatively new within the health care team for the same reasons as the NP role (as cited earlier), and is continually being broadened and reinvented as experience and opportunity allows. Maximizing the PCN's scope of practice creates opportunities for the PCN and PHCNP to work in tandem in the provision of patient care, specifically beneficial for primary prevention and with chronic disease presentations.

Formal interprofessional collaboration may occur in the form of daily "team huddles" or weekly team meetings, or with ad hoc meetings involving outside agencies to discuss complex case management. This may involve the team directly caring for the patient, or may be an opportunity for other health professionals to hear the challenges with a patient's condition and provide input based on their professional background and expertise.

Informal collaboration is more often the reality of primary care and patient management for the PHCNP: PHCNP to PCN, PHCNP to physician or support staff, or vice versa. Informal collaboration is necessary to expedite patient management inherent in the day-to-day interaction. It may occur as an informal hallway huddle between an NP, PCN, and physician, or some mix thereof. These consults usually involve a patient currently in the clinic who requires change management.

A cornerstone feature of NP practice is collaboration, and it is embedded into the core competencies (CNA, 2010a). Given the nature of funding of NP roles, collaboration with other health care professionals is essential. It allows for more comprehensive health care for the patient and results in high-quality, cost-effective outcomes (Cowan et al., 2006; Pohl & Kao, 2014).

Consultation

Consultation or referral to other health care professionals in the primary care clinic such as a referral to the PCN, counsellor, or dietitian may be indicated in circumstances where more comprehensive, interdisciplinary care is required. Consultation may also occur to the larger system outside the clinic. A PHCNP requests consultation via the referral mechanism for those situations they identify as outside their scope of practice in order to optimize patient care. The PHCNP's comfort with consultation enhances patient care and provides for more comprehensive care (CNA, 2010a). Examples of how consultation is actualized by the PHCNP include a referral for surgical consult for cholelithiasis; to gynecology for uterine fibroid complications; or to psychiatry for mental health assessment, diagnosis, and management suggestions.

There are circumstances when another of the health care providers may consult the PHCNP within the clinic. The physician may seek the PHCNP's opinion for example, regarding reproductive health or contraceptive management. There may be some role evolution occurring, whereby as the NP role becomes further integrated and embedded within the health care system, physician understanding and acceptance continues to grow, and respect for the role enhances the collaborative relationship.

CASE STUDY

The Story of Ayana

Ayana is a 52-year-old Somalian woman who has been in Canada for two years. She is relatively new to the clinic and to the PHCNP, Lori. She is accompanied by her daughter Fatmata who translates for Ayana, even though Fatmata's command of English is poor.

Through Fatmata's translation, Lori is able to glean the following history: as a recent immigrant to Canada, Ayana lives with her two daughters and infant granddaughter in an apartment complex in the downtown area. She has been widowed for 10 years; her husband was killed due to political unrest in Somalia. Ayana and her children spent the previous eight years in a refugee camp prior to coming to Canada. She does not work as she does not feel confident with her language and feels she will be discriminated against for both gender and race; the thought of having to enter the workforce makes her very anxious. In Somalia, Ayana had been a self-employed businesswoman operating her own vegetable stand. Her source of income is through Employment and Income Assistance and she is attending daily language classes to improve her English. Health care prior to coming to Canada was limited to seeking care as needed for episodic situations, such as childbirth or breathing problems. Ayana is unfamiliar with and suspicious of primary and secondary prevention strategies that are commonplace in Canada. She has never had a complete physical examination.

Her current health concern is that she is having "trouble breathing." Today she has had trouble catching her breath since being outside in the cold. She experiences similar episodes a few times a week but they usually pass within an hour or two. She was told in Somalia that she has asthma and should carry a puffer to help her, but she couldn't afford it and felt she didn't need it as the episodes usually passed on their own. She feels a bit better in the office now that she is warm. On examination, Ayana's BP is 154/92, R = 24, P = 80, T = 37.1(oral), O2 saturation 91% room air, S1/S2RRR, no S3/S4/M; air entry decreased to bases, expiratory wheezes throughout; no increased work of breathing observed. Lori's working diagnosis is asthma exacerbation.

Lori's management plan is comprehensive, reflecting not only the acute presentation of Ayana's, but other multi-dimensional needs that have been identified: long-term asthma management; primary and secondary prevention application such as immunizations, mammography, colorectal cancer screening, cervical cytology, diabetes and cholesterol screening; exploration of anxiety; and further assessment of psychosocial needs.

In order to implement the management plan, Lori addresses Ayana's asthma exacerbation by ordering a chest X-ray, WBC & differential, and prescribing a short-acting bronchodilator and an inhaled corticosteroid. She requests that the primary care nurse see Ayana and Fatmata before leaving the clinic to review correct inhaler technique and to discuss immunizations. She requests follow-up in 48 hours with both herself and the PCN. At that time, the asthma management plan can be adjusted accordingly, but will also afford Lori and the PCN an opportunity to discuss with Ayana the importance of regular health surveillance strategies.

After Ayana leaves the clinic, Lori speaks with the clinic social worker regarding community resources for immigrant women for both job entry and counselling, with the intention of exploring Ayana's receptiveness to support at the next visit. Lori is also able to make arrangements for a health authority translator to be present for the next visit, as Fatmata is unable to attend.

At her next visit, Ayana is feeling much better. She is resistant to having any further physical exam take place, or any further blood work as she doesn't see the need. She is receptive to speaking with the social worker regarding counselling and community supports.

Non-Clinical Primary Health Care Nurse Practitioner Domains of Practice

Reflective Practice

The benefits of reflection for professional practice are increasingly being recognized in Canada. The CNA (2004) and CASN advocate for the development of reflective practitioners. Reflection encourages practitioners to review an experience of practice in order to describe, analyze, evaluate, and so inform learning about practice (Reid, 1993). Continuing competency is a requirement of many regulatory bodies for NP registration and incorporates elements of self-reflection. It allows the NP opportunity to assess areas of strength and weakness, and the professional obligation to self-identify areas of weakness and create a self-learning plan for change (CNA, 2010a).

Reflective practice is inherent to growth as a PHCNP, regardless of whether one is a novice or an expert (Tracy, 2014). Direct clinical practice requires the integration of standards of care, awareness of scope of practice, and evidence-based management through a level of expertise acquired through educational preparation, a supportive work environment, and self-reflection (Pohl & Kao, 2014). A novice NP may initially be more task-oriented with patient presentations, but as they gain confidence and expertise with the role they will integrate "critical thinking and skillful interviewing" (Pohl & Kao, 2014, p. 407). Reflective practice allows the NP to explore experiences to critically analyze and improve practice (Tracy, 2014).

Research

Research is one domain considered foundational throughout most APN models and is often an expectation cited in job descriptions (CNA, 2011; Spross, 2014). "Research-sensitive practice" (Tracy, 2014, p. 164) is an approach that incorporates research in an unstructured manner for the APN. The PHCNP is well positioned to evaluate practice and clinical outcomes, to benchmark and identify best practices, and to lead efforts designed to improve quality and patient safety. Research may be actualized at the clinic level through quality improvement projects, or at a more systemic level with research contributions to the science of nursing as a whole. It is within the professional obligation of the PHCNP to stay current with evidence-based information and build opportunities into the role for either engaging in research or reviewing research, which is instrumental to fulfilling this responsibility.

Leadership

There is no noteworthy definition of leadership. Leadership is generally explained as the art and science of influencing a group toward the achievement of a goal. The NP role is derived from a strong base of clinical experience and education, which develops both extensive and extended skills and a critical awareness of the place of nursing in health service delivery. Consequently, the NP role is a leadership role in clinical practice (Carryer, Gardner, Dunn, & Gardner, 2007). Key elements of clinical leadership include the need to guide and influence care delivery systems, act as a change agent, and effectively deal with conflict by the use of skills in communication, negotiation, collaboration, and evaluation. Thus, the PHCNP lead both in the immediate clinical environment and in the wider context of health service delivery.

The leadership domain is essential to the emerging role in Canada where acting as a resource, consultant, or collaborating to shape policy or educate organizations is necessary to advance the NP role (CNA, 2010a). The PHCNP may actualize this by providing leadership in the clinical area through initiation of research, or assuming the lead as a role model for the PCNs by challenging them to maximize their scope of practice. Leadership is also demonstrated by being an educator or a preceptor to the public and other health care providers. Primary health care nurse practitioners should also advocate for quality, accessible, and cost-effective health care and ensure that clinical practice, as a whole, reflects evidence-based standards (CNA, 2010a; Pohl & Kao, 2014). The PHCNP's role as a leader in the community through memberships on boards of health and education, and as an influential policy-maker, is based primarily on the competency of collaboration.

Barriers to Practice

The integration of PHCNPs into the Canadian health care system has not been without its challenges and there continue to be barriers to practice. Barriers prevent full role integration and sustainability, affect continuity of care, and jeopardize safe and effective care.

Inconsistencies in legislation and education standards have led to lack of role clarity and challenges with credibility and portability (Donald et al., 2010). Restrictions to scope of practice such as prescriptive authority and medication management interfere with seamless patient care. Medication lists appropriate for the PHCNP may not be suitable for the NP working in a personal care home or in the emergency department setting. Health and social policy review is necessary to remove barriers, such as the signing of death certificates or completion of passport applications (Donald et al., 2010).

Perceived hierarchical roles also present ongoing challenges interprofessionally between PHCNPs and other health care professionals (Dinh, 2012b). Settings that lack a strong governance and understanding of the NP role can lead to failure of role implementation or suboptimal utilization of the PHCNP. Insufficient structure for collaboration has also been cited as a barrier, as has lack of evaluation of NP role implementation. A national tracking system has been suggested to monitor the trend of PHCNP activity (Donald et al., 2010). National level guidance would serve to further integrate and promote the role and allow for a more cohesive voice in addressing the barriers that continue to exist.

Conclusion

The PHCNP role is the fastest growing APN role in the country, as the benefits of the role to accessibility and quality care are increasingly recognized by the public and various levels of governments. PHCNPs provide comprehensive health care to individuals and families across the life continuum in a multi-dimensional approach consistent with the domains of APN. Operationalization of the role is supported by the CNA's NP core competencies, which provide guidance and structure for the role. It is expected that the PHCNP role will continue to experience integration and acceptance into the health care system.

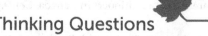

Critical Thinking Questions

1. In what manner is collaboration demonstrated in the role of the PHCNP?
2. Discuss incentives for developing and supporting interprofessional practice teams either in an NP-led clinic or in a general primary health care practice group.
3. If you were advocating for the PHCNP role, what would you consider to be the strengths and contributions of the role in improving health care for Canadians?

References

Ackerman, M., Norsen, L., Martin, B., Wiedrich, J., & Kitzman, H. (1996). Development of a model of advanced practice. *American Journal of Critical Care, 5*(1), 68–73.

Bryant-Lukosius, D., DiCenso, A., Browne, G., & Pinelli, J. (2004). Advanced practice nursing roles: Development, implementation and evaluation. *Journal of Advanced Nursing, 48*(5), 519–529. doi: 10.1111/j.1365-2648.2004.03234.x

Canadian Association of Schools of Nursing (CASN). (2011). *Nurse practitioner education in Canada: Final report.* Ottawa, ON: CASN.

CASN. (2012). *Nurse practitioner education in Canada: National framework of guiding principles & essential components.* Ottawa, ON: CASN.

Canadian Nurses Association (CNA). (2004). *Joint position statement: Promoting continuing competency for registered nurses.* Ottawa, ON: CNA.

CNA. (2008). *Advanced nursing practice: A national framework.* Ottawa, ON: CNA.

CNA. (2010a). *Canadian nurse practitioner core competency framework.* Ottawa, ON: CNA.

CNA. (2010b). *Meeting the challenges: CNA's response to promoting innovative solutions to health human resources challenges, a report of the standing committee on health.* Ottawa, ON: CNA.

CNA. (2011). *Collaborative integration plan for the role of nurse practitioners in Canada 2011–2015.* Ottawa, ON: CNA.

Canadian Nurse Practitioner Initiative (CNPI). (2006a). *Nurse practitioners: The time is now. An integrated report.* Retrieved from http://www.npnow.ca/docs/tech-report/section1/01_Integrated_Report.pdf

CNPI. (2006b). *Nurse practitioners: The time is now. A solution to improving access and reduction wait times in Canada.* Ottawa, ON: CNPI.

Carryer, J., Gardner, G., Dunn, S., & Gardner, A. (2007). The core role of the nurse practitioner: Practice, professionalism and clinical leadership. *Journal of Clinical Nursing, 16*(10), 1818–1825.

Cowan, M., Shapiro, M., Hays, R., Afifi, A., Vazirani, S., & Ward, C. (2006). The effect of a multidisciplinary hospitalist/physician and advanced practice nurse collaboration on hospital costs. *Journal of Nursing Administration, 36*(2), 79–85.

de Leon-Demare, K., MacDonald, J., Gregory, D., Katz, A., & Halas, G. (2015). Articulating nurse practitioner practice using King's theory of goal attainment. *Journal of the American Academy of Nurse Practitioners, 27*(11), 631–636. doi: 10.1002/2327-6924.12218

DiCenso, A., Auffrey, L., Bryant-Lukosius, D., Donald, F., Martin-Misener, R., Mathews, S., & Opsteen, J. (2007). Primary health care nurse practitioners in Canada. *Contemporary Nurse, 26*(1), 104–115.

DiCenso, A., Bryant-Lukosius, D., Martin-Misener, R., Donald, F., Abelson, J., Bourgeault, I., ... & Harbman, P. (2010). Factors enabling advanced practice nursing role integration in Canada. *Nursing Leadership, 23*(Special Issue December), 211–238.

Dinh, T. (2012a). Improving primary health care through collaboration: Briefing 1—current knowledge about interprofessional teams in Canada. *Canadian Alliance for Sustainable Health Care.* Retrieved from http://www.conferenceboard.ca/e-library/abstract.aspx?did=5157

Dinh, T. (2012b). Improving primary health care through collaboration: Briefing 2—Barriers to successful interprofessional teams. *Canadian Alliance for Sustainable Health*

Care. Retrieved from http://www.conferenceboard.ca/temp/3ed162fc-0144-47e3-80e1-e1020d5dfa45/13-146_primaryhealthcare-briefing-2.pdf

Donald, F., Martin-Misener, R., Bryant-Lukosius, D., Kilpatrick, K., Kaasalainen, S., Carter, N., ... & DiCenso, A. (2010). The primary healthcare nurse practitioner role in Canada. *Nursing Leadership, 23*(Special Issue December), 88–113.

Donovan, D. (n.d.). *AFMC primer on population health: A virtual textbook on public health concepts for clinicians*. Ottawa, ON: The Association of Faculties of Medicine of Canada. Retrieved from http://phprimer.afmc.ca/inner/about_the_primer

Gardner, A., Hase, S., Gardner, G., Dunn, S.V., & Carryer, J. (2007). From competence to capability: A study of nurse practitioners in clinical practice. *Journal of Clinical Nursing, 17*(2), 250–258.

Jones, M.L. (2005). Role development and effective practice in specialist and advanced practice roles in acute hospital settings: Systematic review and meta-synthesis. *Journal of Advanced Nursing, 49*(2), 191–209.

Kaasalainen, S., Martin-Misener, R., Kilpatrick, K., Harbman, P., Bryant-Lukosius, D., & Donald, F. (2010). A historical overview of the development of advanced practice nursing roles in Canada. *Nursing Leadership, 23*(Special Issue December), 35–60.

Mick, D.J., & Ackerman, M.H. (2000). Advanced practice nursing role delineation in acute and critical care: Application of the strong model of advanced practice. *Heart & Lung, 29*(3), 210–21.

Pohl, J., & Kao, T. (2014). The primary care nurse practitioner. In A. Hamric, C. Hanson, M. Tracy, & E. O'Grady (Eds.), *Advanced practice nursing: An integrative approach* (pp. 396–428). St. Louis, MO: Elsevier.

Pohl, J., Savrin, C., Fiandt, K., Beauchesne, M., Drayton-Brooks, S., Scheibmeir, M., & Werner, K. (2009). Quality and safety in graduate nursing education: Cross-mapping QSEN graduate competencies with NONPF's NP core and practice doctorate competencies. *Nursing Outlook, 57*(6), 349–354.

Pulcini, J., Jelic, M., Gul, R., & Loke, A.Y. (2010). An international survey on advanced practice nursing education, practice, and regulation. *Journal of Nursing Scholarship, 41*(1), 31–39.

Reid, B. (1993). But we're doing it already! Exploring a response to the concept of reflective practice in order to improve its facilitation. *Nurse Education Today, 13*(4), 305–309.

Ruel, J., & Motyka, C. (2009). Advanced practice nursing: A principle-based concept analysis. *Journal of the American Academy of Nurse Practitioners, 21*(7), 384–392.

Spross, J. (2014). Conceptualizations of advanced practice nursing. In A. Hamric, C. Hanson, M. Tracy, & E. O'Grady (Eds.), *Advanced practice nursing: An integrative approach* (pp. 27–61). St. Louis, MO: Elsevier.

Tracy, M. (2014). Direct clinical practice. In A. Hamric, C. Hanson, M. Tracy, & E. O'Grady (Eds.), *Advanced practice nursing: An integrative approach* (pp. 147–182). St. Louis, MO: Elsevier.

Venning, P., Durie, A., Roland, M., Roberts, C., & Leese, B. (2000). Randomised controlled trial comparing cost effectiveness of general practitioners and nurse practitioners in primary care. *British Medical Journal, 320*(7241), 1048–1053.

Williams, A., & Jones, M. (2006). Patients' assessments of consulting a nurse practitioner: The time factor. *Journal of Advanced Nursing, 53*(2), 188–95.

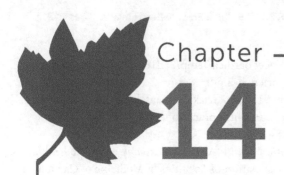

Chapter 14

The Nurse Practitioner: Adult

Rosemary Wilson

Rosemary Wilson is an Assistant Professor at Queen's University, School of Nursing in Kingston, Ontario. She is also an NP–Adult in chronic pain management at Kingston General and Hotel Dieu Hospitals.

KEY TERMS

acute care nurse practitioner (ACNP)

advanced practice nurse (APN)

clinical nurse specialist/nurse practitioner (CNS/NP)

nurse practitioner-adult (NP–Adult)

specialty nurse practitioner (SNP)

tertiary care nurse practitioner (TCNP)

OBJECTIVES

1. Describe the NP roles in adult acute and specialty care practice.
2. Explore the NP practice competencies in NP–Adult roles in Canada.
3. Discuss the barriers and facilitators of NP–Adult practice.
4. Explore the evidence of the effectiveness of NP–Adult roles in the Canadian context.

Introduction

This chapter discusses the role of the nurse practitioner (NP) in the adult patient care stream. The **nurse practitioner–adult (NP–Adult)** is an **advanced practice nurse (APN)** who provides specialized health care to adolescents, adults, older adults, and their families with particular health conditions. Direct clinical care occupies the largest domain of NP–Adult practice while the domains of research, leadership, consultation, and collaboration also contribute to the foundation of this largely hospital-based NP role (DiCenso et al., 2010). As is the case with other NP roles, the *Canadian Nurse Practitioner Core*

Competency Framework developed by the Canadian Nurses Association (CNA, 2010) guides the operationalization of NP–Adult across the continuum of care. Core competencies for the NP–Adult role are: professional role responsibility and accountability (clinical practice, collaboration, consultation and referral, research, leadership); health assessment and diagnosis; therapeutic management; and health promotion and prevention of illness and injury.

The NP–Adult role began its evolution in the 1980s and 1990s as a blended **clinical nurse specialist/nurse practitioner (CNS/NP)** role as a response to increases in patient complexity and a shortage of physician coverage (DiCenso et al., 2010; Kilpatrick et al., 2010). In the years since, role titles across Canada have included **acute care nurse practitioner (ACNP), tertiary care nurse practitioner (TCNP), specialty nurse practitioner (SNP)**, and CNS/NP. The role titles ACNP and NP–Adult will be used interchangeably to be consistent with the literature presented.

NP–Adult Education

NP–Adult education has consistently been at the graduate level since its early inception through the CNS/NP titled role (DiCenso et al., 2010; Martin-Misener, 2010). Educational programs are offered either as a combined graduate or post-graduate NP certificate or diploma. Educational programs for the NP–Adult role provide a combination of theoretical and clinical learning consistent with the preparation for APN, providing essential content for practice in all domains. In combined programs, core graduate-level courses in nursing theory, research methods, statistics, and health policy are taken along with NP courses. NP courses include pathophysiology, pharmacotherapeutics, advanced health assessment and clinical reasoning, advanced health assessment and therapeutic management, and NP roles and issues. Practicum experience hours are required in each of the programs.

The Canadian Association of Schools of Nursing (CASN) recommends the entry requirement for NPs be a graduate education with a minimum of 700 hours of direct clinical practice (excluding laboratory time), regardless of stream (CASN, 2012). All NP–Adult education programs are generalist in nature, except for those offered in Quebec, where the specialties of cardiology and nephrology are supported by Ordre des Infirmières et Infirmiers du Québec (OIIQ). (Table 14.1 presents the various NP–Adult programs in Canada.) At successful completion of an NP–Adult program, students are eligible to write either the Adult-Gerontology Primary Care Nurse Practitioner Certification Examination offered by the American Academy of Nurse Practitioners Certification Program (AANPCP), or the Adult Nurse Practitioner Exam offered by the American Nurses Credentialing Center (ANCC) for provincial or territorial registration. The CASN Task Force on NP Education (2012) recognized that there is a paucity of doctorally prepared NPs in faculty roles, and that recruitment of NPs into doctoral studies is an issue in Canada.

TABLE 14.1:   NP–Adult Education Programs by School

School	Length of Program (years)	Degree
Memorial University of Newfoundland	2	MN
Université de Montréal	2	MSc
Université Laval	2	MSc
University of Toronto	2	MN/NP
University of Alberta	2.5	MN/NP
University of Calgary	2	MN/NP
British Columbia Institute of Technology	1.5	Certificate only

MN = Master of Nursing; MSc = Master of Science; MN/NP = Master of Nursing/Nurse Practitioner

Source: Canadian Institute for Health Information (CIHI), 2010.

Overall, NP–Adult education programs are designed to meet entry to practice competencies set out by individual provincial regulatory bodies (CASN, 2012). It is important to note that, similar to the primary health care nurse practitioner (PHCNP), the NP–Adult's knowledge, skills, and ability expands with practice experience. As such, there is variability in scope of practice enactment. In addition, although clinical practice within educational programs may be specialty-based, the context and detail required for autonomous specialty practice beyond entry to practice competency often requires additional effort by the NP–Adult in the early part of their career.

There can be a mismatch between the educational stream taken, the NP stream of registration, and the ultimate practice/employment setting (CASN, 2012; DiCenso et al., 2010). For example, PHCNPs may be employed in acute care settings and ACNPs may be employed in primary care settings as a result of position and resource availability in the area, although Almost and Laschinger (2002) found that 90.5% of ACNPs in Canada were working in acute care settings and 82.5% were employed full-time.

NP–Adult Role and Scope of Practice in Canada

The NP–Adult/ACNP contributes to patient care by utilizing an expanded scope of clinical practice, with activities that fall within both traditional medical and nursing disciplines (Sidani & Doran, 2010). Consistent with the early blended roles of CNS/NP, NP–Adults in Canada practice within the established competencies of APN in the broad domains of clinical, research, education, and administration (Kilpatrick et al., 2010). The NP–Adult role can be found in a multitude of specialty settings ranging from in-patient service-based groups (e.g., neurosurgery, orthopedics, cardiac surgery, cardiology) and outpatient service-based groups (e.g., oncology, asthma) to consultative/concurrent care management teams in both in-patient and outpatient settings (e.g., palliative care, acute and chronic pain management, anticoagulation, diabetes) (Spross, 2009). Overall, the NP–Adult provides specialty care to meet the needs of specialty populations (DiCenso et al., 2010). NPs in most Canadian provinces and territories are authorized to diagnose diseases or conditions, order and interpret diagnostic testing, and prescribe medications and treatments. The level of legislated autonomy to perform these functions varies across Canada, depending on provincial and territorial regulations.

The NP–Adult role has been found to be associated with greater clinical responsibilities than the CNS role, with as much as 80% of work time spent providing clinical care (Sidani et al., 2000). Individuals in these roles have described their practice as including consultation, support, and education for both physicians and nurses in specialty areas (DiCenso et al., 2010). The hallmark of this role is its interprofessional and collaborative practice with diverse groups of health professionals in a team-based approach (Bryant-Lukosius & DiCenso, 2004; Hurlock-Chorostecki, Forchuk, Orchard, van Soeren, & Reeves, 2014).

In a study of a combined group of ACNPs, physicians, administrators, and staff nurses, van Soeren and Micevski (2001) found that most staff nurses agreed that the role was an important clinical resource in their practice. Hurlock-Chorostecki et al. (2015) conducted a survey of NPs in acute and long-term care settings to assess the processes of implementing interprofessional care that included interdependence, partnership and collaboration, collective problem solving, professional relationships, communication, and shared decision-making. In the study, more than 50% of NPs in acute care engaged in all of the elements of interprofessional care. Partnership and collaboration, and collective problem solving, had the broadest range of activity engagement, while more than 75% of NPs reported engaging in shared decision-making, communication, and interdependence. In non-clinical activity, ACNPs reported engaging in more research and academic activities than PHCNPs (DiCenso et al., 2010).

However, individual NP–Adult practice is variable in role enactment as patient care demands and existing support usually dictate workflow. Kilpatrick et al. (2012b), using a mixed methods time and motion study, found that ACNPs in an in-patient cardiology specialty experienced a faster pace of work in the morning, reflective of patient care demands. The interaction with physician colleagues and the clarity of administrative structures in place for this group were related to participants' engagement in both clinical and non-clinical activities. For example, ACNPs with more institutional support from administration and medicine spent more time in the domain of research.

Interestingly, those with greater practice autonomy spent less time on indirect clinical care activities, but were identified as the first responder and as having an important role as the professional presence with patients. In the two cases studied, ACNPs spent between 73% and

61.5% of time in clinical practice, 4.4% and 12.3% in educational activity, 4.2% and 16% in administrative activity, and 10.2% and 0.9% in research activity. Both groups spent between 8% and 9% on activities associated with personal time. In a related examination of the same group, Kilpatrick (2013b) observed the processes surrounding patient care, decision-making, and communication within direct and indirect clinical care. ACNPs were observed to have initiated 40% of communications with team members and patients, roughly double the amount of time spent by the physician on service. The average number of communication behaviours per minute recorded in the two cases were 9.5 and 13.8. This finding illustrates the importance of the ACNP role as central to team functioning in coordination of care.

The reliance of the clinical specialties on the presence of the NP–Adult has, however, been found to come at a price for nurses in some of these roles. Rashotte and Jensen (2010) conducted a qualitative study of ACNPs in specialty practice ($n = 26$). Informants described feeling adrift in the early part of their practice, particularly when mentoring with physicians rather than other ACNPs. For participants in the latter part of their practice, the theme of being spread too thin was an aspect of addressing the needs of the clinical environment. Overall, the notion was that ACNPs felt they were pioneers within the context of their institutional environment.

Barriers and Facilitators to NP–Adult Practice

Barriers and facilitators to NP practice exist regardless of stream of registration. The effect these factors have is variable, and largely depends on the structure and functional aspects of the practice environment. DiCenso et al. (2010) found that certain features of the role, such as initial role development, clarity, awareness and implementation, and intraprofessional and interprofessional relationships, could act as either barriers or facilitators.

A discrepancy between administration and physician specialists regarding the amount of time ACNPs should spend in direct patient care can contribute to both inter- and intraprofessional conflict. In some cases, physicians want ACNPs to spend more time in clinical practice while administrators want time protected for non-clinical activities of leadership, education, and research to ensure the role is more aligned with nursing. Risking alignment to other disciplines continues with the predisposition for some roles to be implemented with reporting structures to non-nursing program level administrators or physicians. The additional impact of inconsistent titling in organizations (NP versus APN) complicates awareness and understanding of the role, as well as the achievement of role clarity. Physicians, administrators, staff nurses, and ACNPs all cited role clarity as essential to the successful implementation of the ACNP role (van Soeren & Micevski, 2001).

Physician receptivity to the role has been found to be related to the physician remuneration systems in place. Dimeo and Postic (2012) identified a fee-for-service billing structure to be one of the greatest barriers to role implementation in emergency room settings, while alternative or salary-based funding systems were facilitators of success. In addition, physicians were found to prefer a complementary rather than a replacement role with activities of coordination of care, patient self-management facilitation, and discharge planning being key for a value-added role in clinical service (DiCenso et al., 2010). The understanding of the line between independent NP–Adult practice and autonomous practice can affect the impact "overlapping scopes of practice of NPs and physicians" (DiCenso et al, 2010, p.25) has on improving patient access to care. Relationships with collaborating physicians and administration have been associated with the achievement of autonomous practice and successful role implementation (Almost & Laschinger, 2002; Dimeo & Postic, 2012; Kilpatrick, Lavoie-Tremblay, Ritchie, Lamothe, & Doran, 2012a). Kilpatrick et al. (2012a) identified the need for an administrative and medical champion, and Almost and Laschinger (2002) reported a statistically positive association between ACNP empowerment and collaboration with physicians that was similar to collaboration with managers. The role of management as a conduit for organizational communication is an important link, allowing ACNPs to function within the broader context of the organization in addition to providing the resources required for patient care.

A related barrier to successful role implementation and enactment is the job strain associated with empowerment in ACNP practice (Almost & Laschinger, 2002). Almost half of the variance in job strain associated with workplace empowerment was accounted for by the combined effect of collaboration with physicians and managers. Trust between team members is essential for collaboration, and was reported as a factor in successful role implementation and enactment in emergency room (ER) and cardiology settings (Dimeo & Postic, 2012; Kilpatrick et al., 2012a). For example, Dimeo and Postic (2012) assert that the traditional hierarchical relationship between physicians and the NP dissipated with the development of a collaborative and trusting professional relationship. The researchers make recommendations for ensuring NPs hired are the right fit for the clinical team and the population served. They also suggest that a 12-week orientation is ideal for implementation success, as time is required to complete the boundary work necessary for collaboration and role fluidity, and to work toward the improvement of patient care and achievement of team objectives (Kilpatrick et al., 2012a). Such boundary work also included creating space to help to adjust to interpretation of the role in daily activities, loss of valued interactions between experienced nurses and physicians, creating trust between team members, and paying attention to interpersonal dynamics, such as taking time to listen to others, being available to staff, setting appropriate limits, and promoting work of other team members (Kilpatrick et al., 2012a).

Evidence of NP–Adult Role Effectiveness

The impact of NP–Adult practice on continuity of care has been noted by physicians, administrators, staff nurses, and ACNPs, and may be related to its clinical focus (van

Soeren & Micevski, 2001). The role of the NP–Adult has been examined for effectiveness in improving functional outcomes, length of hospital stay, testing and associated costs, team effectiveness, and processes of care and associated patient satisfaction (Kilpatrick, 2013a; Sarkissian & Wennberg, 1999; Sidani et al., 2005; Sidani & Doran, 2010). In two cities in Southern Ontario, Sidani et al. (2005) investigated, in a cross-sectional design, the outcomes of patients (n = 123) who did and did not receive care by an ACNP, and who were admitted for orthopedic, cardiac, and spinal surgery. Patients who received ACNP care reported higher levels of physical and social functioning, and less role limitations due to physical and mental health.

In epilepsy care service, Sarkissian and Wennberg (1999) found a reduction in length of hospital stay and decreased use of laboratory testing and associated costs after the implementation of an ACNP. The monitoring activities of this ACNP role included diagnostic functions, care planning and delivery, patient assessment, assessment of home and community resources, and patient and family education, along with the indirect activities of coordination of care, staff education, quality improvement, research consultation with attending and specialist staff, referrals, and discharge planning. Kilpatrick (2013a) found an improvement in team effectiveness, and reported that an increase in the team's ability to meet patient needs, complete follow-up, and facilitate communication made an important contribution to care coordination and patient/family focused care. Additionally, ACNPs in this study were found to have a more global view of patient care that resulted in medical issues being addressed more quickly. Similarly, Sidani and Doran (2010) found that patients who reported higher levels of care coordination also reported improvement in mental health. Moreover, patients in this study who reported higher levels of counselling and education also reported improvements in physical function and social functioning respectively. Overall, most patients reported satisfaction with care and a reduction in the number and severity of symptoms during the study period.

CASE STUDY

The Story of Martha

Martha is a 42-year-old woman with long-standing, chronic widespread pain. Martha has been newly referred to the Chronic Pain Clinic by the NP–PHC from her Family Health Team, which is closer to her home in the extreme northern boundary of the Local Health Integration Network, 120 kilometres away. Leanne, the NP–Adult who first sees Martha, has many years of experience caring for patients with chronic pain not related to cancer.

Leanne has planned to spend extra time assessing Martha, as the very comprehensive referral letter she received documents the many challenges Martha has experienced prior to coming to the clinic. Martha had a musculoskeletal injury 10 years ago while working as a registered practical nurse (RPN) in a long-term care facility. At the time of her injury, Martha was assessed for a vertebral fracture and intervertebral disc prolapse using X-rays and a lumbar spine MRI. The imaging results were negative and Martha expressed being particularly frustrated with these findings stating, "I still have pain."

Since the injury, Martha has been unable to continue working as sitting, standing, and lifting cause increased pain. She had been receiving assistance from the Workplace Safety and Insurance Board (WSIB) several months after her workplace disability coverage ceased. Martha's treatment has included physiotherapy and massage therapy, neurofeedback, and medications such as muscle relaxants and pain/adjunctive pain medications, including opioids and non-steroidal medications. Martha reported that the only treatments she received that were of benefit were the massage therapy, neurofeedback, and baclofen. Martha's health history included hypothyroidism and depression (for which she had received treatment), and smoking around 30 packs of cigarettes per year. She denies alcohol or other substance use. Martha is financially stable, although she finds covering the costs of transportation for clinic visits difficult. Martha lives with her husband and two teenaged sons in a rural community. Her husband works as a farm hand. Her home relationships are solid and supportive and she has some household assistance from her mother-in-law two days a week. Martha's current medications are as follows: acetaminophen 325 mg po prn; oxycodone 5 mg two tablets po qid prn (average 8/day); L-thyroxine 0.025 mg po daily; duloxetine hydrochloride 40 mg po daily; and colace 200 mg po bid prn.

Using her knowledge of the evidence-informed recommendations, as well as the guidelines for the assessment and management of chronic, non-cancer pain, Leanne asked Martha to complete a number of questionnaires to provide a baseline picture of her pain. The results revealed that Martha has moderate to severe pain-related interference with activity, the absence of depression, and a low rating on the Pain Catastrophizing Scale for opioid risk. Descriptions of her pain were aching, tiring, gnawing, and throbbing, all occurring in the lower back area with no radiation. Martha rated her overall pain intensity as 7/10. Her focused physical examination revealed an antalgic gait and tested negative for any neurologic findings or red flags. Leanne noted that Martha had some trigger point tenderness in her erector spinae muscles, as well as in the bilateral musculature above her iliac crests.

Leanne's initial plan of care included ordering baseline blood work (CBC, electrolytes, magnesium) and a referral to social work, with Martha's consent, for support and assistance with covering travel costs. Leanne called the referring NP–PHC from Martha's Family Health Team to assess whether the imaging reports required new imaging. Recognizing that a review of the imaging would be required prior to referral for additional physiotherapy, or to one of her physician colleagues for consideration of interventional pain management techniques, Leanne used the visit to establish a trusting relationship with Martha and develop a comprehensive understanding of her current situation. Leanne collaborated with Martha to choose a date for her next clinic appointment, which would include the social worker, Leanne, and her physician colleague. It was also scheduled at a time when Martha's husband could drive her. Leanne promised to ensure that any additional imaging required could be performed at the same time.

Martha left the clinic expressing a sense of relief that she had been "listened to and valued," and stated she was hopeful that working with the chronic pain team could help ease her pain and improve her quality of life.

Conclusion

The NP–Adult (also referred to as CNS/NP, ACNP, TCNP, and SNP) provides care to patients with complex health challenges in the context of collaborative teams, typically in acute care institutional settings. Practice characteristics of the role are variable and dependent on the needs of the specialty population and available organizational supports, but it includes activities in both clinical and non-clinical domains. The number of these types of APN roles is growing in the face of increased needs for chronic disease management within a fiscally constrained health care system. Essential to the successful scope of practice enactment of the NP–Adult role is the individual practitioner's ability to realize their own potential.

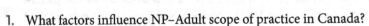

Critical Thinking Questions

1. What factors influence NP–Adult scope of practice in Canada?
2. What steps should be taken to increase role success when implementing an NP–Adult role in a specialty practice area?
3. What are the main practice differences between the PHCNP and NP–Adult roles?

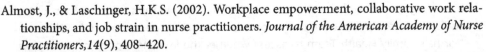

References

Almost, J., & Laschinger, H.K.S. (2002). Workplace empowerment, collaborative work relationships, and job strain in nurse practitioners. *Journal of the American Academy of Nurse Practitioners,14*(9), 408–420.

Bryant-Lukosius, D., & DiCenso, A. (2004). A framework for the introduction and evaluation of advanced practice nursing roles. *Journal of Advanced Nursing, 48*(5), 530–540. Retrieved from http://aipsq.com/_pdf/Bryant-Lukosius%20DiCenso%20A%20framework%20for%20

the%20introduction%20and%20evaluation%20of%20advanced%20practice%20nursing%20 roles.pdf

Canadian Association of Schools of Nursing (CASN). (2012). *Nurse practitioner education in Canada: National framework of guiding principles and essential components.* Ottawa, ON: CASN.

Canadian Institute for Health Information (CIHI). (2010). *Nurse practitioners: Education requirements.* Retrieved from https://www.cihi.ca/en/spending-and-health-workforce/ health-workforce/nurse-practitioners#eduReq

Canadian Nurses Association (CNA). (2010). *Canadian nurse practitioner core competency framework.* Ottawa, ON: CNA. Retrieved from http://www.cno.org/globalassets/for/rnec/ pdf/competencyframework_en.pdf

DiCenso, A., Bryant-Lukosius, D., Borgeault, I., Martin-Misener, R., Donald, F., Abelson, J., ... Harbman, P. (2010). *Clinical nurse specialists and nurse practitioners in Canada: A decision support synthesis.* Ottawa, ON: CHSRF/FCRSS. Retrieved from http://www.cfhi-fcass.ca/ Libraries/Commissioned_Research_Reports/Dicenso_EN_Final.sflb.ashx

Dimeo, M., & Postic, M. (2012). Lessons learned in developing and implementing the nurse practitioner role in an urban Canadian emergency department. *Journal of Emergency Nursing, 38*(5), 484–487.

Hurlock-Chorostecki, C., Forchuk, C., Orchard, C., van Soeren, M., & Reeves, S. (2014). Hospital-based nurse practitioner roles and interprofessional practice: A scoping review. *Nursing & Health Sciences, 16*(3), 403–410. doi: 10.1111/nhs.12107

Hurlock-Chorostecki, C, van Soeren, M., MacMillan, K., Sidani, S., Collins, L., Harbman, P., ... Reeves, S. (2015). A survey of interprofessional activity of acute and long-term care employed nurse practitioners. *Journal of the American Association of Nurse Practitioners, 27*(9), 507–513. doi: 10.1002/2327-6924.12213

Kilpatrick, K. (2013a). How do nurse practitioners in acute care affect perceptions of team effectiveness? *Journal of Clinical Nursing, 22*(17–18), 2636–2647.

Kilpatrick, K. (2013b). Understanding acute care nurse practitioner communication and decision-making in healthcare tams. *Journal of Clinical Nursing, 22*(1–2), 168–179.

Kilpatrick, K., Harbman, P., Carter, N., Martin-Misener, R., Bryant-Lukosius, D., Donald, F., ... DiCenso, A. (2010). The acute care nurse practitioner role in Canada. *Nursing Leadership, 23*(Special Issue December), 114–139. doi: 10.12927/cjnl.2010.22272

Kilpatrick, K., Lavoie-Tremblay, M., Ritchie, J., Lamothe, L., & Doran, D. (2012a). Boundary work and the introduction of acute care nurse practitioners in healthcare teams. *Journal of Advanced Nursing, 68*(7), 1504–1515.

Kilpatrick, K., Lavoie-Tremblay, M., Ritchie, J.A., Lamothe, L., Doran, D., & Rochefort, C. (2012b). How are acute care nurse practitioners enacting their roles in healthcare teams? A descriptive multiple-case study. *International Journal of Nursing Studies, 49*(7), 850–862.

Martin-Misener, R. (2010). Will nurse practitioners achieve full integration into the Canadian health-care system? *Canadian Journal of Nursing Research, 42*(2), 9–16.

Rashotte, J., & Jensen, L. (2010). The transformational journey of nurse practitioners in acute-care settings. *Canadian Journal of Nursing Research, 42*(2), 70–91.

Sarkissian, S., & Wennberg, R. (1999). Effects of the acute care nurse practitioner role on epilepsy monitoring outcomes. *Outcomes Management for Nursing Practice, 3*(4), 161–166.

Sidani, S., Doran, D., Porter, H., LeFort, S., O'Brien-Pallas, L., Zahn, C., & Sarkissian, S. (2005). Outcomes of nurse practitioners in acute care: An exploration. *The Internet Journal of Advanced Nursing Practice, 8*(1). Retrieved from https://ispub.com/IJANP/8/1/12232

Sidani, S., & Doran, D. (2010). Relationships between process and outcomes of nurse practitioners in acute care: An exploration. *Journal of Nursing Care Quality, 25*(1), 31–38.

Sidani, S., Irvine, D., Porter, H., O'Brien-Pallas, L., Simpson, B., McGillis Hall, L., ... Redelmeir, D. (2000). Practice patterns of acute care nurse practitioners. *Canadian Journal of Nursing Leadership, 13*(3), 6–12.

Spross, J. (2009). Conceptualizations of advanced practice nursing. In A. Hamric, J. Spross, & C. Hanson (Eds.) *Advanced practice nursing: An integrative approach* (4th ed.), (pp. 27–66). St. Louis, MO: Saunders Elsevier.

van Soeren, M., & Micevski, V. (2001). Success indicators and barriers to acute nurse practitioner role implementation in four Ontario hospitals. *AACN Clinical Issues, 12*(3), 424–437.

Chapter 15

The Nurse Practitioner: Pediatrics

Kristina Chapman

Kristina Chapman is an NP–Pediatrics in Hematology/Oncology at the IWK Health Centre in Halifax, Nova Scotia.

Kristina Chapman is an NP–Pediatrics in Hematology/Oncology at the IWK Health Centre in Halifax, Nova Scotia.

KEY TERMS

family-centred care
pediatric nurse practitioner (NP)
transition

OBJECTIVES

1. Review the history of the pediatric nurse practitioner (NP) role.
2. Identify concepts in implementing new pediatric NP roles.
3. Review the role of the pediatric NP in providing family-centred care.
4. Discuss the NP role in preparing pediatric patients for transitions in their health care experience.

Introduction

The **pediatric nurse practitioner (NP)** works with infants, children, adolescents, and their caregivers to provide advanced health care services. They assess, diagnose, and treat patients with acute, episodic, or chronic health care conditions, and consult and collaborate with other health care team members to provide **family-centred care**. As well, a unique part of the pediatric NP's role is preparing patients and families for the **transition** from pediatric to primary or adult care while building capacity in the patient to take responsibility for their own health management. In this chapter, the pediatric NP role will be reviewed. In the context of this chapter, the pediatric NP role discussion excludes the role of the neonatal nurse practitioner (NNP).

History of the Pediatric Nurse Practitioner Role

The first pediatric NP role began in the US at the University of Colorado, where a program was developed in 1965 (Wilson, 2005). NPs graduating from this program were educated to provide well-child care and to manage common health problem seen in childhood. Later, programs for pediatric NPs working in acute care were subsequently developed.

In Canada, pediatric NPs originated as one of a number of acute care nurse practitioner (ACNP) roles developed in the early 1990s (Kaasalainen et al., 2010). ACNPs were graduate-prepared and practiced in acute care settings with specialized populations. The first acute pediatric NP program was offered by the University of Toronto in 1993 (Hurlock-Chorostecki, van Soeren, & Goodwin, 2008). Pediatric NPs were educated to provide comprehensive advanced practice nursing care to patients and their families in general pediatrics or in subspecialty settings.

In Ontario during the 1990s, there was a decrease in the number of medical residents along with an increase in the number of acute care admissions (Sidani et al., 2000). The severity of illness of those hospitalized had increased, and the NP role was identified as part of the solution to address the health care needs of hospitalized patients. Subsequently, NPs were introduced to improve continuity of care for medically complex patients who required prolonged hospitalizations (Pringle, 2007). During this time, health care reforms were occurring that set out to ensure more efficient use of health care resources (Kaasalainen et al., 2010). The introduction of ACNPs occurred as a result of these changes and helped to meet the needs of hospitals and patient populations. Pediatric NPs were one of the roles introduced at that time; this role has been developed in many other provinces since it was first introduced in Ontario. Today, most tertiary pediatric centres in Canada utilize NPs in both the in-patient and the ambulatory settings.

Role Implementation and Integration

Pediatric NP roles in Canada are often incorporated within interprofessional (IP) teams and successful role implementation is essential for the success of the NP. Introducing the NP role into a complex health care system can be challenging, and several factors can impact role implementation. Barriers to role implementation may occur at the system, organization, or practice setting levels (Sangster-Gormley, Martin-Misener, Downe-Wamboldt, & DiCenso, 2011). A review of Canadian NPs identified three concepts associated with the process of role implementation.

The first concept, involvement in the implementation of the NP role from the initial stages, indicates that various health provider stakeholders should be involved in NP role implementation. This includes managers, physicians, nursing staff, and allied health care providers. Team members may mentor new NPs, introduce the NP to other team members, and work with the team to identify how the NP role may fit into the practice setting. The pediatric NP will work with nursing and medical staff to meet the health care needs of the patient. Pharmacists and dietitians may be involved in ensuring these needs are met. Social work, child life specialists, and psychologists may also be involved in ensuring the psychosocial needs of the family are addressed. The pediatric NP must understand how the NP role will interact and overlap to provide care to the patient and the family. Prior to implementing the NP role, the NP must understand the patient population needs, the gaps in care, and how the role will integrate with the other roles to ensure optimal patient care.

The second concept is the acceptance of the NP role. The pediatric NP improves the chances of role success if the team understands the NP role, engages and collaborates with the NP, and is open to working with the NP. The NP's ability to work in the full scope of the role may be affected by how well the team accepts the NP role. The pediatric NP must be able to clearly articulate their role description and what they bring to the team. As well, they must understand the other team members' roles and how the NP role will incorporate into the team function.

The final concept, intention, impacts on the success or failure of the NP role. Clear NP role intentions will assist in defining the NP role, having set expectations, developing goals for the role, and having a plan for role implementation. Defining NP integration with the other health care provider roles and establishing role expectations, such as defining the patient population, is more readily achieved if the intentions of the NP role are clearly defined. Pediatric NPs work in a complex system where health care providers not only work with the patient, but also with the family unit to optimize the health and well-being of the patient. Clear goals for the role assist in identifying how the role will be placed into this complex system.

Understanding how processes, systems, and health care personnel interact can inform the integration of a new NP into the health care team. The central process dimensions of ACNP role enactment, team effectiveness, and boundary work are impacted by the structural dimensions described in the framework by Kilpatrick, Lavoie-Tremblay, Lamothe, Ritchie, and Doran (2013). Many process dimensions in the framework are interconnected, such as the patient-level structure through to the health care system level. As one moves from the patient-centred focus to incorporate reciprocal relationships with other stakeholders and the organization, this can impact outcomes. The framework's authors suggest that the inner dimensions are associated with boundary work, perception of team effectiveness, and ACNP role enactment, which can form the basis of how identified multi-level influences can result in structure, process, and outcome changes.

Having someone to champion the role, whether from the nursing or medical field, can help the NP enact their role. Trust among team members was identified as the key component of boundary work. The NP can improve team function by providing timely care, improving team communication, support of team members, and the addition of interventions that increase team communication.

Collaboration with other team members, joint problem solving of patient issues, and the sharing of workloads can help to bring team members together when the NP role is implemented. Measurement of outcome indicators can also help assess the implementation of the new NP. Indicators that may be used include staff knowledge, timely care, improved patient follow-up, and improved discharge planning.

NP role integration is reliant on four factors:

1. full utilization of role components
2. scope of practice
3. team acceptance
4. funding issues (Kilpatrick et al., 2010)

NP practice is primarily clinical, which can limit the NP's ability to incorporate the other role competencies of educator, leader, and researcher into daily practice. Clear articulation of the NP's non-clinical practice and stakeholder involvement in establishing role priorities can assist in diminishing conflicting demands and facilitate successful role implementation. Jurisdictional and/or organizational regulations can also limit the NP's scope of practice, thereby impacting the optimization of the role. Stakeholder participation in the development and ongoing evaluation of the NP role can also facilitate agreement on the NP's role expectations, and secure and stable funding for NP roles ensures long-term security of the position.

The Pediatric Nurse Practitioner Role

In Canada, pediatric NPs work primarily in pediatric acute care facilities. Roles may include general pediatrics or in one of a number of pediatric medical and surgical subspecialties, including hematology/oncology, cardiology, respirology, palliative care, general surgery, and orthopedics, and several other areas. Care is provided along the continuum from diagnosis, acute care management, and chronic illness management to palliative care or transition to primary or adult care.

The Canadian Nurses Association (CNA) (2010) describes the following core competencies categories required for NPs: professional role, responsibility and accountability, health assessment and diagnosis, therapeutic management, and health promotion and prevention of illness and injury. The core competencies within the professional role, along with responsibility and accountability categories, are divided into clinical practice, research, leadership, consultation, and collaboration. NP roles in Canada are developed using this framework (CNA, 2010).

The Pediatric Nurse Practitioner's Clinical Role

In a survey of ACNPs in Ontario, 20% identified themselves as working in pediatric hospitals (Hurlock-Chorostecki et al., 2008). Thirty percent of respondents reported that they worked with infants and children younger than 12 years of age and 24% worked with adolescents. All respondents had hospital-based practices and saw patients in the in-patient and/or ambulatory settings. Overall, respondents indicated that 75% of their work time was spent providing direct patient care, with the remainder of the time divided between teaching, research and scholarly activity, administration, and other responsibilities. NPs provided continuity of care to patients, for example, by following them from the in-patient unit to follow-up in the ambulatory clinic, or through multiple hospital admissions. NPs perceive themselves as being part of a collaborative practice providing direct patient care.

An Ontario survey examining NP roles in hospital settings included NPs from two pediatric hospitals (van Soeren, Hurlock-Chorostecki, & Reeves, 2011). Pediatric NPs reported that they spent 38% of their time in the clinical domain, but the majority of their time was spent in the consultation domain. Pediatric NPs reported working closely with the interprofessional team, physician collaborators, and specialists to provide care to vulnerable patient populations. Health care colleagues reported that NPs were approachable, provided continuity of care, and had a good knowledge of the patient with a deep understanding of their issues, which they were able to share with colleagues, patients, and their families. It was concluded that patient safety was improved because NPs were able to ensure that details of care were not missed. The majority of consultations by the NP were with physicians or nurses. Allied health care professionals, residents, specialty clinics, and other professionals accounted for the remainder of the NP consultations. The NP role supports communication among team members across health disciplines, which was appreciated by the other professionals. The pediatric NPs spent the remaining 20% of their time equally divided between the leadership, research, and other work categories.

As an example, a pediatric NP practicing in an in-patient oncology unit collaborates with an interprofessional team to provide care for a variety of oncology patients, including those newly diagnosed with cancer, receiving treatment, requiring supportive care, or receiving palliative care (Maloney & Volpe, 2005). Using the Strong Model of Advanced Practice Nursing (see Chapter 4), NP practice was described in the five domains of advanced nursing practice: direct comprehensive care, support of systems, education, research, and publication and professional leadership (Ackerman, Norsen, Martin, Wiedrich, & Kitzman, 1996). In addition to direct patient care, the NPs provide nursing advocacy, collaborate on multidisciplinary research, and contribute to quality improvement initiatives.

In a survey that examined the role function of advanced practice nurses (APN) in a tertiary pediatric centre, 80% were working in NP or CNS/NP roles (Kotzer, 2005). Their practice primarily provided care to patients at risk for significant health problems, with most patients having a chronic health problem. Approximately three-quarters of their patients often or sometimes had acute health conditions. Patient education, guidance and counselling, assessment, diagnosis, and development of a treatment plan were the direct patient care functions most often performed in this group. Consultation with other health professionals was the coordination task most commonly identified by APNs to be part of their role. Ninety-five percent of respondents stated that they sometimes or often incorporated research findings into their practice.

The NP role in a level II pediatric trauma management unit was implemented to improve the emergency department (ED) length of stay, with the goal that patients would be discharged from the ED or admitted to the hospital within three hours of arrival (McManawy & Drewes, 2010). The role of pediatric NPs in a pre-operative setting was examined by Frisch, Johnson, Timmons, and Weatherford (2010), who found that NPs were associated with improved patient satisfaction, decreased pre-operative assessment time, decreased operating room delays, and cost savings for the institution. Another review of the role of NPs in the pre-operative setting identified pre-operative education of patients and their family as an integral part of the NP role (Frisch et al., 2010).

Pediatric NPs provide education to patients, families, students, and staff as part of their role (Maloney & Volpe, 2005; McCarty & Rogers, 2012). NPs educate patients and families, nurses, residents, and fellows; precept graduate nursing students; and provide guest lectures at their local school of nursing. In one hospital, NPs direct an in-patient asthma education program, promoting self-management by patients and their parents (McCarty & Rogers, 2012). In addition to teaching individual patients and families, they provide group education to families. Education to health care staff is provided in both formal and informal settings. The NPs' expertise supplements the day-to-day care of the patient by RNs and medical trainees.

Family-Centred Care

Family-centred care provides an approach to health care that incorporates the needs and wishes of both the patient and their family members. Pediatric health care centres work with both the patients and their families to address the health care needs of the patient. Decisions about the patient's diagnosis, workup, treatment, and overall plan impact not only the patient but their family unit as well. The pediatric NP works in a position where they can engage with the patient and the family to identify a plan of care that works best for the entire family. The NP forms a partnership with the patient and their caregivers to guide the patient's care. Health care planning, delivery, and evaluation are performed in collaboration with patients, families, NPs, nurses, physicians, and other care providers (American Academy of Pediatrics, 2012). The care team takes into consideration the family's cultural, ethnic, and socioeconomic background when developing care plans for patients and their families.

Policies, procedures, and organizational practices need to factor in patients' and families' needs, beliefs, and cultural values. Patients and families should have all the information needed to effectively participate in care and decision-making, and they should be able to choose their level of involvement. For hospitalized patients, the effective NP and team regularly communicate with the family so they are able to make informed decisions. Both formal and informal supports should be in place to help the child at all stages of development. Collaboration with patients and families should take place at all levels. Patient and family representatives should be involved in policy-making, committee work, and education, and should sit on advisory councils. Patients and families need to be empowered in order to participate in the care of the patient and contribute to decision-making. The pediatric NP must incorporate family-centred care into their practice by communicating regularly with the family and understanding their needs and concerns; they must also be able to provide this information to other health care team members and act as an advocate for the family.

CASE STUDY

The Story of Jamal

Chief Complaint: Jamal is a 12-year-old male with moderate persistent asthma. He was seen in the respirology clinic for follow-up evaluation after a recent emergency department (ED) visit for an acute asthma flare.

History of Present Illness: Two weeks prior to the ED visit, Jamal had a respiratory tract infection that lasted approximately seven days. He developed a cough on day two of the infection, which persisted after the other respiratory tract infection symptoms had resolved. The symptoms progressed and three days prior to his ED visit Jamal developed wheezing. He was unable to attend gym class and didn't want to participate in activities with his friends. He was using his rescue inhaler, salbutamol, several times per day and woke with nighttime symptoms on two occasions. Subsequently, Jamal presented to the ED with an acute asthma exacerbation.

In the ED, his RR was 36, HR 120. His O2 sats were 88% on room air. Peak expiratory flow was 60% of value expected for age. Jamal was treated with nebulized salbutamol, oxygen, and started on prednisone. His symptoms improved and he was discharged from the ED six hours later.

Past Medical History: Seasonal allergies, asthma, bronchiolitis at one year of age, and two previous ED visits for asthma flares in the past 10 months.

Social History: Lives with parents and six-year-old sister. Attends public school, and is in the sixth grade. Jamal has no pets.

Family History: Both parents and sister have atopic dermatitis; father has diagnosed asthma.

Physical Examination: HR 84, RR 22, BP 105/72, O2 sat 97% on room air. Chest has bilateral air entry to bases, with occasional expiratory wheeze. Remainder of exam within normal limits.

Pertinent Diagnostic Tests:
Chest X-ray: no consolidation, no evidence pneumonia.
Pulmonary Function Testing: FEV1 74%, FEV1/FVC 76%.

Allergies: Pollen, grass, dust, ragweed. No drug allergies.

Medications: Salbutamol 100 mcg/puff, one to two puffs, q4h prn; Fluticasone 100 mcg/puff, two puffs, bid; Prednisone 30 mg po for five days, day four of five.

Review of Systems: Occasional cough, which Jamal states is improving. No fever, no rhinorrhea. No shortness of breath. Able to walk and participate in after-school activities with friends. Fatigue experienced with sports, but improving. GI and GU normal. When reviewing medications, it is discovered that parents have recently allowed patient to take responsibility for his asthma medications. Jamal reports that he "usually" takes his fluticasone, but sometimes forgets. Despite being advised to continue with fluticasone while on prednisone, he has stopped.

Plan: Jamal is to return to the clinic in two weeks for follow-up assessment. At the end of this visit, Jamal's asthma action plan was reviewed with him and his parents. Repeat PFTs were ordered to be completed in three months once he had recovered from this exacerbation. The importance of not missing fluticasone doses was reinforced. The child life specialist was consulted and in discussion with Jamal and his parents, strategies were identified to improve medication compliance. In this case, Jamal continued to take responsibility for taking his medication and was provided a calendar to record his doses. His parents were to review the calendar daily with Jamal to ensure compliance. If he remembers all of his doses for a week, a reward has been identified to celebrate his success.

Transitioning From Pediatric to Adult Health Care

Many pediatric patients undergo several transitions in their health care experience. Transition, defined as the move from one level of health care to another, may occur at one or several time points. Successful transition may require advanced preparation and engagement of the patient, their family, and involved health care providers. Intervals for transitions include transition at diagnosis, from childhood to adolescence to young adulthood, from pediatric tertiary care to adult tertiary care, and from tertiary care to primary care. Pediatric NPs work with their patients to prepare them for these transition points. In order to ensure the successful transition of patients, the health care team requires a structured approach to the transition process (O'Sullivan-Oliveira, Fernandes, Borges, & Fishman, 2014). The developmental stage of the patient must be considered when implementing transition planning.

Children, adolescents, and young adults with chronic illness, or who have had childhood illnesses with potential for future complications as a result of the diagnosis or treatment, require preparation as they transition to adult care. Transition is the process of preparing adolescents and young adults for the move from one point in the health care system to another.

Clear goals on transition are needed to ensure the best outcomes for the patient (Moreno, 2013). This includes policies on the timing of transfer from the pediatric service, the preparation and education of the patient, and the integration of primary care providers in the transfer process. Pediatric NPs can participate in developing transition policies and programs, and engaging stakeholders in the process. As well, they can work with patients to ensure they have self-advocacy skills by providing the patient with education related to their treatment plan, its potential short- and long-term side effects, and the need for lifelong monitoring that facilitates the development of self-advocacy skills. When preparing a patient for transition from pediatrics, the NP participates in creating a summary of recommendations for the team taking on the care of the patient by engaging the patient, family, and primary care or adult care providers to ensure a successful transition.

Several factors need to be taken into consideration; these include timing the patient's needs, while also being flexible. The patient needs to understand their treatment plan, be aware of the risks for short- and long-term effects as a result of their disease and/or treatment, have the skills to manage their own health care, and understand the importance of lifelong risk-based monitoring (Wilkins, D'Agostino, Penney, Barr, & Nathan, 2014). The NP, in preparing the patient for transition, should assess the patient's capacity to engage in the process, including the patient's knowledge, skills/self-efficacy, beliefs and expectations, goals, relationships, and psychosocial functioning. The NP, in their encounters with the patient, should evaluate the patient's physical health and function, sexual/reproductive health, mental health, social competence, health behaviours, and health education (Nathan, Hayes-Lattin, Sisler, & Hudson, 2011).

Transition assessment tools should be implemented early in the patient's continuum of care and be reassessed at defined developmental time points (O'Sullivan-Oliveira et al., 2014). Psychosocial and transitional needs have to be factored in when deciding to transition a patient. The NP can play a role in alleviating parental and patient concerns around transition, developing institutional recommendations for transition, and providing the health care providers to whom the patient is being transitioned with relevant information on the patient, their management, and their treatment on follow-up recommendations. As well, they can work with their care team to develop transition guidelines and identify research priorities for the population. The NP can act as the liaison with the patient, the pediatric, and the adult service by identifying patient, family, and health care provider barriers, as well as act as facilitators to transition and create potential solutions (Jallkut & Allen, 2009). Anticipatory guidance should be used to engage the patient and to prepare them for the adult health care experience. The conversation should include a review of the patient's disease and treatment, discussion about career planning, lifestyle review, and care recommendations.

Conclusion

Pediatric NPs in Canada practice primarily in pediatric tertiary care centres. They practice as part of an interprofessional team in providing family-centred care to pediatric patients and their families. Pediatric NP roles require team engagement, role integration, and intention to be successfully implemented. The pediatric NP may be involved in the patient's care from diagnosis, throughout treatment, and to transition to adult or primary care. They provide education on illness, management, and best practices to patients, families, colleagues, and health care learners. They practice collaboratively with health care team members and consult with other health care professionals to ensure optimal pediatric patient care is provided.

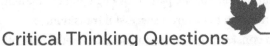

Critical Thinking Questions

1. A new NP role is being developed in a pediatric asthma clinic. What steps should be taken to ensure that the role is successfully implemented?
2. As a pediatric NP in a diabetes clinic, you see a 12-year-old patient with type I diabetes who admits that she doesn't always remember to check her blood glucose and give herself insulin before meals. How do you approach this problem and address it with the patient and her family?
3. You are seeing a 15-year-old male with hemophilia in the hematology clinic. What needs to be done to prepare the patient for transition to adult hematology service?

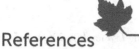

References

Ackerman, M.H., Norsen, L., Martin, B., Wiedrich, J., & Kitzman, H.J. (1996). Development of a model of advanced practice. *American Journal of Critical Care, 5*(1), 68–73.

American Academy of Pediatrics Committee on Hospital Care and Institute for Patient and Family-Centered Care. (2012). Policy statement: Patient- and family-centered care and the pediatrician's role. *Pediatrics, 129*(2), 393–404. doi: 10.1542/peds.2011-3084.

Canadian Nurses Association (CNA). (2010). *Canadian nurse practitioner core competency framework*. Ottawa, ON: CNA.

Frisch, A.M., Johnson, A., Timmons, S., & Weatherford, C. (2010). Nurse practitioner role in preparing families for pediatric outpatient surgery. *Pediatric Nursing, 36*(1), 41–47.

Hurlock-Chorostecki, C., van Soeren, M., & Goodwin, S. (2008). The acute care nurse practitioner in Ontario: A workforce study. *Nursing Leadership, 21*(4), 100–116.

Jalkut, M.K., & Allen, P.J. (2009). Transition from pediatric to adult health care for adolescents with congenital heart disease: A review of the literature and clinical implications. *Primary Care Approaches, 35*(6), 381–387.

Kaasalainen, S., Martin-Misener, R., Kilpatrick, K., Harbman, P., Bryant-Lukosius, D., Donald, F., … DiCenso, A. (2010). A historical overview of the development of advanced practice nursing roles in Canada. *Nursing Leadership, 23*(Special Issue December), 35–60.

Kilpatrick, K., Harbman, P., Carter, N., Martin-Misener, R., Bryant-Lukosius, D., Donald, F., … DiCenso, A. (2010). The acute care nurse practitioner role in Canada. *Nursing Leadership, 23*(Special Issue December), 114–139.

Kilpatrick, K., Lavoie-Tremblay, M., Lamothe, L., Ritchie, J.A., & Doran, D. (2013). Conceptual framework of acute care nurse practitioner role enactment, boundary work, and perceptions of team effectiveness. *Journal of Advanced Nursing, 69*(1), 205–217. doi: 10.1111/j.1365-2648.2012.06046.x

Kotzer, A.M. (2005). Characteristics and role functions of advanced practice nurses in a tertiary pediatric setting. *Journal for Specialists in Pediatric Nursing, 10*(1), 20–28.

Maloney, A.M., & Volpe, J. (2005). The inpatient advanced practice nursing roles in a Canadian pediatric oncology unit. *Journal of Pediatric Oncology Nursing, 22*(5), 254–257. doi: 10.1177/1043454205279290

McCarty, K., & Rogers, J. (2012). Inpatient asthma education program. *Pediatric Nursing, 38*(5), 257–263.

McManaway, C., & Drewes, B. (2010). The role of the nurse practitioner in level II trauma at Nationwide Children's Hospital. *Journal of Trauma Nursing, 17*(2), 82–84.

Nathan, P.C., Hayes-Lattin, B., Sisler, J.J., & Hudson, M.M. (2011). Critical issues in the transition and survivorship of adolescents and young adults with cancer. *Cancer, 117*(10 supplemental), 2335–2341.

Moreno, M.A. (2013). Transition of care from pediatric to adult clinics. *Journal of American Medical Association Pediatrics, 167*(7), 684. Retrieved from http://archpedi.jamanetwork.com/article.aspx?articleid=1703907. doi: 10.1001/jamapediatrics.2013.2657

O'Sullivan-Oliveira, J., Fernandes, S.M., Borges, L.F., & Fishman, L.N. (2014). Transition of pediatric patients to adult care: An analysis of provider perceptions across discipline and role. *Pediatric Nursing, 40*(3), 114–121.

Pringle, D. (2007). Nurse practitioner role: Nursing needs it. *Nursing Leadership, 20*(2), 1–5.

Sangster-Gormley, E., Martin-Misener, R., Downe-Wamboldt, B., & DiCenso, A. (2011). Factors affecting nurse practitioner role implementation in Canadian practice settings: An integrative review. *Journal of Advanced Nursing, 67*(6), 1178–1190.

Sidani, S., Irvine, D., Porter, H., O'Brien-Pallas, L., Simpson, B., McGillis Hall, L., … Redelmeir, D. (2000). Practice patterns of acute care nurse practitioners. *Nursing Leadership, 13*(3), 6–12. doi: 10.12927/cjnl.2000.1630

van Soeren, M., Hurlock-Chorostecki, C., & Reeves, S. (2011). The role of nurse practitioners in hospital settings: Implications for interprofessional practice. *Journal of Interprofessional Care, 25*(4), 245–251.

Wilkins, K.L., D'Agostino, N., Penney, A.M., Barr, R.D., & Nathan, P.C. (2014). Supporting adolescents and young adults with cancer through transitions: Position statement from the Canadian Task Force on adolescents and young adults with cancer. *Journal of Pediatric Hematology/Oncology, 36*(7), 545–551. doi: 10.1097/MPH.0000000000000103

Wilson, K. (2005). The evolution of the role of nurses: The history of nurse practitioners in pediatric oncology. *Journal of Pediatric Oncology Nursing, 22*(5), 250–253.

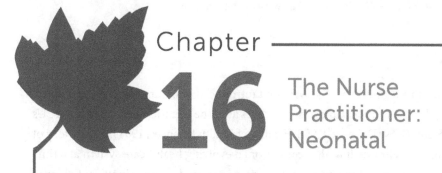

Chapter 16

The Nurse Practitioner: Neonatal

Marilyn Ballantyne, Mary McAllister, and Amanda Symington

Marilyn Ballantyne is an NP–Pediatrics and Chief Nurse Executive & Clinician Investigator at the Holland Bloorview Kids Rehabilitation Hospital in Toronto, Ontario. She has extensive clinical experience as an NP–Pediatrics in acute and outpatient settings. Marilyn has held academic positions at McMaster University in Hamilton, Ontario, the Lawrence S. Bloomberg Faculty of Nursing, University of Toronto in Toronto, Ontario, and clinical/research positions at SickKids Hospital in Toronto, Ontario.

Mary McAllister is the Associate Chief, Nursing Practice at SickKids in Toronto, Ontario. It was there she began her career and later acted as a CNS. Mary has held academic positions at Ryerson University, the Lawrence S. Bloomberg Faculty of Nursing, and the University of Toronto in Toronto, Ontario, and the Edith Cowan University School of Nursing in Perth, Australia. Mary has been actively involved in nursing professional organizations, contributing to advances in nursing practice, and being a champion for evidence-informed practice provincially, nationally, and internationally.

Amanda Symington is an NP–Pediatrics in the Neonatal Intensive Care Unit at McMaster Children's Hospital and Assistant Clinical Professor, McMaster University, School of Nursing in Hamilton, Ontario.

KEY TERMS

advanced practice nursing (APN)

clinical nurse specialist/nurse practitioner (CNS/NP)

expanded role nurse (ERN)

neonatal nurse practitioner (NNP)

OBJECTIVES

1. Summarize the historical development of the neonatal nurse practitioner (NNP) role in Canada.
2. Understand the evolution of NNP education.
3. Characterize the role, credentialing, and scope of practice of NNPs.
4. Examine the available evidence evaluating NNP impact.
5. Construct a vision for the future of NNPs in Canada.

Introduction

Neonatal nurse practitioners (NNPs) were first introduced into Canadian neonatal intensive care units (NICUs) in 1988, almost two decades after the role was introduced in NICUs in the United States (US) (DiCenso, 1998; Faculty of Health Sciences, 1991). The history of the NNP role offers a glimpse into the realities of an evolving health care system at a time when medical education and the health care system were undergoing significant change. This chapter explores the origins of the NNP role in Canada and its evolution, with emphasis on education, scope of practice, and evaluation.

Historical Development of the Neonatal Nurse Practitioner Role in Canada

While introduced in Canada later than in the US, the impetus for introducing the NNP role into tertiary-level NICUs was similar on both sides of the border. Proposed changes in medical education would result in reductions in the number of funded pediatric trainees who traditionally rotated through NICUs and provided care to critically ill and premature newborns (Faculty of Health Sciences, 1991; Honeyfield, 2009). Given this emerging reality, the Ontario Minister of Health asked the Ontario Council of Administrators of Teaching Hospitals (OCATH) and the Council of Ontario Faculties of Medicine (COFN) to explore resident alternatives for teaching hospitals. A neonatal subcommittee was established to consider two alternatives: an expanded nursing role and a physician assistant role. The subcommittee agreed that nurses, with appropriate preparation, would be well positioned to assume responsibilities traditionally designated to pediatric residents; this decision was consistent with the College of Nurses of Ontario's (CNO) position. Introduction of physician assistants at that time was viewed as costly duplication of education and services, with the potential for fragmentation in care and potential role confusion and overlap among care providers (Faculty of Health Sciences, 1991; School of Nursing, McMaster University, 1987). The Ontario Ministry of Health subsequently funded a pilot project to study the need for nurses in an expanded role to fill service gaps in tertiary-level care.

The feasibility of the development and implementation of an **expanded role nurse (ERN)** in Ontario NICUs, funded by the Ontario Ministry of Health, was explored by a team of researchers from McMaster University in Hamilton, Ontario (Mitchell, Pinelli, Patterson, & Southwell, 1993; School of Nursing, McMaster University, 1987). Broad consultation with key stakeholders ($n = 655$) was completed, including surveying post-graduate residency program directors in Ontario as well as all Ontario tertiary-level NICU medical directors and nursing leaders. Surveys were also sent to Alberta as they were exploring NNP roles as alternatives to resident care in NICUs, and to established US centres. The results of these surveys informed the decision to develop the NNP role, indicating that workload in NICUs exceeded medical staff availability and there was an openness to pursue an expanded nursing role as a suitable alternative to resident care (Paes et al., 1989). Key stakeholders envisioned a professional role that included high levels of technical expertise, autonomous decision-making, and leadership skills. In the US, NNPs were already assuming responsibility for the care of a caseload of infants, as well as having educational, research, and leadership responsibilities. This stakeholder consultation led to the definition of a new nursing role to be deployed in Ontario NICUs (Faculty of Health Sciences, 1991; Hunsberger et al., 1992; School of Nursing, McMaster University, 1987).

The nature of the ERN role was explored and defined in an early, unpublished background paper (School of Nursing, McMaster University, 1987) and careful attention was paid to the characteristics of basic, extended, and expanded nursing practice. At the time, basic nursing practice was characterized as diploma or bachelor's educational preparation and possession of generalist skills. Extended nursing practice included the same basic educational preparation with the addition of specialty preparation (formal or informal) in a specific practice area. Extended nursing practice was described as incorporating specific skills, some of which might be seen as traditionally performed by other disciplines. Expanded nursing practice was differentiated from basic practice by requiring a graduate degree in nursing, and was characterized by expertise in a clinical nursing specialty with knowledge and skills grounded in theory and research. The attributes of the expanded role nurse were consistent with those of **advanced practice nursing (APN)** roles. Given the experiences of the US, and to be consistent with the findings of the stakeholder analysis and the review of the levels of nursing practice, it was agreed that the proposed ERNs be prepared at the graduate level, in alignment with the role definition of an APN (Faculty of Health Sciences, 1991; McAllister et al., 1993; School of Nursing, McMaster University, 1987).

To prepare for the first graduates of McMaster University's ERN program, regulatory organizations were required to review specific delegated medical acts that this new type of clinician would require authorization to perform (e.g., endotracheal intubation, umbilical arterial and venous line insertion, lumbar puncture). The Advisory Committee on Special Procedures of the College of Physicians and Surgeons, with membership from the CNO, the Registered Nurses' Association of Ontario (RNAO), Ontario Medical Association (OMA), and Ontario Hospital Association (OHA), reviewed and approved the delegation of these specific acts to neonatal ERNs. Later, as roles proliferated in other acute care environments and with the proclamation of the Regulated Health Professions Act (1991) in Ontario as a new regulatory framework, medical directives were used as the mechanism to authorize qualified clinicians to perform controlled acts considered outside their discipline-specific scope of practice.

Once the NICU ERN role was implemented, clinicians, regulators, and professional association representatives began work to regulate this new APN role. As other acute care nurse practitioner (ACNP) roles were introduced, more attention was paid to the development of regulation to authorize the full scope of nurse practitioner practice across all specialties, beginning with the practice of primary health care NPs (PHCNPs) and then those practicing with specific populations.

By the time the first three graduates completed their graduate program (1988) at McMaster University, the role had been renamed **clinical nurse specialist/nurse practitioner (CNS/NP)**. These graduate-prepared clinicians pioneered this new, expanded neonatal nursing role in three Ontario tertiary NICUs with a vision of developing a clinical leadership role. As the program continued, the number of graduates increased, and by 1992 there were 15 CNS/NPs practicing in five Ontario NICUs and related practice environments (e.g., neonatal follow-up programs) (Hunsberger et al., 1992). By 1989, interest in this advanced nursing practice role was emerging in other parts of the country, with Alberta and Manitoba establishing their first positions at that time (Evanochko, 2011). Other parts of the country, including Nova Scotia and Quebec, followed suit, piloting the development and integration of this expanded nursing role in NICUs.

However, a discussion of the history of the NNP role in Canada would not be complete without acknowledging a controversy that emerged along the way. In its early iterations, the ERN role was described by some as an assistant to physicians. Expanding the scope of nursing practice was conceptualized by some authors as taking on medically delegated tasks and they questioned the need for nurses to assume such tasks when there seemed to be no shortage of physicians in Canada (Mitchell & Santapinto, 1988). These authors concluded that the ERN concept did not represent the advancement of nursing, rather the extension into medicine, thus diluting nursing impact with medical model–dependent practice. Those opposed to the ERN suggested that it was not necessary for nursing to own the problems arising from medical residency shortages (Mitchell & Santapinto, 1988). Those practicing in expanded roles offered a different perspective, presenting the development of the ERN as an opportunity to enhance the nursing role in order to improve the quality of patient care. The role was presented as holistic, complementary, and capable of advancing the profession of nursing, encompassing clinical care, education, and research responsibilities (Rubin, 1988).

A final historical focus is that of funding for this new role. In Ontario, the provincial Ministry of Health provided funding for the establishment of the first neonatal ERN positions. This allowed employing organizations to embed the role in their structures and provided a unique opportunity to evaluate the impact of the role in practice settings (Mitchell et al., 1993). However, over time and as NNP teams were established, the responsibility for securing funding to employ additional NPs has been borne by NICUs. Presently, hospitals employing NNPs are required to source funding from within their allocated budgets. This can be challenging given the large number of competing financial and clinical priorities faced by hospitals.

Evolution of Neonatal Nurse Practitioner Education in Canada

In the 1970s, hospital-based "in-house training" programs were developed in the US in response to the urgent need in neonatology for expanded nursing roles. Over time, the need for a more standardized approach to nursing education became apparent. Hospital-specific neonatal education lacked connection with university programs in nursing that created barriers for nursing mobility and career advancement. Preparation at the graduate level was increasingly viewed as essential to achieve the level of standardization and in-depth knowledge and skills required for expanded nursing practice in an academic interprofessional NICU context. Highly influential was the concurrent success of graduate-level NNP education in the US, programs that started in the early 1970s. The appropriateness of the NNP role for academically prepared nurses was controversial. NNP education was viewed as moving away from nursing core curricula to embrace the medical model. Graduate nursing education traditionally grounded in administration, education, and research was evolving to include advanced practice nursing curricula to the exclusion of NP-specific content.

In Canada, a multidisciplinary group at McMaster University conducted an initial feasibility study that verified the need for expanded role neonatal nurses in Ontario (Paes et al., 1989; Hunsberger et al., 1992). The program admission criteria, program objectives, course descriptions and content, educational resources, length of program, supervision, and staffing were developed based on the findings of the interprofessional role definition study (Hunsberger et al., 1992) and through faculty consultation, surveys, and site visits to existing graduate-level NNP programs in the US. Graduate-level education prepared NNPs for clinical practice with knowledge based on theories, concepts, and research, and facilitated the development of leadership, education, and research skills.

In 1986, McMaster University launched the first graduate-level program to prepare advanced neonatal nurses in Canada. The neonatal stream was incorporated into the existing 16-month Master of Health Sciences (MHSc) degree program. The neonatal component included 600 hours of theory-specific problem-based tutorials and 720 hours of supervised clinical practice. The course content included advanced physical assessment, diagnostic reasoning, therapeutic management, pharmacology, and pathophysiology. In 1994, the program was integrated into the new thesis-based Master of Science (MSc) program. In 1997, McMaster University recognized the neonatal courses as highly specialized and approved the creation of a separate Graduate Diploma in Advanced Neonatal Nursing (ANN). The program length was 10 months and included three theory-specific courses and 720 hours of clinical practice. To enrol in the Graduate Diploma program, students required a graduate degree in nursing or near completion of a graduate degree. In 2011, McMaster University began to offer the program via distance education to increase access to students from across

Ontario and other provinces. Education was offered using a hybrid format of synchronous on-campus and off-campus problem-based learning via web-conferencing, three innovative one-week residency periods, clinical practica completed at home, and NICU sites with local qualified NNP preceptors.

The education program for advanced neonatal nursing founded at McMaster University was evaluated extensively. Mitchell and colleagues demonstrated in a before/after study that graduating NNPs from the first three programs (1987 to 1989) acquired the expected competencies and scored higher than first year students and scored similarly in a cohort study with pediatric residents on knowledge, problem solving, examination, communications, and clinical skills in the NICU (Mitchell et al., 1995; Mitchell et al., 1991). The positive findings validated the educational preparation of NNPs that ultimately led to the expansion of programs across Canada and set the foundation for the subsequent successful establishment of acute care advanced practice NP education in pediatrics and adults (Mitchell et al., 1995). Table 16.1 provides an overview of Canadian NNP programs, program status, and number of graduates since inception.

In Alberta, the first NNP education program was established in 1992 as a certificate of Advanced Neonatal Nursing Practice at the University of Alberta. The certificate program courses were offered in addition to the required Master of Nursing (MN) degree courses and thesis. The NNP courses included pathophysiology and clinical management curricula

TABLE 16.1: Canadian Neonatal Nurse Practitioner Programs

University Name and Location	Year of Program Start	Program Status	Type of Program	Length of Program	Number of Graduates n = 121
McMaster University Hamilton, Ontario	1986	Active*	Post MSc diploma	Full-time, 10 months	75
University of Alberta Edmonton, Alberta	1992	Closed 2012	MN	Full-time, 2 years	27
			Post-MN	1 year	
Dalhousie University Halifax, Nova Scotia	1998	Not active	MN	Full-time, 2 years	7
McGill University Montreal, Quebec	2004	Active	MSc(A) and Diploma	Full-time, 2.5 years	12
			Post-graduate certificate	11 months	

MSc = Master of Science; MSc(A) = Master of Science in Nursing (Applied); MN = Master of Nursing

Note: *No intake in 2014/2015, 2015/2016, and 2016/2017 academic years due to low enrolment numbers.

and 600 hours of supervised clinical practice. The overall program length was two full years plus thesis. The program changed in 1996 to a course- or thesis-based MN in Advanced Nursing Practice degree including three NNP-specific pathophysiology, advanced physical assessment, and clinical management courses and 800 hours of clinical practice. The overall program length was two years including the MN courses. In addition, a post-MN option was offered that included the same courses completed over a one-year period. In 2012, the University of Alberta program closed due to low student enrolment (Evanochko, 2015).

In Nova Scotia, the first NNP program was established in 1998 through the Dalhousie University School of Nursing's Master of Nursing program. The program length was two years with 760 clinical practice hours. The MN with integrated NNP courses was offered twice in response to the health human resources needs in the NICU at the affiliated IWK Health Centre. The program is currently inactive (M. Campbell-Yeo, personal communication, March 12, 2015).

In Quebec, the first NNP education program started in 2004 at McGill University's Ingram School of Nursing. Students complete the non-thesis Master of Science in Nursing (applied; MSc[A]) degree over a one and one-half year period followed by a Graduate Diploma in Neonatology. The MSc(A) program consists of 45 credits (21 of 45 credits are neonatal-specific courses) and a clinical internship. The diploma program includes 30 credits with additional pathophysiology content and clinical internship. Overall, the combined master's and diploma program is completed over a two-and-a-half year period with 75 credits and 1,100 clinical practice hours. McGill offers the option of a post-master's certificate in the theory of neonatology. Once completed, students transition to complete the diploma program. The McGill program curriculum extends beyond the NICU to include antenatal consultation and neonatal follow-up care (L. Morneault, personal communication, March 11, 2015).

Since 2010, there has been a steady decline in the number of available and active Canadian NNP education programs (see Table 16.1). Some programs run every other year during periods of low enrolment and/or fiscal restraint. For the 2014 to 2015 academic year, the McGill NNP program is the only active program. There is a similar trend reported in the US of a declining number of NNP education programs and concurrent decline in the number of new NNPs entering practice based on the annual survey results of NNP program directors (Bellini, 2013). Since 2005, a total of 19 US NNP programs have closed, and, since 2012, the number of online programs has decreased by 10% (Bellini, 2013). Overall, the number of NNPs graduating from US programs has decreased by 23% over a five-year period (2009 to 2013). At the same time, both in Canada and the US, the demand for NNPs has grown due to increasing NICU admissions per year, expanded bed capacity, and the aging of the current NNP workforce.

To address the emerging gap in the supply and demand of NNPs, McMaster University conducted an education needs survey of Canadian tertiary care NICUs (94% response rate) in June 2014 (Ballantyne, 2014). Respondents indicated that 40 full-time NNPs will be needed, taking the current clinical activities, total volume of patients, staffing patterns, and impending retirements into consideration. At the time of the survey, 79% of the NICUs indicated that the current numbers of NNPs were not sufficient to provide service needs and 57% reported vacant NNP positions. Furthermore, one-third of the existing national NNP workforce reported they intend to retire over the next 10-year period (11 within zero to three years; 10 within three to six years; and 9 within seven to ten years). Should education programs continue to decline, the supply of new NNP graduates will not adequately meet the emerging needs for new NNPs.

As of March 2015, there were 109 NNPs working in neonatology (Level 3 NICU, Level 2, and Neonatal Follow-up) in seven provinces across Canada. There are 21 in Alberta, 6 in Saskatchewan, 3 in Manitoba, 54 in Ontario, 16 in Quebec, 8 in Nova Scotia, and 1 in Newfoundland. NPs in the neonatal specialty represent approximately 3% of the estimated 3,655 NPs working in Canada in 2013 (CIHI, 2013).

Titling, Scope of Practice, and Credentialing

Titling and Scope of Practice

Even though they completed an ERN program, the first graduates from McMaster University were never called ERNs but rather clinical nurse specialist/nurse practitioners (CNS/NP). Graduate preparation, while still controversial, was deemed necessary in order to develop advanced practitioners who were able to make autonomous decisions in the care of critically ill newborns and their families (Mitchell et al., 1993).

At that time, graduate-prepared nurses who focused on advancing clinical practice, predominantly in acute care, were employed as CNSs. While there were similarities between the CNS and the new CNS/NP roles, there were also differences. Both CNSs and CNS/NPs were expected to generate and use research and incorporate clinical practice, consultation, education, and leadership activities. However, while the CNS scope of practice focused on improving patient care in an issue-driven way (e.g., focusing on improvement of pain management for a patient population), CNS/NPs were expected to provide and manage patient care and had a population-driven clinical practice (e.g., providing comprehensive care for specific patients). Both roles incorporated expanded nursing knowledge and skills and leadership responsibilities, but this new neonatal role also included extended knowledge and skills (e.g., medical diagnosis, prescriptive authority) (Pinelli, 1997; Wright, 1997). The CNS has always been identified as an APN role and, as the CNS/NP in neonatology incorporated the three essential elements that characterized advanced nursing practice, including graduate education, client focus, and specialized knowledge and skills within a clinical specialty, it was deemed an APN role (Giovannetti, Tenove, Stuart, & van den Berg, 1996).

The merged role of CNS/NP has been controversial and the analysis has featured prominently in the literature (Kaasalainen et al., 2010). Fenton and Brykczynski (1993) reported three distinct perspectives regarding the education of CNSs and NPs. The first advocated merging the roles, a second suggested that they be kept separate, and a third proposed that core educational content become the basis for both roles with distinct content focusing on role-specific knowledge and skill development. While the analysis of the merged CNS/ NP role was presented long after the title was used for the new neonatal role, the third perspective reflects the intention at the time the McMaster University curriculum was developed. The CNS/NP title acknowledges shared and unique competencies, as well as the core characteristics of an APN role (Pinelli, 1997).

Given the deliberate adoption of the CNS/NP title, early position descriptions reflected the current role domains characteristic of advanced nursing practice: clinical practice, education, research, consultation, and leadership. These new neonatal clinicians used "advanced knowledge and skills to ensure optimal care to high-risk neonates and their families in collaboration with the health care team" (The Hospital for Sick Children, 1987, p. 1).

In their clinical role, they assumed responsibility for managing the care of neonates and their families from admission to discharge, including neonatal and delivery room issues, infant resuscitation, and assessment and initiation of diagnostic investigations and therapies, in collaboration with a neonatologist. Initially, controlled acts traditionally authorized to physicians were delegated to CNS/NPs but supervision was required before these acts could be performed independently. These controlled acts included making a medical diagnosis, ordering medications, performing procedures such as intubations, lumbar punctures, and insertion of chest drains (Mitchell et al., 1991; DiCenso, 1998). In addition, all diagnostic and treatment orders required co-signature by a physician. Despite these restrictions, these early clinicians evolved a role that offered care that was provided by traditional clinicians such as clinical nurses and physicians (Canada West Foundation, 1998). They spent 80% of their time in clinical care, and established themselves as leaders in advancing clinical care and quality improvement and research (DiCenso, 1998). They practice in a variety of practice sites focusing on neonatal care, including NICUs, level II neonatal units, neonatal follow-up clinics, and even breastfeeding support services. Currently, credentialed NNPs no longer require authorization mechanisms for many aspects of care management, including communicating a diagnosis, ordering diagnostic investigations, and prescribing medications and other treatment options.

As APNs, neonatal CNS/NPs were viewed as mentors and role models by front-line nursing colleagues and they collaborated with other nursing leaders to provide leadership, and support and encouragement for nurses' development. Their consultation role often involved responding to requests from within their organizations, or to those from external organizations or the community, for information about the specialized needs of neonates. Their research role included critical appraisal of evidence as it related to clinical decision-making, identifying researchable questions, and participating or leading research teams. Leadership responsibilities included the development of policies and procedures to guide practice, as well as participating in or leading quality improvement initiatives (Mitchell-DiCenso, Pinelli, & Southwell, 1996).

As the CNS/NP role was established as an advanced role in nursing, their position within hiring organizations reflected their nursing roots. From the first introduction of the role, neonatal CNS/NPs were hired as APNs, reporting directly to a senior nursing leader (Director, Chief Nursing Officer, etc.) for professional practice with a matrix reporting line to neonatal medicine for the medical dimensions of their role. This reporting structure has been implemented consistently across Canada, a role feature that differentiates it from similar roles in the US where approximately half of the NNP respondents to a survey stated they reported directly to medicine (Ruth-Sanchez, Lee, & Bosque, 1996; Samson, 2006). Medical recognition of the importance and complementary nature of APN roles in neonatal care was galvanized in 2000 with the publication of a position statement by the Canadian Paediatric Society (CPS) (Fetus and Newborn Committee, 2000). Reaffirmed by CPS in 2001, this statement offers strong support for the continued development and implementation of APN roles at the graduate level to support the provision of care for critically ill newborns and their families.

As NPs became increasingly well recognized in the health care system and regulated as legitimate health care providers across Canada, the merged role title of CNS/NP faded and NPs practicing in the neonatal field transitioned to the title of NNP, the same title used for many years in the US. The roles and responsibilities of these advanced clinicians continue to evolve, in alignment with the establishment of national advanced nursing practice frameworks and standards (CNA, 2008, 2010).

Credentialing

In Ontario, the CNS/NP title was used for approximately 10 years, when, as a result of changes to provincial legislation, the scope of practice of NPs was defined (Nurse Practitioners Association of Ontario [NPAO], n.d.). In keeping with the early evolution of NP roles, PHCNPs were the first to be regulated, but that left practicing NNPs in regulatory limbo, requiring the use of physician-approved medical directives to authorize their practice. In Alberta, legislative changes to authorize NP practice were proclaimed in 2000, including NP title protection, but regulations for the Child (Neonatal Specialty) stream were not introduced until 2004 (College and Association of Registered Nurses of Alberta [CARNA], 2011). It wasn't until 2008 when NP title protection was enacted in Ontario and three streams of NPs (Primary Health Care, Adult, and Pediatrics) now qualified for registration in the extended class (EC). While a positive step forward, title protection left practicing NNPs unable to use the NP title while pursuing new and unclear regulatory requirements to be credentialed and recognized as NPs in a subspecialty of pediatrics (NPAO, n.d.). Initially, NPs practicing in neonatology had several examination options to be credentialed provincially, but in 2010, when the National Certification Corporation in the US no longer allowed Canadian educated neonatal NPs access to their NNP examination, a made-in-Canada alternative was sought. As of 2015, the only examination available to credential NNP program graduates is offered in Quebec by the Ordre des Infirmières et Infirmiers du Québec (OIIQ) on a limited basis and it has not been deemed a national examination. This reality has the potential to limit the availability of credentialed NNPs in the future.

Evaluation of the Neonatal Nurse Practitioner Role in Canada

The introduction of the NNP role was comprehensively evaluated in Canada. A prospective randomized controlled trial (RCT) was conducted by Mitchell-DiCenso and colleagues to determine safety and effectiveness, quality of care, satisfaction with care, and associated costs of the role (Mitchell-DiCenso et al., 1996). All infants admitted to the tertiary-level NICU at McMaster Children's Hospital ($n = 821$ infants) over a one year period were randomized to care by an NNP ($n = 414$) or a pediatric resident ($n = 407$) team. The study findings indicated that NNP care met practice standards and was equivalent to pediatric resident care on all measures of performance including neonatal mortality, morbidity, length of stay, quality of care, parent satisfaction, long-term developmental outcomes, and costs (Mitchell-DiCenso et al., 1996). NNPs scored significantly better in two of seven quality-of-care indicators for documentation and the care of neonates with jaundice. Neonatologists reported statistically lower time spent with NNPs than residents. Staff nurses reported overall increased job satisfaction and an increased sense of autonomy, as well as increased participation in decision-making with NNP care (Mitchell-DiCenso et al., 1996). US-based studies using less rigorous research designs (e.g., retrospective chart review) similarly found that NNPs provided safe, cost-effective, and equivalent to or superior quality of care as compared to pediatric residents (Aubrey & Yoxall, 2001; Bissinger, Allred, Arford, & Bellig, 1997; Carzoli, Martinez-Cruz, Cuevas, Murphy, & Chiu, 1994; Karlowicz & McMurray, 2000; Schultz, Liptak, & Fioravanti, 1994). To date, the study conducted by Mitchell-DiCenso and colleagues is the only clinical trial to validate the NNP role in tertiary-level NICUs (Donald et al., 2014). The findings from the NNP comparison studies are remarkably consistent with the broader NP literature that has demonstrated no difference in health outcomes of patients across the lifespan with NP care as compared to physician care (ibid.).

Future research is needed to ascertain the "current state" of NNPs' contributions, quality of care, and cost-effectiveness. The initial trial was conducted when the NNPs were still in the novice phase of their roles and development (i.e., one to three years post-graduation). A similar study done today, when many of the NNPs have more than 20 years of practice experience, would capture the richness of their expertise and highlight their unique role in comparison to any other health care providers in the NICU.

Future Implications

The NNP role has been effectively integrated into the Canadian health care system for almost three decades, despite its controversial start. However, if this important and effective clinical role is to be sustained in current and future health care systems, there are a number of issues that must be considered, including supply and demand, credentialing, access to education programs, role satisfaction, role effectiveness, and, ultimately, role sustainability.

NNP supply and demand has been identified as an issue throughout the role's history and is multi-faceted in nature (Honeyfield, 2009). Quantifying the number of practicing NNPs, unfilled NNP positions, and NNPs joining and leaving the workforce in a given year is challenging. In Canada, we have not explored these issues consistently and, with regulation being a provincial jurisdiction, the task is even more complicated. However, anecdotally we know that many of the NNPs who pioneered this role beginning in the late 1980s and early 1990s are still practicing, meaning that the average age of NNPs is likely rising, a reality similar to that of the US (Honeyfield, 2009).

The demand for NNPs persists as NICUs continue to provide care to smaller and more critically ill infants and their families. Recruitment, education, and credentialing of NNPs are influenced by provincial funding; provincial and organizational priorities; availability of seats in education programs; accessibility of credentialing processes that accurately reflect the knowledge, skills, and abilities of entry-level NNPs; and acceptance of the role in the clinical environment. As most nurses now enter the profession with an undergraduate nursing degree, the pool of nurses qualified to enter a graduate NNP program is large. However, nurses who choose to pursue this career path must see that there are employment opportunities for them. Many have been positively influenced by their experiences working with NNPs and see the role as an opportunity to remain directly involved in clinical care, while also developing their leadership abilities as an APN.

Credentialing issues require attention and NNPs must be considered as part of the national NP workforce. While NPs are regulated provincially, a national body, the Canadian Council of Registered Nurse Regulators (CCRNR), began an analysis of NP entry to practice knowledge, skills, and abilities for all three NP categories: Family/All Ages, Adult, and Pediatrics (CCRNR, 2013). While NNPs are registered or licensed in a pediatric or child category, there is a risk that, given NNPs' sub-specialized clinical practice, they will not be included as CCRNR develops a national examination and credentialing strategy. As of 2015, the exam offered by OIIQ in Quebec is the only examination available to credential graduates from Canadian NNP education programs. As this examination was not developed as a national examination, it is essential that the credentialing of NNPs be considered within the national NP practice review process. Failure to do so may reduce credentialing options and further reduce the supply of NNPs to meet a sustained and even increasing need for these specialized APNs.

Access to education programs is also important to consider. As described earlier, there are currently only two active programs preparing NNPs in Canada. Graduates of US programs can apply to have their credentials reviewed at the provincial level, but completion of a US program doesn't expose graduates to issues relevant to the Canadian context. Given the ongoing supply and demand issues, the availability of NNP education programs must be closely monitored and assessed on a regular basis to ensure there are enough seats to meet the demand for this role.

A reduced supply of NNPs may also be a stimulus for organizations to look at other roles to address their NICU human resource needs. Physician assistants (PAs) have been introduced in several provinces and their numbers are growing, although they are not currently practicing in NICUs in Canada. US sources report that some NICUs have explored PA or pediatric hospitalist models, but the majority continue to seek NNPs to support their human resource strategy (Honeyfield, 2009). Given that these alternatives were considered when the NNP role was first established, it may seem unlikely that these options would be pursued, but attention must be paid to the possibility.

The NNP role has evolved as a full advanced practice role with the majority of the NNP's time focused on direct clinical practice. However, there is a clear expectation from NNPs and employers alike that NNPs actively engage in activities that reflect all elements of advanced nursing practice. Most NNPs have approximately 20% of their time allocated to these other dimensions of the role. However, when there are staff shortages or surges in patient census, this time can shrink, compromising NNP impact as nursing leaders who are charged with advancing quality improvement initiatives, leading research, teaching, and mentoring. This can lead to frustration on the part of NNPs because they are unable to achieve broader professional goals. As well, the talents and expertise of these advanced clinicians may not be leveraged and their impact may not be maximized.

With respect to NNP effectiveness, well-designed Canadian studies have confirmed that NNPs are safe and effective care providers in NICUs. However, there are opportunities to continue to evaluate the current impact of this role. Given recent attention to lengths of stay, patient safety, quality, and hospital-acquired conditions (such as central line–associated infections), NNPs can consider how they might collaborate to evaluate their impact on patient outcomes. Nurse-sensitive outcomes, such as readiness for discharge, might be explored to further substantiate the value NNPs bring to the care of critically ill newborns and their families. There may also be opportunities to align NNP research and evaluation efforts with the priorities of clinical programs and organizations, strengthening interprofessional collaborative efforts.

The NNP role has been well established and sustained for almost 30 years in the majority of Canadian provinces, but it cannot be assumed that its sustainability is guaranteed. While the role is thriving across the country and these neonatal nursing leaders are well respected and valued in their regions, there may be value in developing a national community of practice for NNPs so that they can share innovative practices, research, patient safety initiatives, recruitment/retention efforts, and their collective wisdom in order to strengthen the NNP presence nationally. The power of the NNP collective could be leveraged to advance the role further and cement it within the health care system.

CASE STUDY

The Story of Jonathan

Jonathan, a twin, was born at 27 weeks gestation to Mrs. G, a 32-year-old G4P0 mother. Jonathan received surfactant at birth, and then required positive pressure ventilation to support his respiratory status. His sister, Emily, also received surfactant and required a short period of positive pressure ventilation, but quickly weaned to non-invasive ventilation. Upon admission, both Jonathan and Emily were admitted to the neonatal nurse practitioner (NNP) team in the Neonatal Intensive Care Unit (NICU).

Shortly after their admission, the admitting NNP met with the twins' parents. The NNP confirmed the antenatal and perinatal history with them, explained what they might expect during the twins' first few days of life, and answered the parents' questions. The NNP also asked them how they had planned to feed the twins, discussing the advantages of providing breast milk. Mr. and Mrs. G told the NNP that they planned to breastfeed. As the twins were not able to do so immediately, Mrs. G was anxious to get started with milk expression. The NNP introduced Mr. and Mrs. G to one of the NICU's breastfeeding nurse champions, who accompanied them to a private room, and oriented them to the breast pump so they could get started with milk expression.

Over the next few weeks of life, Emily continued to do well with non-invasive ventilation but Jonathan continued to require significant oxygen and ventilator support. He experienced many desaturation and bradycardic episodes, requiring frequent adjustments in his oxygen. Jonathan's mother was very worried about him, and talked to the NNP about her concerns. She didn't understand why Emily was doing so well while Jonathan was having such trouble. The NNP listened to Mrs. G's concerns, completed a thorough physical assessment, reviewed all of Jonathan's recent investigations and clinical data, and then sat down to discuss Jonathan's care with her.

Given Jonathan's evolving chronic lung disease, and his labile respiratory status, the NNP decided to discuss a trial of diuretics to target his chronic lung disease. With the intent to partner with Mrs. G in treatment planning, the NNP outlined how a three-day course of furosemide might help to clear excess fluid in Jonathan's lungs, and possibly reduce his need for oxygen and ventilator support. The NNP asked Mrs. G what she thought about this option; Mrs. G seemed surprised by this question, and then asked the NNP what they thought. The NNP described the benefits and risks associated with the treatment option. The NNP also discussed how they would know if the strategy was effective for Jonathan, specifically by seeing that his oxygen requirements would stabilize and/or decrease, resulting in a decrease in ventilator support and fewer desaturation and bradycardic episodes. After thoughtful consideration Mrs. G agreed that they should try the course of furosemide, and the NNP wrote the orders for the three-day course at 2 mg/kg/day.

The next day, while the NNP was making rounds on the patients in their care, they met a very excited Mrs. G in the hall who stated that she thought the furosemide was working, that Jonathan had experienced far fewer desaturation and bradycardic episodes overnight, his oxygen had come down by 10%, and his ventilator rate had also been reduced. The NNP was enthusiastic when they told Mrs. G that this sounded very positive and that they would come and see Jonathan shortly. The NNP reflected on the partnership that they had cultivated between themselves and Mrs. G, and was pleased that Jonathan had a solid team of nurses, respiratory therapists, physicians, NPs, and his parents on his side, monitoring his response to the treatment plan, so that the best decisions could be made to support him in his recovery.

Conclusion

In summary, the NNP role has been a positive addition to the Canadian health care system, emerging at a time when changes were being made within the medical education system. The development of the role was done in a thoughtful and planned way, ensuring that key stakeholders were engaged. The number of NNPs deployed in NICUs and related clinical environments has grown steadily, their effectiveness has been confirmed, and professional organizations have published position statements that advocate for the role in practice settings. Access to education programs and appropriate national credentialing standards are recent challenges that must be addressed. However, the NNP role was the right role at the right time, providing care to the right population in the right way and, today, it continues to be an essential advanced nursing practice role across the country. These nursing leaders will continue to be intellectually curious, creative, and courageous as they solidify this role within the national health care landscape.

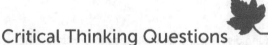

Critical Thinking Questions

1. What factors should be considered when deciding how to address a gap in clinical care, and what type of role might best address the gap?
2. When considering the CNS and NP roles, what are the advantages and disadvantages of a merged CNS/NP role?
3. What are the barriers and facilitators that influence the successful integration of a new role in health care?
4. Is graduate preparation necessary to provide care to critically ill newborns? Why or why not?
5. What issues should be considered in relation to sustainability of the NNP role in the Canadian health care system?

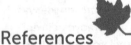

References

Aubrey, W.R., & Yoxall, C.W. (2001). Evaluation of the role of the neonatal nurse practitioner in resuscitation of preterm infants at birth. *Archives of Diseases Child Fetal and Neonatal Edition, 85*(2), F96–99.

Ballantyne, M. (2014). Education needs survey of Canadian tertiary care NICUs. Unpublished raw data.

Bellini, S. (2013). State of the state: NNP program update 2013. *Advances in Neonatal Care, 13*(5), 346–348.

Bissinger, R.L., Allred, C.A., Arford, P.H., & Bellig, L.L. (1997). A cost-effectiveness analysis of neonatal nurse practitioners. *Nursing Economics, 15*(2), 92–99.

Canada West Foundation. (1998). *Nurse practitioners and Canadian health care: Toward quality and cost effectiveness.* Retrieved from http://cwf.ca/pdf/docs/publications/December1998-Nurse-Practitioners-and-Canadian-Health-Care-Toward-Quality-and-Cost-Effectiveness.pdf

Canadian Council of Registered Nurse Regulators (CCRNR). (2013). *CCRNR announces national nurse practitioner practice analysis.* Retrieved from http://www.cno.org/Global/new/CCRNR/NP-Practice-Analysis-CCRNR.pdf

Canadian Institute for Health Information (CIHI). (2013). *Regulated nurses, 2013 summary report.* Ottawa, ON: CIHI. Retrieved from https://secure.cihi.ca/estore/productFamily.htm?locale=en&pf=PFC2646&lang=en

Canadian Nurses Association (CNA). (2008). *Advanced nursing practice: A national framework.* Retrieved from https://www.cna-aiic.ca/~/media/cna/page-content/pdf-en/anp_national_framework_e.pdf

CNA. (2010). *Canadian nurse practitioner core competency framework.* Retrieved from http://www.cno.org/Global/for/rnec/pdf/CompetencyFramework_en.pdf?epslanguage=en

Carzoli, R.P., Martinez-Cruz, M., Cuevas, L.L., Murphy, S., & Chiu, T. (1994). Comparison of neonatal nurse practitioners, physician assistants, and residents in the neonatal intensive care unit. *Archives in Pediatric and Adolescent Medicine, 148*(12), 1271–1276.

College of Registered Nurses of Alberta (CARNA). (2011). *Scope of practice for nurse practitioners (NPs)*. Retrieved from http://www.nurses.ab.ca/content/dam/carna/pdfs/DocumentList/Standards/NP_ScopeOfPractice_Sep2011.pdf

DiCenso, A. (1998). The neonatal nurse practitioner. *Current Opinion in Pediatrics, 10*(2), 151–155.

Donald, F., Kilpatrick, K., Reid, K., Carter, N., Martin-Misener, R., Bryant-Lukosius, D., … DiCenso, A. (2014). A systematic review of the cost-effectiveness of nurse practitioners and clinical nurse specialists: What is the quality of the evidence? *Nursing Research and Practice, 2014.* Article ID 896587. Retrieved from http://dx.doi.org/10.1155/2014/896587

Evanochko, C. (2011). "Growing your own" … Creating a neonatal nurse practitioner team. *Neonatal Network, 30*(5), 289.

Faculty of Health Sciences, McMaster University (1991). *Expanded role nurses in neonatology.* Hamilton, ON: Unpublished.

Fenton, M.V., & Brykczynski, K.A. (1993). Qualitative distinctions and similarities in the practice of clinical nurse specialists and nurse practitioners. *Journal of Professional Nursing, 9*(6), 313–326.

Fetus and Newborn Committee, Canadian Paediatric Society. (2000). Advanced practice nursing roles in neonatal care. *Paediatrics and Child Health, 5*(3), 178–82.

Giovannetti, P., Tenove, S., Stuart, M., & van den Berg, R. (1996). *Report of the CAUSN working group on advanced nursing practice.* Ottawa, ON: CAUSN.

Honeyfield, M.E. (2009). Neonatal nurse practitioners: Past, present, and future. *Advances in Neonatal Care, 9*(3), 125–128.

The Hospital for Sick Children. (1987). *Job description – clinical nurse specialist – nurse practitioner (neonatal).* Toronto, ON: The Hospital for Sick Children.

Hunsberger, M., Mitchell, A., Blatz, S., Paes, B., Pinelli, J., Southwell, D., … Soluk, R. (1992). Definition of an advanced nursing practice role in the NICU: The clinical nurse specialist/neonatal nurse practitioner. *Clinical Nurse Specialist, 6*(2), 91–96.

Kaasalainen, S., Martin-Misener, R., Kilpatrick, K., Harbman, P., Bryant-Lukosius, D., Donald, F., … DiCenso, A. (2010). A historical overview of the development of advanced practice nursing roles in Canada. *Nursing Leadership, 23*(Special Issue December), 35–60.

Karlowicz, M.G., & McMurray, J.L. (2000). Comparison of neonatal nurse practitioners' and pediatric residents' care of extremely low-birth-weight infants. *Archives in Pediatric and Adolescent Medicine, 154*(11), 1123–1126.

McAllister, M., Fryers, M., Campbell, H., Avery, S., Haddad, M., Booth, M., Sabo, K., … Doyle, S. (1993). *The Hospital for Sick Children position paper: Enhancing, extending and expanding the role of the nurse.* Toronto, ON: The Hospital for Sick Children.

Mitchell, A., Watts, J., Whyte, R., Blatz, S., Norman, G., Guyatt, G., … Paes, B. (1991). Evaluation of graduating neonatal nurse practitioners. *Pediatrics, 88*(4), 789–794.

Mitchell, A., Pinelli, J., Patterson, C., & Southwell, D. (1993). *Utilization of nurse practitioners in Ontario (Paper 93–4).* Hamilton, ON: Unpublished.

Mitchell, A., Watts, J., Whyte, R., Blatz, S., Norman, G.R., Southwell, D., … Pinelli, J. (1995). Evaluation of an educational program to prepare neonatal nurse practitioners. *Journal of Nursing Education, 34*(6), 286–289.

Mitchell-DiCenso, A., Guyatt, G., Marrin, M., Goeree, R., Willan, A., Southwell, D., … Baumann, A. (1996). A controlled trial of nurse practitioners in neonatal intensive care. *Pediatrics, 98*(6 Pt 1), 1143–1148.

Mitchell-DiCenso, A., Pinelli, J., & Southwell, D. (1996). Introduction and evaluation of an advanced nursing practice role in neonatal intensive care. In K. Kelly (Ed.), *Outcomes of effective management practice,* (pp. 171–186). Thousand Oaks, CA: SAGE Publications.

Mitchell, G., & Santopinto, M. (1988). The expanded role nurse: A dissenting viewpoint. *Canadian Journal of Nursing Administration, 1*(4), 8–10, 14

Nurse Practitioners' Association of Ontario (NPAO). (n.d.). *Nurse practitioner history in Ontario.* Retrieved from http://npao.org/nurse-practitioners/history

Paes, B., Mitchell, A., Hunsberger, M., Blatz, S., Watts, J., Dent, P., … Southwell, D. (1989). Medical staffing in Ontario neonatal intensive care units. *Canadian Medical Association Journal, 140*(11), 1321–1326.

Pinelli, J.M. (1997). The clinical nurse specialist/nurse practitioner: Oxymoron or match made in heaven? *Canadian Journal of Nursing Administration, 10*(1), 85–110.

Rubin, S. (1988). Expanded role nurse. Part 1. Role theory concepts. *Canadian Journal of Nursing Administration, 1*(2), 23–27.

Ruth-Sanchez, V., Lee, K.A., & Bosque, E.M. (1996). A descriptive study of current neonatal nurse practitioner practice. *Neonatal Network, 15*(5), 23–29.

Samson, L.F. (2006). Perspectives on neonatal nursing: 1985–2005. *Journal of Perinatal and Neonatal Nursing, 20*(1), 19–26.

School of Nursing, McMaster University. (1987). *Background paper for position-statement on the "expanded role" in nursing.* Hamilton, ON: School of Nursing, McMaster University.

Schultz, J.M., Liptak, G.S., & Fioravanti, J. (1994). Nurse practitioners' effectiveness in NICU. *Nursing Management, 25*(10), 50–53.

Wright, J. (1997). *Commonalities and diversity between acute care CNSs and ACNPs.* Toronto, ON: Unpublished.

SECTION IV

Critical Issues in Advanced Practice Nursing in Canada

This section provides the reader with an understanding of the current and future critical issues affecting advanced practice nursing (APN) within Canada and globally, including sustainability of roles. Issues relating to APN roles, education, interprofessional practice, evaluation of APNs and outcomes of practice, and the influence of health policy within a changing health care environment are also discussed.

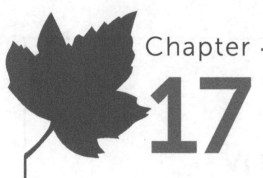

Chapter

17

The Advanced Practice Nurse and Interprofessiona Collaborative Practice Competence

Carole Orchard

Carole Orchard is a Professor at the Arthur Labatt Family School of Nursing and Coordinator for the Interprofessional Health Education and Research Office at Western University in London, Ontario. She developed an instrument to assess collaboration in teams that is widely used and has been translated into several languages, and was also the co-lead in developing the Canadian Interprofessional Health Collaborative (CIHC) national framework for IP competencies that is used internationally.

Introduction

In most countries, advanced practice nurses (APNs), and in particular nurse practitioners (NPs), are required to achieve a level of competence in licensing examinations and competence in enacting their roles. Others, such as clinical nurse specialists (CNSs), complete advanced practice programs before entering into their roles. However, the competence all APNs achieve is generally focused on their specific practice in the NP or CNS role. The requirement for competence within interprofessional (IP) team-based practice necessitates effective working relationships with a variety of other health professionals. This practice is not necessarily a standardized norm of competence development in present APN programs.

In reality, an APN has three levels of competence requirements: at the professional role implementation level, as an individual APN within an IP collaborative team, and as a collaborating partner within an IP team.

This chapter will open the discourse around the meaning of competence and competency, and then focus on the second and third levels of competence and how they are used to define APN practice. This will be followed by a discussion of how APNs may assess their capacity to demonstrate competence in IP client-centred, collaborative practice through the application of the Canadian Interprofessional Health Collaborative's (CIHC) *A National Interprofessional Competency Framework* (2010). Finally, the chapter will provide a brief discussion of how APNs can demonstrate their competence in collaborative teamwork practice.

Competence and Competency

What constitutes competence in practice? Competence is often associated with the demonstration of competencies. Competencies are characterized in a variety of ways and are linked to professional roles and practice domains, as well as work processes and outcomes. They can also be associated with minimal performance and linked to entry-to-practice competence (Govaerts, 2008). Competencies are considered to contain five dimensions: "cognitive knowledge (know-that), functional skills (know-how), personal behaviours (know how to behave), ethical values, and meta-competencies (ability to cope with uncertainty)" (Le Deist & Winterton, 2005, p. 35). Competency can be used by employers to address performance expectations in job roles, by professional regulators to specify required performance by professionals in their practice, and to determine how to assess the impact of care on patient outcomes or when to provide care to patients (Axley, 2008). Competency is therefore viewed in a variety of ways, such as an outcome demonstrated by a set of behaviours, a process leading to outcomes, a shared approach in arriving at care decisions, and a means to determine when performance is at an acceptable level in a job role. (Rarely is *competence* viewed consistently by those who use the term.) Competence is focused not at the team level, but on the individual's performance and may also be considered as minimal, not exceptional, performance (Cowan, Normal, & Coopamah, 2005). The complexity of care for many patients today necessitates the interdependence of knowledge (knowing that), skills (knowing how to), and expertise of all members in a team of health professionals (coping with uncertainty), along with the patient as a contributing member of the team (Adams, Orchard, Houghton, & Ogrin, 2014). Considering competence within a set of outcome behaviours limits its focus, and excludes an understanding of processes adopted in arriving at care decisions. Team competence necessitates attention to assessing the integrated knowledge and tasks of each member (Garavan & McGuire, 2001).

Teamwork is dependent on building relationships among team members. Team relationships act as a "glue," connecting the members into a unified whole. Team competence, then, is a measure of the effectiveness of team relationships and requires a multi-dimensional (processes and outcomes) approach that addresses both the processes used and the outcomes achieved from the team's relational work to determine their practice competency (Garavan & McGuire, 2001). Roegiers (2007) provides one approach through an integrative pedagogy perspective that proposes that the demonstration of IP collaborative practice is dependent on judgments made by a group of IP practitioners, based on an integration of their combined knowledge, skills, and attitudes arrived at through shared competencies. Roegiers (2007) also suggests that making team judgments requires use of their combined resources, which comprise each member's knowledge, know-how (skill enactment), and life skills (experiential learning) to address complex patient situations. Team members confronting patient situations are dependent on their chosen thinking processes, arising from application of their collective resources associated with professional standards of practice, evidence-based knowledge, experiential practice, and procedures for assessing, defining, and interpreting patient care needs. The integration of team resource contributions helps the team at a shared plan to enact care (make judgments) (Roegiers, 2007).

Therefore, health professionals' capacity to work collaboratively in teams is dependent on the complexity of the situation, the team's ability to share and use additive application of resources, integration of resources into care planning, and members' developmental capacity to work within the team (Tardiff, 1999). Individual team members' capacity to work collaboratively is evolutionary, and depends upon their familiarity with the practice context and previous experience with teamwork. Thus, each team member's competence in IP collaborative client-centred practice is always changing. Team members are in a constant and self-directed learning cycle, enacting their collaborative team practice competence.

Collaborative teamwork is a form of practice where all team members, including NPs, are constantly striving to achieve competency. Collaboration is both a process and an outcome of teamwork. Competencies can be associated with behavioural measure of NPs and other members' performance outcomes, or with judgments measuring the processes used by both NPs and group members. What comprises IP team collaboration competence will be explored in the next section.

Interprofessional Collaboration Competency Framework

The Canadian Interprofessional Health Collaborative's (CIHC) *A National Interprofessional Competency Framework* (2010) is one of the only frameworks that focuses on the processes teams utilize to achieve collaborative practice. The framework's goal of **IP collaboration**, defined as "a partnership between a team of health professionals and a client in a participatory, collaborative and coordinated approach to shared decision-making around health and social issues" (Orchard, Curran, & Kabene, 2005, p. 1), provides the outcome or goal for competence. The foundational outcome components that together assist in achieving the goal are identified. The overall direction is on patient/client/family-centred care and services, which require demonstration of IP communications between health professionals. This necessitates an understanding of each other's roles that is inclusive of each person's knowledge, skills, and expertise, and how their team functions together through adoption of collaborative (shared) leadership, as well as their ability to address and resolve any IP conflicts (see Figure 17.1). Each of these competencies will be discussed below.

FIGURE 17.1:   The National Interprofessional Competency Framework

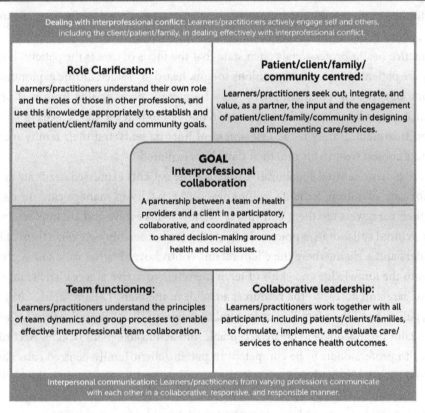

Dealing with interprofessional conflict: Learners/practitioners actively engage self and others, including the client/patient/family, in dealing effectively with interprofessional conflict.

Role Clarification:

Learners/practitioners understand their own role and the roles of those in other professions, and use this knowledge appropriately to establish and meet patient/client/family and community goals.

Patient/client/family/ community centred:

Learners/practitioners seek out, integrate, and value, as a partner, the input and the engagement of patient/client/family/community in designing and implementing care/services.

**GOAL
Interprofessional collaboration**

A partnership between a team of health providers and a client in a participatory, collaborative, and coordinated approach to shared decision-making around health and social issues.

Team functioning:

Learners/practitioners understand the principles of team dynamics and group processes to enable effective interprofessional team collaboration.

Collaborative leadership:

Learners/practitioners work together with all participants, including patients/clients/families, to formulate, implement, and evaluate care/ services to enhance health outcomes.

Interpersonal communication: Learners/practitioners from varying professions communicate with each other in a collaborative, responsive, and responsible manner.

Source: Adapted from Canadian Interprofessional Health Collaborative (CIHC), 2010. Reprinted with permission.

Patient/Client/Family/Community-Centred Care

Patients (or clients) and their families are responsible for managing their health care. Health professionals provide episodic, expert input into how patients and their family members (or chosen caregivers) can address identified health care issues. Actual outcomes of health care are dependent on what patients choose to act on to address their current state of health. It is, therefore, the self-care management that patients adopt that determines their health outcomes—albeit with expert guidance of health professionals.

As adults, patients or their family members are problem-focused. The likelihood of moving beyond what they view as current problem(s) for which they seek health professionals' advice acts as the outer boundary of what can be achieved. While the effectiveness of IP collaborative teamwork is dependent on its impact in improving clients' health outcomes, the likelihood of positive outcomes is greatly increased when patients share the responsibility of shaping their own care. The current predominance in thinking that all care should be based on best practices arising from evidence-informed research tends to minimize the role of patients and their family members. At the same time, there is only limited evidence of positive outcomes when patients are directly involved in their care (Adams et al., 2014; Reeves et al., 2009).

Practice health professionals often state that the focus of care is the patient; however, rarely are patient viewpoints or opinions sought, heard, or valued during exploration and creation of care and treatment plans. More frequently, plans arising from best practice evidence are presented to patients who are requested to make a "quick" selection of their chosen treatment. Rarely is the assessment of how patients and their family members integrate chosen treatments into their daily lives explored.

In IP patient-centred collaborative practice, the patients expressed needs act as "drivers" for care planning. Patients' willingness and capacity to manage care needs along with their caregivers are then "controllers" of how plans evolve and are implemented. IP client-centred collaborative practice is defined as "a partnership between a team of health providers and a client where the client retains control over his/her care and is provided access to the knowledge and skills of team members to arrive at a realistic team shared plan of care and access to the resources to achieve the plan" (Adams et al., 2014, p. 1). Thus, patients and their families are integral members of IP collaborative teams, and work with health professionals to create acceptable and achievable plans of care. Accordingly, for health professionals to be competent in patient/client/family-centred care, they are required to negotiate with patients and their families, and to adapt care to the realities of their situation (see Box 17.1).

There is evidence that when CNSs/NPs/physicians involve other health care providers in discussions around patient care and respect their input, it results in shared planning of care (Gair & Hartery, 2001). Patients' active participation in their care results in high levels of satisfaction and feelings of empowerment, and is believed to result in higher self-care management of health (Adams et al., 2014; Hibbard, Mahoney, Stock, & Tusler, 2007). To achieve the above competency necessitates that APNs and other health providers reassess their assumptions underpinning current approaches to patient and family interactions, as well as inclusions in their own care. Using effective communication between health team members, patients, and families is key to achieving IP collaboration.

BOX 17.1

Patient/Client/Family/Community-Centred Care/ Service Competence

Statement: Health practitioners are expected to "seek out, integrate and value, as a partner, the input, and the engagement of the patient/client/family/community in designing and implementing care/services" (CIHC, 2010).

This is achieved by

- supporting the participation of patients/clients, their families, and/or community representatives as integral partners alongside health care personnel;
- sharing information with patient/clients (or family and community) in a respectful manner, and in such a way that it is understandable, encourages discussion, and enhances participation in decision-making;
- ensuring that appropriate education and support is provided to patient/ clients, family members, and others involved with care or service; and
- listening respectfully to the expressed needs of all parties when shaping and delivering care or services.

Interprofessional Communication

Collaborative, interactive communication is "a continuous transactional process involving participants' exchange of messages, many of which are affected by external physiological and psychological noise" (Adler & Proctor II, 2010, p. 11). Hence, in any transaction, people have a strong likelihood of occupying different environments and using varying communication channels in which a degree of "noise" is always present. Communication channels comprise two components: content and relational. The content of communications relates to what is to be discussed, while the relational aspect reflects how parties feel about each other. The relational aspect of interactions in IP teams can be further affected by four factors: affinity (connection to one another), immediacy (the interest or attention to what is being said), respect (the amount of respect shared between team members), and control (the degree of control one team member exerts over the other during any interaction) (Adler & Proctor II, 2010).

The ability to effectively use the combined knowledge, skills, and expertise of all team members is associated with the team's collaborative communication skills. The patterns health professionals use in professional communications are unique within each profession and are an outcome of their uni-educational professional identity formation. Within their own professional learning, health care providers accumulate unique language and patterns of communications, as well as profession-specific approaches to patient/client care. This education model limits learning beyond one's own profession, adds barriers to the effectiveness of interactions, and leads to barriers across professions long associated with untoward patient events and errors in care decision-making (Institute of Medicine [IOM], 2003; Robinson, Forman, Summer, & Yudkowsky, 2010).

IP communications are only as effective as the quality of the information being shared between parties. IP communication is associated with each member's personality, and professional and personal approaches to interaction. Ultimately, effective IP communication is about ensuring that shared understandings exist between team members involved in a transaction. Effective communication is reported to occur when messaging has: clarity and precision and relies on verification; collaborative problem solving; is delivered through a calm, supportive demeanour when under stress; and when parties maintain mutual respect arising from an authentic understanding of each other's unique role (Robinson et al., 2010). In contrast, ineffective communication occurs when interactions make someone feel undermined, when one party depends solely on electronic systems to convey clinical information, or when linguistic and cultural barriers exist (Robinson et al., 2010).

Chances of miscommunication are high if team members do not create a shared set of communication guidelines. These guidelines must identify the level of importance (i.e., degree of urgency), what means are to be used to convey each level (e.g., email, pager), what the content should be, and to whom the message is to be conveyed. Traditionally, most health professionals depend on established forms that organizations use; however, this negates attention to the relational and most important aspect of IP communications.

The accuracy achieved in IP communication has also been reported to be dependent on verification and confirmation of informational understanding between the parties. When attention is not taken in creating shared communication structures and processes within IP teams, there is a greater chance for communication errors that have negative consequences for patients. Competence in IP communication is essential for effective interactions with health professionals, and for ensuring patient safety (see Box 17.2).

In spite of research findings that almost three-quarters of untoward patient events are due to poor communications among team members, there is limited continuing professional education to develop effective IP communications among health practitioners (Baker et al., 2004; IOM, 2001). Moreover, there is little research to assist in determining the content and processes needed for such training.

BOX 17.2

Interprofessional Communication Competence

Statement: Practitioners from different professions communicate with each other in a collaborative, responsive, and responsible manner.

This can be achieved by

- establishing teamwork communication principles;
- actively listening to other team members, including patients/clients/ families;
- ensuring common understanding of care decisions;
- developing trusting relationships with patients/clients/families and other team members; and
- effectively using information and communication technology to improve interprofessional patient/client/community-centred care.

Role Clarification

Limited attention has been paid in health care practice to the importance of understanding each other's roles. Assumptions can be made, and while health professionals learn about their own roles, they also compare them to those of their colleagues. This comparison often leads to the misperception of roles, gleaned from both the media and society as a whole. Hence, many health professionals practice without clarity about their own roles and with misinterpretations about those of their colleagues. Attention to accurate depictions of health professionals' roles is only a recent phenomenon in health professional education.

Profession-specific learning further reinforces the continuance of role confusion across professions. Learning only within one's own profession creates strong in-group affiliation to their profession, and colours perceptions of others as out-group members who cannot perform at the same level of competence. Social psychologists associate this in-group bias with social contact theory. To overcome this in-group bias necessitates IP team members to: learn about the knowledge, skills, and expertise of previous out-group members; change their misperceptions about others and recognize their value to the team; and generate effective ties to each other by valuing all contributions. The IP group reappraisal necessitates the introduction of three sequential mediating activities: helping team members decrease their anxiety about working across professions and moving into a new IP in-group; helping all IP group members develop empathy and understanding on a personal level; and helping all IP group members learn about the roles, knowledge, skills, and expertise that each member of the team brings (Pettigrew & Tropp, 2008). Together, these activities can enhance a higher quality of care than would be realized if approached by each team member independently.

Role learning assists in addressing perceptions of role intrusions through overlaps across professions, such as those occurring with NPs and physicians, and also what unique and shared roles are brought by colleagues. In this way, each team member learns how shared areas of knowledge, skills, and expertise can benefit in balancing workloads across collaborative teams. The regulated or licensed role of each professional reflects their *generic* team role. At the same time, each health professional negotiates how they will enact components of their generic role within the situational context of team or patient care practice; this is termed their *focal* role (Orchard & Rykhoff, 2015). Furthermore, when a health professional is functioning within an IP collaborative team, there are team roles that members assume to achieve set goals; each health professional also accepts this as their *functional* role. Thus, role clarification comprises three levels of team roles: generic, focal, and functional. Enactment of role clarification competence is essential in order for trust to develop among team members (see Box 17.3). The importance of role clarification is highlighted when interprofessional teams function as collaborative groups.

BOX 17.3

Role Clarification Competence

Statement: Practitioners understand their own role and the roles of those in other professions, and appropriately use their knowledge to establish and achieve patient, client, family, and community goals.

This is achieved by

- describing their own role and that of others;
- recognizing and respecting the diversity of other health and social care roles, responsibilities, and competencies;
- performing their own roles in a culturally respectful way;
- communicating roles, knowledge, skills, and attitudes using appropriate language;
- appropriately accessing others' skills and knowledge through consultation; and
- considering the roles of others in determining their own professional and interprofessional roles, as well as integrating competencies/roles seamlessly into models of service delivery.

Team Functioning

Members working within IP collaborative teams must understand and employ team dynamics to develop competence in team functioning. There is often confusion as to what a team is, and who comprises this team. A team, therefore, is defined as "a collection of individuals who are interdependent in their tasks, who share responsibility for outcomes, who see themselves and who are seen by others as an intact social entity embedded in one or more larger social systems, and who manage their relationships across [clinic] boundaries" (Cohen & Bailey, 1997, p. 241). In collaborative teams, responsibility for team functioning is held by all members. The World Health Organization (WHO) identifies key elements for collaborative teamwork as follows: understanding the role of each member in carrying out the team's responsibilities, the extent of overlap in team members' roles, identifying necessary working processes, and acknowledging the part played by the team in the overall delivery of care (WHO, 1988). The components associated with team functioning include: team context/structure, team processes, and team outcomes (Deneckere et al., 2011).

Team Context/Structure

The structure or context of a team is composed of its culture and climate for team organization, team interdependence, resources, and coordinating mechanisms (Deneckere et al., 2011). IP collaborative teams can be found in any health care setting, and are composed of any number of members. The longer members remain on a team, the greater their capacity to work together. Team structure is also associated with the supportive environment or climate created by its members. West and Poulton (1997) identify five concepts found to be associated with team effectiveness: team participation, team objectives, task orientation and clarity of role, support for innovation, and commitment to teamwork. Team task orientation focuses on creating an atmosphere in which all members can seek each other for advice, and to collectively and critically explore generated knowledge and skills that can be applied to address complex patient care situations. Team structures support care performance ideas identified from set goals and criteria for outcomes, and from criteria used to judge the quality of patient care provided by the team. A positive team environment supports peer and group performance monitoring and evaluation for achievement of collaborative patient care outcomes (West & Poulton, 1997).

Team Processes

Processes used by teams are necessary to support positive working environments. Teamwork processes include: learning to work across health provider groups to achieve "meaningful task interdependencies; holding shared and valued objectives across the team; consistently using multiple information sources available both within the team and from other sources; creating team shared process adaptive mechanisms to achieve their teamwork; and developing the ability to work together in performing through intensive communication processes" (Salas, DiazGranados, Weaver, & King, 2008, p. 1002).

Team Outcomes

Team outcomes are achieved through coordination of care processes, team effectiveness, perceived communication with client/family, satisfaction, perceived follow-up of care, and professional agreements on best practices (Deneckere et al., 2011). The focus of collaborative teamwork is always on the achievement of shared goals associated with how their team functions and reflects on its own ability to work together, or on how their team functions in working with patients and their families to reach improved health states. Team maturity is a key ingredient in relationship building, or what Howarth, Warne, and Haigh (2012) called reciprocal respect and trust of members. Shared confidence between members is dependent on their creation of team credibility, and evolves as members gain skills in using their collective efficacy to work towards a shared goal of patient-centred care. Team credibility only occurs through members' negotiated time (length they work together) and space (setting and work environment), allowing for formation of conditional partnerships. The outcome is achievement of shared goals and effective team functioning (see Box 17.4).

Collaborative teamwork cannot be achieved without members taking time away from patient care to develop skills related to effective teamwork. If IP collaborative teams are

---

BOX 17.4

Team Functioning Competence

Statement: Practitioners understand the principles of teamwork dynamics and group/team processes to enable effective interprofessional collaboration.

This is achieved by

- understanding the process of team development;
- developing a set of principles for working together that respects the ethical values of members;
- effectively facilitating discussions and interactions among team members;
- respecting all members' participation in collaborative decision-making;
- regularly reflecting on their functioning with team practitioners;
- establishing and maintaining effective and healthy working relationships with practitioners, patient/clients, and families, whether or not a formalized team exists; and
- respecting team ethics, which includes confidentiality, resource allocation, and professionalism.

to function effectively, they require group training that reflects team-building activities associated with goal-setting, interprofessional relationships, role clarification, and problem solving leading to shared decision-making (Adams et al., 2014; Salas et al., 2008). Getting to team conditional partnerships necessitates teams addressing how to be competent within their shared leadership.

Collaborative/Shared Leadership

The complexity of patient care needs necessitates the decentralization of leadership, and the importance of placing it in the hands of those who interact directly with patients. No longer can health professionals wait until administrative decision-making processes are provided to affirm care decisions. Today, decision-making must occur within IP teams through collaborative or shared leadership that occurs "when all members of a team are fully engaged in the leadership of the team and are not hesitant to influence and guide their fellow team members in an effort to maximize the potential of the team as a whole" (Pearce, 2004, p. 48).

Achievement of shared leadership can only be realized once team members are able to feel respected and valued; ensure that they can trust others and be trusted in turn; have a say in the planning, implementation, and evaluation of teamwork and care; and participate as valued members in shared work outcomes. The capacity of a collaborative team to share resources is just one outcome of effective teamwork. Carson, Tesluk, and Marrone (2007) suggest that collaborative leadership is enacted within two forms: focused and distributed. "Focused leadership occurs when leadership resides within a single individual, whereas distributed leadership occurs when two or more individuals share the roles, responsibilities, and functions of leadership" (p. 1218). No matter which form of collaborative leadership is chosen within a team, effectiveness of their teamwork necessitates "development and shaping of team processes generating shared goal commitment, and shaping a constructive climate" (Balthazard, Waldman, Howell, & Atwater, 2004, p. 7).

Collaborative or shared leadership is usually supported through a formal organizational leader, referred to by Pearce and Sims (2002) as the *vertical leader*. The collaborative team then interacts with the vertical leader to ensure their teamwork "fits" within the overall organization. Orchard and Rykhoff (2015) proposed a Complementary Leadership Framework (see Figure 17.2) that integrates Pearce and Sims' (2002) concepts of vertical and shared leadership. These are incorporated through a reciprocal building of relationships between the vertical leader's transformative, transactional, and empowering leadership (Pierce, 2004). The team members' shared leadership is connected through relational coordination, as proposed by Gittell, Godfrey, & Thistlewaite (2013). The vertical leaders' transformational leadership includes modelling the way (clarifying their own values, and validating and connecting actions to the team's shared values), inspiring a shared vision (helping the team see a desired future), enabling others to act (seeking opportunities for themselves to innovate and take risks), challenging the process (seeking innovative ways to change, grow, and inspire), and encouraging the heart (recognizing contributions of others) (Kouses & Posner, 2006) (see Figure 17.2).

FIGURE 17.2:   The Complementary Leadership Framework

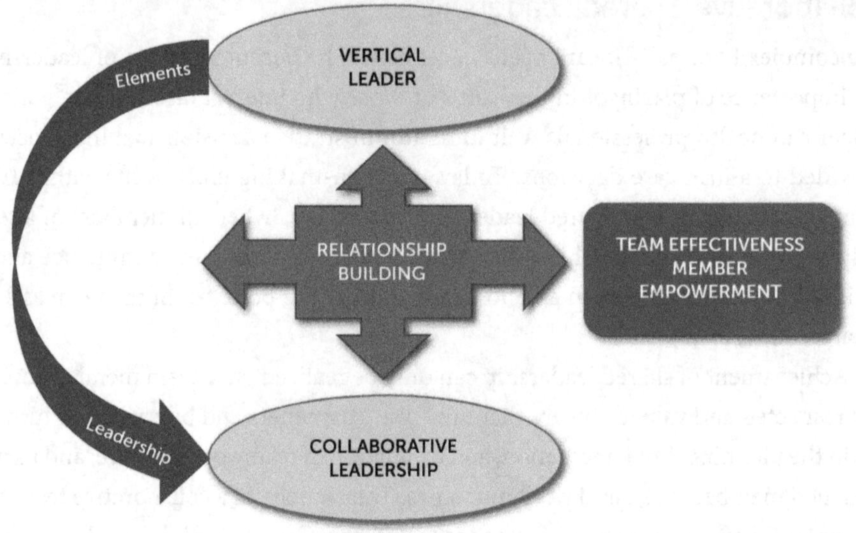

Source: Orchard & Rykhoff, 2015. Reprinted with permission.

The team then complements these leadership elements as a coherent whole in its practice. Team members model leadership when they demonstrate knowledge of their personal values and how these enhance or interfere in working with others, as well as when they help the team stay focused on patients' care and their own well-being. The team creates a shared vision by focusing on patient-specified goals, brought about by collaboratively bringing their shared ideas together. Team members enable others to act by being respectful of each other, and ensuring that goals are shared with their patients. Enabling others to act is shown when team members encourage other colleagues to assume, and support, the team coordination role. Team members test this process by reflecting on their effectiveness at working together, and the inclusion of patients and family members in planning, implementing, and evaluating their care. Finally, the team recognizes each other's and their patients' work by celebrating successes, "encouraging the heart" (Kouzes & Posner, 2012). When the shared leadership elements are operationalized in practice, there is a greater likelihood that the competency of collaborative or shared leadership will be demonstrated (see Box 17.5).

BOX 17.5

Collaborative (Shared) Leadership Competency

Statement: Practitioners understand and apply leadership principles that support a collaborative practice model.

This is achieved by

- working with others to enable effective patient/client outcomes, and advancing interdependent working relationships among all participants;
- facilitating effective team processes, such as decision-making;
- establishing a climate for collaborative practice among all participants;
- co-creating a climate of shared leadership and collaborative practice;
- applying collaborative decision-making principles;
- integrating the principles of continuous quality improvement to work processes and outcomes; and
- demonstrating shared decision-making, as well as leadership and continued individual accountability for one's own actions, responsibilities, and roles as explicitly defined within one's professional/disciplinary scope of practice.

Interprofessional Conflict Resolution

Effective team functioning and shared leadership is essential for IP collaborative team competence. However, the inherent differences in language and approaches to care across professions within a team provide the fuel that can lead to disagreements. How members react to disagreements or conflicts is dependent on their "relationship within the team (power dynamics); the situation the team is addressing; how other people in the team respond; and whether members are seeking to achieve their own personal or the team's goal" (Adler & Proctor II, 2010, p. 347). Key IP team skill development should focus on each member's capacity to negotiate and work towards collaborative decision-making. Team members own profession-specific norms of communication and practice are adopted, negotiated, and renegotiated in exchanges between themselves (Conn et al., 2009). These profession-specific norms and practices are likely to come into conflict when cross-disciplinary approaches to a patient's care are being discussed. While professionals often perceive conflicts as "troublesome," they are actually healthy and allow for a variety of perspectives to be shared. When handled well, conflicts can result in a high quality of comprehensive and collaborative patient care planning. To achieve a healthy outcome from

IP conflicts, team members need to strive towards finding a "win-win" solution to the disagreement. Other options might include deferring to the other person or compromising with other team members. This, however, may lead to residual anger or feelings of being unvalued by the person who is perceived to have lost the argument (see Box 17.6). To arrive at a collaborative "win-win" decision, the team must use a conflict resolution process, which includes the following elements:

- Create an open space where all views can be heard
- Consider all views within individual perspectives
- Consider biases that may exist in individual viewpoints
- Consider justification for these biases, and how one can come to terms with other viewpoints
- Weigh alternating individual views, based on the viewpoints of others and in the context of the patient's safety
- Share thinking with other team members
- Hear each other's viewpoints
- Come to a shared agreement (Orchard, 2010)

An assumption underpinning the above is that the contributions made by each member of a team add substantive value to the discussion. If members listen to each other and consider the value of what each team member suggests, and then compare it to their own position on the issue, all parties should be able to see merit in at least some aspects of other viewpoints. These merits can help reshape individual viewpoints into one that incorporates the richness of all members' ideas.

BOX 17.6

Interprofessional Conflict Resolution Competency

Statement: Practitioners actively engage self and others, including the client/patient/family, in positively and constructively addressing disagreements as they arise.

This is achieved by

- valuing the potential positive nature of conflict;
- recognizing the potential for conflict to occur, and taking constructive steps to address it;

- identifying common situations that are likely to lead to disagreements or conflicts, including role ambiguity, power gradients, and differences in goals;
- knowing and understanding strategies to deal with conflict;
- setting clear guidelines for addressing disagreements;
- effectively working to address and resolve disagreements, including analyzing the causes of conflict and working to reach an acceptable solution by establishing a safe environment in which to express diverse opinions; and
- developing a level of consensus among those with differing views by allowing all members to feel their viewpoints have been heard, no matter what the outcome.

Advanced Practice Nurses as Members of Interprofessional Collaborative Teams

The Canadian Advanced Practice Nurses Framework states that APN core competencies "are based on an appropriate depth, breadth and range of nursing knowledge, theory, and research, enhanced by clinical experience" (CNA, 2008, p. 21). Within the core competency framework is a set of competencies associated with consultation and collaboration. Several of these competencies relate to interprofessional practice, including: "consult and collaborate with members of the health care team to develop quality improvement and risk-management strategies; practice collaboratively and build effective coalitions; apply theories related to group dynamics, roles, and organizations; demonstrate knowledge and skills in communication, negotiation and conflict resolution including the ability to analyze, manage and negotiate conflict; and clearly articulate the contribution of advanced nursing practice within the interprofessional health care team" (CNA, 2008, pp. 26–7). Comparing the APN competencies with the CIHC IP collaboration competencies there are many similarities, as shown below in Table 17.1 (CIHC, 2008). However, the expectation of APNs understanding the roles of other health professionals, which is a key component in IP teamwork, is not clearly stated. Furthermore, attention to consultations, referrals, and collaboration with other health care providers is well articulated, but what is absent is how the patient and their family are viewed by APNs as key members of the health care team within the core competency for consultation and collaboration (see Table 17.1).

The APN, whether a CNS or NP, has the potential to influence the effectiveness of an IP collaborative team as a collaborative leader within the group. The NP role has been described as a bridge in interprofessional teams because of their ability to diagnose patients and order treatments and drugs (van Soeren, Hurlock-Chorostecki, & Reeves, 2011). The CNS role provides a level of expertise in practice, based on theories and research that enhance how an

TABLE 17.1: CIHC IP Collaboration Competencies with CNA and APN Competencies for Consultation and Collaboration

CIHC Interprofessional Collaboration Competencies	CNA Advanced Practice Nursing Core Competencies for Consultation & Collaboration
Patient/client/family/community-centred care	Advocate for changes in health policy at regional, provincial/territorial, and federal levels.
Interprofessional communication	Work with others to gather and synthesize qualitative and quantitative information on determinants of health from a variety of sources. (See IP conflict resolution.)
Role clarification	Clearly articulate the contribution of advanced practice nurses within the interprofessional health care team.
Team functioning	Apply theories related to group dynamics, roles, and organizations. Practice collaboratively and build effective coalitions. Consult and collaborate with members of the health care team to develop quality improvement and risk-management strategies.
Collaborative (shared) leadership	Initiate timely and appropriate consultations, referrals, and collaborations with other health care providers.
Interprofessional conflict resolution	Demonstrate knowledge and skills in communication, negotiation, and conflict resolution, including the ability to analyze, manage, and negotiate conflicts.

IP team considers their collaborative care. However, there is also danger in APNs assuming power in the team based on their advanced education. This can be mitigated by participating collaboratively with other health professionals in the team who have complementary and enriched knowledge, skills, and experiences to that of their own. Hence, more attention to learning about the roles, knowledge, skills, and expertise of other health professionals is required for APNs to truly become collaborative partners in health care teams. No matter what health professional role is assumed within IP teams, it must be remembered that the controller is the patient and how much they are prepared to work with the team to enhance their health. APNs, like other health professionals, are simply expert advisors to patients and their families. This is the essence of interprofessional patient-centred collaborative practice.

Conclusion

Competence in practice has long been touted as key for APNs being accepted into teams. However, understanding the meaning of competence from a variety of perspectives may have led to differing views of what competence and competency in roles means. In this chapter we have reviewed the various ways in which competence is perceived, and discussed the application of competence into IP collaborative practice using the CIHC IP Competency Framework as a guide. A brief comparison was also made between the APNs' competencies for consultation and collaboration within IP collaborative teams was also explored. In essence, APNs have a pivotal role in helping to shift practice from provider- and system-centric to being truly patient-centred.

Critical Thinking Questions

1. As a health care provider, consider how to articulate an APN role to another health professional. What is the meaning of the type of communication used? Are there certain words that are not likely to be understood by another health provider, and that might cause lack of understanding of the APN role and message?

2. In your practice as an APN, consider a conflict situation you may have recently experienced. What role did you assume in this conflict? Were you able to transcend your own viewpoint to hear those of team members and come to a positive outcome? Or are you still questioning that outcome?

3. Reflect on how you currently include patients and their chosen caregivers in discussions about their health care. How well have you respected their input when shaping and negotiating their care to fit with their needs?

References

Adams, T.L., Orchard, C., Houghton, P., & Ogrin, R. (2014). The metamorphosis of a collaborative team: From creation to operation. *Journal of Interprofessional Care, 28*(4), 1–6. doi: 10.3109/13561800.2014.891571

Adler, R.B., & Proctor II, R.F. (2010). *Looking out, looking in* (13th ed.). Boston, MA: Wadsworth Cengage Learning.

Axley, L. (2008). Competency: A concept analysis. *Nursing Forum, 43*(4), 214–222. doi:10.1111/j.1744-6198.2008.00115.x

Baker, G.R., Norton, P.G., Flintoft, V., Blais, R., Brown, A., Cox, J., ... Tamblyn, R. (2004). The Canadian Adverse Events Study: The incidence of adverse events among hospital patients in Canada. *Canadian Medical Association Journal, 170*(11): 1678–1686.

Balthazard, P., Waldman, D., Howell, J., & Atwater, L. (2004). Shared leadership and group interactions styles in problem-solving virtual teams. In R.H. Sprague Jr. (Ed.), *Proceedings of the Hawaii International Conference on System Sciences (HICSS)* (Vol. 37), (pp. 693–702). Waikoloa, HI: University of Hawai'i.

Canadian Interprofessional Health Collaborative (CIHC). (2008). *Interprofessional education & core competencies.* Vancouver, BC: CIHC.

CIHC. (2010). *A national interprofessional competency framework.* Retrieved from http://www.cihc.ca/files/CIHC_IPCompetencies_Feb1210.pdf

Canadian Nurses Association (CNA). (2008). *Advanced nursing practice: A national framework.* Ottawa, ON: CNA.

Carson, J.B., Tesluk, P.E., & Marrone, J.A. (2007). Shared leadership in teams: An investigation of antecedent conditions and performance. *Academy of Management Journal, 50*(5), 1217–1234.

Cohen, S.G., & Bailey, D.E. (1997). What makes teams work? Group effectiveness research from the shop floor to the executive suite. *Journal of Management, 23*(3), 239–290. doi: 10.1177/014920639702300303

Conn, L.G., Lingard, L., Reeves, S., Miller, K.L., Russell, A., & Zwarenstein, M. (2009). Communication channels in general internal medicine: A description of baseline patterns for improved interprofessional collaboration. *Qualitative Health Research, 19*(7), 943–953. doi: 10.1177/1049732309338282

Cowan, D.T., Norman, I., & Coopamah, V.P. (2005). Competence in nursing practice: A controversial concept—a focused review of the literature. *Nurse Education Today, 25*(5), 355–362.

Deneckere, S., Robyns, N., Vanhaecht, K., Euwema, M., Panella, M., Lodewijckx, C., ... Sermeus, W. (2011). Indicators for follow-up of multidisciplinary teamwork in care processes: Results of an international expert panel. *Evaluation and the Health Professions, 34*(3), 258–277. doi: 10.1177/0163278710393736

Gair, G., & Hartery, T. (2001). Medical dominance in multidisciplinary teamwork: A case study of discharge decision-making in a geriatric assessment unit. *Journal of Nursing Management, 9*(1), 3–11.

Garavan, T.N., & McGuire, D., (2001). Competencies and workplace learning: Some reflections on the rhetoric and the reality. *Journal of Workplace Learning, 13*(4), 144–164. doi: 10.1108/13665620110391097

Gittell, J.H., Godfrey, M., & Thistlethwaite, J. (2013). Interprofessional collaborative practice and relational coordination: Improving healthcare through relationships. *Journal of Interprofessional Care, 27*(3), 210–213. doi: 10.3109/13561820.2012.73056

Govaerts, M.J.B. (2008). Educational competencies or education for professional competence? *Medical Education, 42*(3), 234–236. doi: 10.1111/j.1365-2923.2007.03001.x

Hibbard, J.H., Mahoney, E.R., Stock, R., & Tusler, M. (2007). Do increases in patient activation result in improved self-management behaviours? *Health Services Research, 42*(4), 1443–1463. doi: 10.1111/j.1475-6773.2006.00669x

Howarth, M., Warne, T., & Haigh, C. (2012). Let's stick together! A grounded theory exploration of interprofessional working used to provide person centred chronic back pain services. *Journal of Interprofessional Care, 26*(6), 491–496. doi: 10.3109/13561820.2012.711385

Institute of Medicine (IOM). (2001). *Crossing the quality chasm: A new health system for the 21st century.* Washington, DC: National Academy Press.

IOM. (2003). *Health professions education: A bridge to quality.* Washington, DC: National Academies Press.

Kouzes, J., & Posner, B. (2006). *Student leadership practices inventory* (2nd ed.). San Francisco, CA: Jossey-Bass.

Kouzes, J., & Posner, B. (2012). The leadership challenge: How to make extraordinary things happen in organizations (5th ed.). San Francisco, CA: Jossey-Bass.

Le Deist, F.D., & Winterton, J. (2005). What is competence? *Human Resource Development International, 8*(1), 27–46. doi: 10.1080/1367886042000338227.10441876

Orchard, C. (2010). Persistent isolationist or collaborator? The nurse's role in interprofessional collaborative practice. *Journal of Nursing Management, 18*(3), 248–257.

Orchard, C.A., Curran, V., & Kabene, S. (2005). Creating a culture for interdisciplinary collaborative practice. *Medical Education Online, 10*(11), 1–13. Retrieved from http://www.med-ed-online.net/index.php/meo/article/viewFile/4387/4569

Orchard, C.A., & Rykhoff, M. (2015). Collaborative leadership in the context of interprofessional patient-centred collaborative practice. In D. Forman, M. Jones, & J. Thistlethwaite (Eds.) *Leadership and collaboration*. Basingstoke, Hampshire, UK: Palgrave MacMillan.

Pearce, C.L. (2004). The future of leadership: Combining vertical and shared leadership to transform knowledge work. *Academy of Management Executive,18*(1), 47–57.

Pearce, C.L., & Sims Jr., H.P. (2002). Vertical versus shared leadership as predictors of the effectiveness of change management teams: An examination of aversive, directive, transactional, transformational, and empowering leader behaviors. *Group Dynamics: Theory, Research, & Practice, 6*(2), 172–197. doi: 10.1037//1089-2699.6.2.172

Pettigrew, T.F., & Tropp, L.R. (2008). How does intergroup contact reduce prejudice? Meta analytic tests of three mediations. *European Journal of Social Psychology, 38*(6), 922–934. doi: 10.1002/ejsp504

Reeves, S., Zwarenstein, M., Goldman, J., Barr, H., Freeth, D., Hammick, M., & Koppel, I. (2009). Interprofessional education: Effects on professional practice and health care outcomes (Review). *The Cochrane Collaboration, 1*, 1–21. Retrieved from http://www.thecochranelibrary.com

Robinson, F.P., Gorman, G., Summer, L.W., & Yudkowsky, R. (2010). Perceptions of effective and ineffective nurse-physician communication in hospitals. *Nursing Forum, 45*(3), 206–216. doi: 10.1111/j.1744-6198.2010.00182.x

Roegiers, X. (2007). Curricular reforms guide schools: But, where to? *Prospects, 37*(2), 155–186. doi: 10.1007/s11125-007-9024-z

Salas, E., DiazGranados, D., Weaver, S.J., & King, H. (2008). Does team training work? Principles for health care. *Academic Emergency Medicine, 15*(11), 1002–1009. doi: 10.1111/j.1553-2712.2008.00254.x

Tardif, J. (1999). *Le transfert des apprentissages*. Montréal, QC: Les Éditions Logiques.

van Soeren, M., Hurlock-Chorostecki, C., & Reeves, S. (2011). The role of nurse practitioners in hospital settings: Implications for interprofessional practice. *Journal of Interprofessional Care, 25*(4), 245–251. doi: 10.3109/13561820.539305

West, M.A., & Poulton, B.C. (1997). A failure of function: Teamwork in primary health care. *Journal of Interprofessional Care, 11*(2), 205–216. doi: 10.3109/1356-1820/97/020205-12

World Health Organization (WHO). (1988). *Learning Together to Work Together for Health*, 1–72. Geneva, CH: WHO. Retrieved from http://whqlibdoc.who.int/trs/WHO_TRS_769.pdf

Chapter

18

Outcomes Evaluation and Performance Assessment of Advanced Practice Nursing Roles

Eric Staples and Joanna Pierazzo

Eric Staples is an Independent Nursing Practice Consultant, who previously worked as an APN. He has served as an Assistant Professor at Dalhousie University in Halifax, Nova Scotia, where he was involved in implementing the Advanced Nursing Practice stream in 1998; at McMaster University, where he worked as NP coordinator in the Ontario Primary Health Care Nurse Practitioner Program; and at the University of Regina. He has served on a number of Canadian Association of Schools of Nursing (CASN) committees related to NP education, preceptorship, prescribing, and the development of the position statement on doctoral education in Canada.

Joanna Pierazzo is an Assistant Professor and BScN Curriculum Chair at McMaster University, School of Nursing in Hamilton, Ontario. She has held APN roles in regional neurosurgery programs in Ontario, including ACNP at Hamilton Health Sciences and APN community outreach at Trillium Health Partners in Mississauga, Ontario. Joanna currently teaches in the graduate program, both nursing and health science education, and her research interests have primarily focused on simulation-based learning, self-efficacy, and learner anxiety.

KEY TERMS

outcomes
outcomes evaluation
peer review
performance
  assessment

OBJECTIVES

1. Discuss approaches to evaluating outcomes in advanced practice nursing (APN).
2. Examine findings across Canada related to APN outcomes research.
3. Identify how evidence-informed practice can be used to enhance the effectiveness of APN roles.
4. Examine issues associated with APN performance assessment.

Introduction

Over the last several years, the integration of advanced practice nursing (APN) roles into health care settings in Canada has required continual growth and development through attention to role clarity and other factors enabling role integration (DiCenso & Bryant-Lukosius, 2010). Through advancing awareness of the need for an organized process, introducing APN roles has strengthened role effectiveness and, more importantly, provided evidence related to research-based outcomes. With this professional growth, measuring outcomes has become mandatory as federal and provincial regulatory bodies, institutional guidelines, employers, and the general public advocate for quality health care with enhanced patient care. As pressures increase to reign in escalating health care costs, outcomes are more actively monitored within health care organizations. Monitoring outcomes is useful to guide quality decision-making, while simultaneously attending to accreditation, certification, and competency requirements.

Greater discussion on enhancing the quality and safety of health care delivery has fuelled debate regarding which measured outcomes are affected by individual providers, technology, education, and health care systems (Doran, 2011). It is important that outcomes are uniformly and systematically examined to both effectively inform health care policy and guide consumers' choices about their care. Today's consumers are well equipped to ask questions related to their care, particularly in terms of health and well-being. In light of this, it is vital for health care professionals to continue gathering outcome data, evaluating interventions, and identifying issues related to care in order to improve the overall quality and efficiency of health care delivery (Friese & Beck, 2004).

APNs impact both direct patient care and processes within the health care systems in which they practice. As the APN role has evolved, the tracking and documentation of outcomes associated with APN practice has become more prevalent and provided greater clarity and attentiveness to changing health care needs. Outcomes evaluation is considered an essential component of most health care systems' initiatives (Kleinpell & Gawlinski, 2005), and as such there have been strengthened pockets of quality research across Canada attending to this very focus. The literature supports that APN roles have known and measurable benefits for patients, families, health care, and professional practice, as well as important influences on relationships with collaborative health professionals (MacDonald et al., 2005). With this value in mind, Burgess and Purkis (2010) affirm that APNs have risen above tensions related to role development and have become effective providers of care within the community.

This chapter will outline important aspects of the APN role related to evaluating outcomes and performance assessment, and discuss the use of quality indicators to demonstrate APN practice outcomes.

Theoretical Outcomes Framework

Today's health care system is expected to provide efficient and effective care delivery that is both cost-effective and has good outcomes. Trends investigating outcomes begin with a central focus on the end result of patient care (Burns & Grove, 2007). In order to comprehensively explain this end result, it is important to understand both the processes and structures that have contributed to the provision of patient care. Health care providers such as APNs are in a unique position to identify outcomes relevant to the goals of care and matters important to receivers of care (Burns & Grove, 2007; Clancy & Esenberg, 1997). Using this approach, outcomes-based research may further enhance our understanding of how APN roles impact society and evolve to a level of inquiry that considers both the structures and processes within health care.

In considering a comprehensive approach to outcomes evaluation, a number of structure-process-outcome frameworks have been acknowledged in this area. In the Medical Outcomes Study (MOS) (Burns & Grove, 2007; Tarlov et al., 1989), the measurement of quality care outcomes evolved from two-year observational research, replicated at three sites, related to the structures and process of care. The study was designed to distinguish if discrepancies in patient outcomes were related to the system of care, provider specialty, and provider technical and interpersonal styles, and from this develop tools for monitoring outcomes in patients with one or more of four chronic diseases common to adults (Tarlov et al., 1989).

The MOS's conceptual framework (see Figure 18.1) depicts structures of care that include elements of organization and administration such as leadership, tolerance of innovativeness, organizational hierarchy, decision-making processes, distribution of power, financial management, and administrative decision-making processes (Burns & Grove, 2007). Describing these structural elements is an important first step to identifying specific goals for outcomes evaluation. Various theoretical approaches to administration and management further contribute to this initial understanding. The second step involves evaluating the impact of these care structures on the process of care (e.g., referrals, test ordering, expenditures, hospitalizations, continuity of care, medications). This step is complicated, as it involves comparing different structures of care that provide the same process or outcomes of care (Burns & Grove, 2007). The third step involves evaluating outcomes of care (e.g., clinical end points, functional status of patient, general well-being, satisfaction with care), including feedback directly from patients, providers, and records that look at the variations between the structure and process of care.

With a theoretical conceptualization in mind, any number of inquiries can guide the evaluation of APN roles. Since NP and CNS roles vary in their scope of practice, it is important to critically understand the structure-process-outcome relationship with respect to both roles before embarking on an evaluation study. The number of CNS roles in Canada

FIGURE 18.1:   The Medical Outcomes Study Conceptual Framework

Structures of Care

1. **System characteristics** (e.g., organization, specialty mix, financial incentives, workload, access/convenience)

2. **Provider characteristics** (e.g., age, gender, specialty training, economic incentives, beliefs/attitudes, job satisfaction, preferences)

3. **Patient characteristics** (e.g., age, gender, diagnosis/condition, severity, comorbid conditions, health habits, beliefs/ attitudes, preferences)

Process of Care

1. **Technical style** (e.g., visits, medications, referrals, test ordering, hospitalizations, expenditures, continuity of care, coordination)

2. **Interpersonal style** (e.g., interpersonal manner, patient participation, counselling, communication level)

Outcomes

1. **Clinical end points** (e.g., signs and symptoms, laboratory values, mortality)

2. **Functional status** (e.g., physical, mental, social, role)

3. **General well-being** (e.g., health perceptions, energy/ fatigue, pain, life satisfaction)

4. **Satisfaction with care** (e.g., access, financial coverage, quality, convenience)

Source: Adapted from Tarlov et al., 1989.

has declined over the last several years, and with this mind, one way to strengthen and promote the existence of and need for more CNS roles would be to increase the amount of evidence examining structure-process-outcome relationships in health care settings where CNS roles exist.

Coupling Role Implementation and Evaluation

Initiating outcomes research and evaluating APN roles has not been an easy feat. With greater attention being given to providing quality, cost-effective care with good outcomes, it is essential for APNs to demonstrate the impact of their roles through outcomes research. Although a theoretical approach to evaluation research has been introduced, it is important to recognize that evaluation is closely coupled with APN role implementation. Often, the question of evaluation is a precursor to successfully implementing an NP or CNS role in a health care setting. Unfortunately, this makes the inquiry process more difficult and complicates the development of a good research design. The participatory, evidence-based, patient-focused framework for optimal utilization of APN roles (PEPPA; see Chapter 4) is helpful with both the implementation and evaluation of APN roles (Bryant-Lukosius & DiCenso, 2004). This framework is composed of various steps, including clarifying the patient population, modifying the model of care, and planning role implementation. Finally, evaluation and long-term monitoring of APN roles reinforces the structure-process-outcome approach. APNs should consider outcomes that are sensitive to APN interventions, and related to safety, efficacy, and processes of care (Bryant-Lukosius & DiCenso, 2004).

Measurement of Outcomes

The majority of the evidence related to measuring outcomes and APN roles has focused on the clinical, consultative, collaborative, and educational dimensions of practice. The body of research has recognized that APNs provide safe and effective health care (DiCenso et al., 2010). Additionally, there are more studies reported for the NP role in Canada than for the CNS role. The following discussion will highlight a number of studies that have reported outcomes research. Although the overview is not exhaustive, it will hopefully provide a comprehensive review of general themes and trends related to measuring outcomes and APN roles.

Since engaging in evaluation research requires the APN to be actively immersed in the process, Ingersoll, McIntosh, and Williams (2000) surveyed APNs to determine which outcomes they felt were relevant indicators of their practice. The 10 highest ranking indicators were "satisfaction with care delivery, symptom reduction or resolution, perception of being well cared for, compliance with treatment plan, knowledge of patient and families, trust in the care provided, collaboration among care providers, frequency and type of procedures ordered, and quality of life" (p. 1279). Although these outcomes exemplify vital aspects of the APN role, they do not capture the breadth or depth of APN practice. The evaluation process should strive to identify concrete and measurable outcomes, however there are disadvantages in using such outcomes to solely evaluate the delivery of health care. Depending on the APN role and health care setting, the choice of relevant outcomes and the time required to measure them may be incompatible. For example, attitudes and satisfaction are two outcomes that cannot be precisely measured, despite the many tools that have been developed precisely to assess this type of outcome variable (Donabedian, 2005). DiCenso et al. (2010) suggested that these underappreciated or even elusive APN contributions "could be made to address important gaps in maximizing the health of Canadians through equitable access to high-quality health care service" (p. 32).

Several literature reviews have documented the contribution and impact of APN roles within both Canadian and American health care contexts (DiCenso & Bryant-Lukosius, 2010; Kleinpell, 2009; Newhouse et al., 2011; Sangster-Gormley, 2014). These resources should be reviewed for a comprehensive understanding of the scope of literature within this field, as they provide an important contribution to advancing knowledge related to

APN roles and the measurement of outcomes. DiCenso et al. (2010) developed a synthesis report examining both CNS and NP roles in Canada. The findings, comprised of over 60 stakeholder interviews and a review of 500 papers, reported on the competencies of these roles and the contexts in which these roles practice, as well as barriers, facilitators, and implications for effective development and utilization of APN roles.

Reported in the findings were a distinct lack of role clarity and ambiguous articulation of the scopes of practice for these APN roles. Furthermore, recommendations included standardizing regulatory and educational standards, developing communication strategies to disseminate the positive outcomes of APN roles, integrating APN roles within human resource planning based on population health needs, and advancing research related to the value of these roles and their impact on health care costs. Bryant-Lukosius, DiCenso, Browne, & Pinelli (2004) identified several factors leading to unsuccessful APN role implementation and evaluation, including the loss of an innovative health system improvement that would benefit all stakeholders from the expertise the APN can provide. In Ontario, unsuccessful APN role implementation in oncology settings has been associated with poor job satisfaction and difficulty recruiting and retaining qualified APNs (Bryant-Lukosius et al., 2007).

The NP role has been well investigated in terms of outcomes research. Sangster-Gormley's (2014) synthesis reports summarized findings related to patient satisfaction with NP care, comparison of NP care with care provided by MDs and other providers, and other health outcomes sensitive to NP interventions. Patient satisfaction and education were found to be the most commonly researched patient-related outcomes related to NP roles (Kleinpell, 2009; Sangster-Gormley, 2014), and patients reported overall satisfaction with care provided by NPs or in collaboration with other health care providers. NPs contribute to reducing care costs, length of stay, and wait times; they have expert communication skills and empower patients when engaged in patient teaching and health promotion. In terms of NP practice, there were similar, less costly outcomes for models of care integrating NPs or NP-led teams compared to physician-led models (Browne, Birch, & Thabane, 2012; Jacobson & HDR Inc., 2012). APNs were particularly noted to provide effective care in chronic disease management, community care, primary care, and mental health settings, while NP-led initiatives were reported to improve access and continuity of care, education, and disease management.

Outside of Canada, the measurement of outcomes has been more extensively discussed, particularly in terms of economic influence. Kleinpell's (2009) textbook of outcome assessment provides a discussion of the literature, addressing both the health and economic impact of APN practice. Studies dating from the 1960s to 2008 are integrated in an examination of care-related, patient-related, and performance-related outcomes. Outcome measurements are studied by conducting evaluation research using a process, searching for reliable instruments and measures for APN assessment, and then engaging in research related to more specialized APN roles such as nurse-midwifery and nurse anesthesia. Outcomes related to clinical end points and patient-specific outcomes are reported, including control of specific diseases, use of diagnostics, cost of care, patient satisfaction, length of stay, complications, prescribing patterns, and quality of life. APN interventions were noted to reduce hospitalization and readmissions, decrease hospital costs, and shorten the average length of stay (Kleinpell, 2009; Sangster-Gormley, 2014).

Another systematic review conducted outside of Canada amalgamated all APN outcome studies published between 1990 and 2008 (Newhouse et al., 2011) where the measurable outcomes were primarily related to clinical endpoints. A synthesis of 37 outcome studies related to the NP role recorded the following outcomes: patient satisfaction, self-reported perceived health, functional status, glucose control, lipid control, blood pressure, ED visits, hospitalizations, duration of mechanical ventilation, length of stay, and mortality. Reported outcomes for NPs showed either similarity to or improvement on those of a physician. Eleven studies of this synthesis investigated the CNS role, collecting data addressing four outcomes: satisfaction, hospital length of stay, hospital costs, and complications.

Performance Assessment

In terms of individual APN performance assessment, health care organizations are challenged to evaluate the practice competencies of APNs at the advanced practice level. Many current performance assessment methodologies continue to blend a combination of basic nursing competencies with APN competencies, or even medical competencies that are based on organizational goals and objectives originating from human resources (HR) departments (Scarpa & Connelly, 2011).

A performance assessment must be a meaningful evaluation of practice that meets the needs of APNs across different roles, care specialties, and practice settings (Kenny et al., 2008). One approach that is both compatible and complementary with the Canadian Nurses Association (CNA), provincial nursing regulators, and nursing, as a profession, is peer review.

Peer review is a key component of self-regulation and professional practice. It has been proposed that APNs with similar positions and expertise should participate in peer review. APN peer review has existed as part of performance assessment, evaluation of practice patterns, compliance monitoring, and the appraisal of quality indicators (Kenny, Baker, Lanzon, Stevens, & Yancy, 2008).

Scarpa and Connelly (2011) utilized a needs analysis approach including stakeholder focus groups to develop an APN job description adapted to the Synergy Model. The job description evolved into a "criterion-based performance assessment" and this process produced better defined APN roles and competencies that were specific to APN practice, ultimately promoting role autonomy, job satisfaction, and quality improvement.

At the Hospital for Sick Children (SickKids) in Toronto, APNs engage in a formal performance review process designed to evaluate APN role development and performance against a number of behaviours that delineate the growth of an APN from novice to expert. Through this process, the APN is able to provide a self-review and reflection on professional growth, establish goals and strategies to denote progress and achievement, and identify strengths and areas for growth using quantitative and peer feedback from nursing and other disciplines (SickKids, n.d.).

The US Department of Veterans Affairs utilizes a yearly APN peer review program designed to monitor performance based on clinical competence, practice behaviour, and the ability to perform under approved privileges (Rivera, 2012). This program is a hybrid model, based on recommendations from the American Association of Nurse Practitioners (AANP), but it incorporates the medical model integrating peer review between both nursing and medicine. APN peers, including physicians, constructively evaluate the candidate on a number of criteria including knowledge of biomedical, clinical, and social sciences, as well as the application of knowledge in providing collaborative patient care and education to stakeholders. Additionally, the APN must demonstrate ongoing professional development and apply research skills that investigate, evaluate, and improve best practices to provide quality, safe, efficient, and effective patient care (Rivera, 2012).

The Yale New Haven Hospital employs 400 APNs who practice in a wide range of roles and settings, including community health centres and the Yale School of Nursing. A peer review process was used to evaluate APN practice, and a peer review program of ongoing professional practice evaluation (OPPE), based on the medical model, was used by physicians. The hospital's APN council conducted two needs surveys, through which it discovered that APNs were practicing under various employment and collaborative practice models. They had little participation in the peer review process, which lacked APN-specific outcome measures, and found that APNs wanted greater peer advocacy and networking (Davies et al., 2014). In response to these findings, the APN council developed a similar OPPE tool based on the hospital's APN competencies framework and enhanced the peer review process that included self-evaluation. This initiative was piloted by oncology APNs and presented to stakeholders hospital-wide. Feedback directed the refinement and alignment of the review process with other hospital-wide processes, making it more APN-friendly prior to its implementation across all hospital divisions.

Historically, physician and nursing peer review have been separate processes. Emphasizing collaborative practice between physicians and NPs, and expanding care coordination including the expansion of clinical privileges of NPs, a unique integrative model for professional peer review was developed in the US in order to assess, measure, and provide continual quality improvement in practices. This shared structure, along with the processes and practices involved in its development, as well as the peer review tool, were designed with the goal of ensuring that NPs and physicians are engaged in exemplary provider performance and patient outcomes (Clavelle & Bramwell, 2013).

Conclusion

In reviewing the literature related to outcomes of care, it is evident there are numerous studies that have investigated outcomes related to APN practice for both NP and CNS roles. Measuring APN outcomes is important in defining the scope and practice of APN roles and the impact APN practice has on patient care, health care, costs of care, and other quality indicators including access, length of stay, and evidence-informed best practices. Through studying various outcomes, strategies can be developed to remove barriers to APN practice by demonstrating its impact on a variety of health care settings and organizations. Promoting the value of APN by implementing new and innovative models of care that evince APN knowledge, skill, and expertise continues to highlight APN roles by identifying their contributions within the health care field.

APNs must ensure that they have a voice in their own performance assessment processes. This will be become more fundamental in Canada as NPs are granted hospital privileges for admission, discharge, and transfer-of-care. Peer review is one approach that provides a means to monitor and improve professional practice competencies though the evaluations of peers practicing in similar roles and specialties. Like outcome measurements, peer review provides the opportunity for APNs to highlight their contributions to patient care within their employment or practice setting. This essential process supports APN practice and self-regulation while promoting quality patient care and interprofessional collaboration that can stimulate further APN research initiatives.

Critical Thinking Questions

1. Describe a systematic approach that might be utilized for outcomes evaluation of APN roles.
2. How does APN role implementation influence outcomes evaluation?
3. What research inquiries related to outcomes evaluation may further demonstrate the impact of APN roles?
4. What opportunities exist for APNs to be involved in the development of APN-sensitive performance assessment processes?
5. Within your organization, identify any outcome evaluation measures in progress or that may be done in the future.

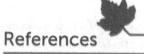

References

Browne, G., Birch, S., & Thabane, L. (2012). *Better care: An analysis of nursing and healthcare systems outcomes.* Ottawa, ON: CHSRF. Retrieved from http://www.cfhi-fcass.ca/sf-docs/default-source/commissioned-research-reports/Browne-BetterCare-EN.pdf?sfvrsn=0

Bryant-Lukosius, D., & DiCenso, A. (2004). A framework for the introduction and evaluation of advanced practice nursing roles. *Journal of Advanced Nursing, 48*(5), 530–540.

Bryant-Lukosius, D., DiCenso, A., Browne, G., & Pinelli, J. (2004). Advanced practice nursing roles: Development implementation, and evaluation. *Journal of Advanced Nursing, 48*(5), 519–529.

Bryant-Lukosius, D., Green, E., Fitch, M., McCartney, G., Robb-Blenderman, L., Bosompra, K., … Milne, H. (2007). A survey of oncology advanced practice roles in Ontario: Profile and predictors of job satisfaction. *Canadian Journal of Leadership, 20*(2), 50–68.

Burgess, J., & Purkis, M.E. (2010). The power and politics of collaboration in nurse practitioner role development. *Nursing Inquiry, 17*(4), 297–308.

Burns, N., & Grove, S.K. (2007). Outcomes Research. In N. Burns & S.K. Grove (Eds.), *Understanding nursing research: Building evidence-based practice* (4th ed., pp. 272–321). Philadelphia, PA: Saunders.

Clancy, C., & Eisenberg, J. (1997). Outcomes research at the Agency of Health Care Policy and Research. *Disease Management and Clinical Outcomes, 1,* 172–180.

Clavelle, J.T., & Bramwell, K. (2013). Nurse practitioner/physician collaborative practice: An integrative model for professional peer review. *Journal of Nursing Administration, 43*(6), 318–320.

Davies, M., Tucker, K., Dest, V., Lyons, C., Fitzsimons, S., & McCorkle, R. (2014). Enhancing peer review to support APN practice. *Oncology Nursing News.* Retrieved from http://nursing.onclive.com/publications/oncology-nurse/2014/October-2014/Enhancing-Peer-Review-to-Support-APN-Practice

DiCenso, A., & Bryant-Lukosius, D. (2010). The long and winding road: Integration of nurse practitioners and clinical nurse specialists into the Canadian health-care system. *Canadian Journal of Nursing Research, 42*(2), 3–8.

DiCenso, A., Martin-Misener, R., Bryant-Lukosius, D., Bourgeault, I., Kilpatrick, K., Donald, F., … Charbonneau-Smith, R. (2010). Advanced practice nursing in Canada: Overview of a decision support synthesis. *Nursing Leadership, 23*(Special Issue December), 15–34.

Donabedian, A. (2005). Evaluating the quality of medical care. *The Millbank Quarterly, 83,* 4.

Doran, D. (2011). *Nursing-sensitive outcomes: State of the science* (2nd ed.). Sudbury, MA: Jones & Bartlett.

Friese, C.R., & Beck, S.L. (2004). Advancing practice and research: Creating evidence-based summaries on measuring nursing-sensitive patient outcomes. *Clinical Journal of Oncology Nursing, 8*(6), 675–677.

The Hospital for Sick Children (SickKids). (n.d.). *APN performance review process.* Retrieved from http://www.sickkids.ca/Nursing/Nursing%20Practice/APN-Performance-Review-Process/index.html

Ingersoll, G., McIntosh, E., & Williams, M. (2000). Nurse-sensitive outcomes of advanced practice. *Journal of Advanced Nursing, 32*(5), 1272–1281.

Jacobson, P.M., & HDR Inc. (2012). *Evidence synthesis for the effectiveness of interprofessional teams in primary care*. Ottawa, ON: CHSRF. Retrieved from http://www.cfhi-fcass.ca/sf-docs/default-source/commissioned-research-reports/Jacobson-Interprofessional-EN.pdf?sfvrsn=0

Kenny, K.J., Baker, L., Lanzon, M., Stevens, L.R., & Yancy, M. (2008). An innovative approach to peer review for the advanced practice nurse: A focus on critical incidents. *Journal of the American Academy of Nurse Practitioners, 20*(7), 376–381.

Kleinpell, R. (Ed.) (2009). *Outcome assessment in advanced practice nursing* (2nd ed.). New York, NY: Springer.

Kleinpell, R., & Gawlinski, A. (2005). Assessing outcomes in advanced nursing practice: The use of quality indicators and evidence-based practice. *AACN Clinical Issues, 16*(1), 43–57.

MacDonald, M., Schreiber, R., Davidson, H., Pauly, B., Moss, L., Pinelli, J., … Hammond, C. (2005). Moving towards harmony: Exemplars of advanced nursing practice for British Columbia. *Nursing Leadership (Online Exclusive), 18*(2). Retrieved from http://www.long-woods.com/content/19030. doi: 10.12927/cjnl.2005.19030

Newhouse, R.P., Stanik-Hutt, J., White, K.M., Johantgen, M., Bass, E.B., Zangaro, G., … Weiner, J.P. (2011). Advanced practice nurse outcomes 1990–2008: A systematic review. *Nursing Economics, 29*(5), 1–29.

Rivera, C. (2012). *Advanced practice nurse (APN) peer review program at the Department of Veterans Affairs*. Retrieved from https://prezi.com/q5qespc0kmmt/advance-practice-nurse-peer-review/

Sangster-Gormley, E. (2014). *Nurse practitioner-sensitive outcomes: A summary report*. Halifax, NS: CRNNS.

Scarpa, R., & Connelly, P.E. (2011). Innovations in performance assessment: A criterion based performance assessment of advanced practice nurses using a synergistic theoretical nursing framework. *Nursing Administration Quarterly, 35*(2), 164–173.

Tarlov, A.R., Ware, Jr., J.E., Greenfield, S., Nelson, E.C., Perrin, E., & Zubkoff, M. (1989). The medical outcomes study: An application of methods for monitoring the results of medical care. *Journal of the American Medical Association, 262*(7), 925–930. Retrieved from http://www.prgs.edu/content/dam/rand/pubs/notes/2009/N3038.pdf

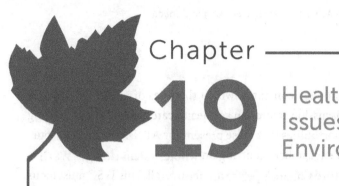

Chapter

19

Health Policy Issues in Changing Environments[1]

Doris Grinspun

Doris Grinspun is the Chief Executive Officer of the Registered Nurses' Association of Ontario (RNAO). Previously, Doris served as Director of Nursing at Mount Sinai Hospital in Toronto, Ontario. She has also worked in practice and administrative capacities in Israel and the United States. Doris holds appointments as an Adjunct Professor in the Lawrence S. Bloomberg Faculty of Nursing at the University of Toronto; Adjunct Professor at York University, School of Nursing; associate member of the Centre for Health Promotion at the University of Toronto; affiliate member of the Centre for Health Studies at York University; and Associate Fellow of the Centre for Research on Latin American and the Caribbean (CERLAC) at York University in Toronto, Ontario. Doris has been featured in major media outlets and publications for her bold and visionary leadership, and, in 2003, was invested with the Order of Ontario.

KEY TERMS

advanced practice nurses
 (APNs)
Canada's performance
health system
nursing
nursing as a body politic
Organisation
 for Economic
 Co-operation and
 Development (OECD)
whole system change
 (WSC)

OBJECTIVES

1. Discuss and compare Canada's health care performance nationally and internationally.
2. Understand nursing and advanced practice nursing (APN) as a key solution for Canada's health system shortfalls.
3. Explore how whole system change happens, and the importance of nursing and nurses' purposeful political engagement to shape healthy public policy.

Introduction

This chapter presents the health policy context in which the roles of advanced practice nurses (APNs) is situated. The discussion centres on key health care challenges confronting Canada, and the threats and opportunities that these present for APNs. The need for purposeful and continuous political engagement centring on whole system change (WSC) is discussed as the only way to improve Canada's performance overall. This WSC must focus on shifting Canada's heavy reliance on illness care towards a robust community care that is anchored in primary care and focuses on health promotion, disease prevention, mental health, and chronic disease prevention and management. Meaningful WSC can only occur if all health professionals work to their optimal scope of practice, in high performing teams that deliver person-centred and evidence-informed care.

Nursing, being the largest segment of the health care workforce, is key to Canada's health system transformation. As the most trusted profession by the public, nursing has a duty to speak out and be heard. This chapter concludes with an urgent call to reclaim nursing as a body politic.

Context: Canada's Health and Health Care Outcomes

International comparisons show that Canada is falling short on key outcome indicators when it comes to delivering health care. For example, the Commonwealth Fund (2014) ranked Canada's health care system 10th out of 11 industrialized countries in terms of quality care, access, efficiency, equity, healthy lives, and expenditures. Canada ranked last in accessing same-day primary care services, last in overall timeliness of care, and eighth for coordinated and patient-centred care (Davis, Stremikis, Squires, & Schoen, 2014).

These results, especially in the areas of equity, healthy lives, and expenditures, can be largely attributed to Canada's lower than average social spending when compared to other Organisation for Economic Co-operation and Development (OECD) nations. In 2013, total health expenditure accounted for 10% of Canada's gross domestic product (GDP) (OECD, 2014a). In 2014, social spending accounted for 17% of Canada's gross domestic GDP, while the OECD average is at 21.6% (OECD, 2015). Simply put, if Canada chooses to spend less on upstream investments indeterminant of health programs (both social and environmental) we will inevitably achieve less equity and healthy lives, and spend more on health care. The solution to improving these specific indicators is investing more in social and environmental programs that will bring increased equity and healthy (or healthier) populations, and decrease the demand for health care services (see Figures 19.1 and 19.2).

It is against this backdrop that nursing holds the key. Through its role as a body politic in the space of public and policy debates about the future of Medicare, and as the largest practice discipline, nursing has much to offer to improve our nation's standing on timely

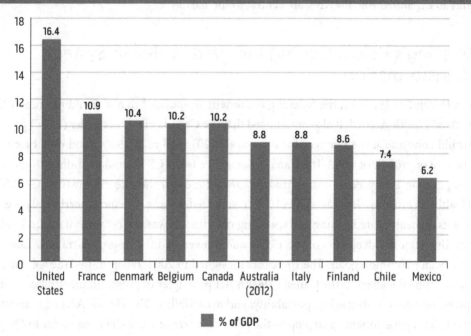

FIGURE 19.1: Total Health Expenditure as a Share of GDP

Source: Adapted from Organisation for Economic Co-operation and Development (OECD), 2015.

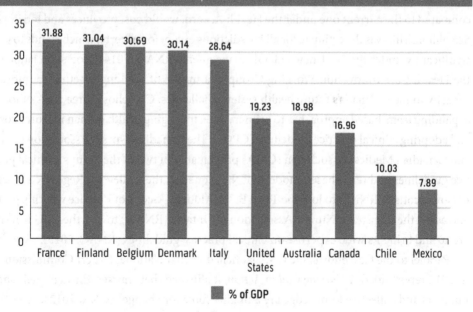

FIGURE 19.2: Public Social Expenditure as a Share of GDP (OECD, 2014)

Source: Adapted from Organisation for Economic Co-operation and Development (OECD), 2014b.

access to quality care, efficiency, and coordinated person-centred care. The role of APNs, and an expanded role for RNs, are central to the narrative.

Nursing's Voice: Getting Involved in Health System Transformation

On December 19, 2011, the federal government announced that it would not renew the Federal Health Accord. It also announced that the Canada Health Transfer (CHT) growth would continue at 6% per year for three years (2014–15 to 2016–17) and then be cut to the rate of growth of GDP. The Canada Social Transfer (CST) would continue to grow at 3% per year. Lastly, equalization transfers would grow at the rate of growth of GDP. The Health Accord was a legal agreement between the federal and provincial/territorial governments on health care funding and spending priorities. It was important as it assured stable funding after the deep cuts of the 1990s, and it leveraged the improved transfer funding to advance common goals. The 10-year plan, signed in 2004, recommitted the federal and jurisdictional leaders to the Canada Health Act principles of public administration, comprehensiveness, universality, portability, and accessibility. The Health Accord mandated the federal government to step up to the plate by increasing the CHT payments to 6% per year. At that time, common goals were set around wait times, team-based primary care, home care, and prescription drugs.

Reacting to the news, the Council of the Federation (CoF), composed of the premiers and leaders of all provinces and territories, confirmed in 2012 that the new arrangement, compared to the current one under the Health Accord, would cost provinces and territories $25 billion. This was the estimate for all jurisdictions except for Alberta, which stands to gain significantly under the 2011 new federal arrangement (RNAO, 2014). CoF soon launched the Health Care Innovation Working Group as a means of working together to improve capacity to meet Canada's future health system challenges. CoF chose three areas of focus: expanding team-based approaches to primary care, managing health human resource costs, and adopting clinical practice guidelines (CPGs). The Canadian Nurses Association (CNA) and Canadian Medical Association (CMA) participated in two of the groups (clinical practice guidelines and team-based models); CNA requested the College of Registered Nurses of Nova Scotia (CRNNS) to join the Team Based Models—Scope of Practice working group and asked the Registered Nurses' Association of Ontario (RNAO) to join the CPG working group and bring its wide expertise on clinical practice guidelines (RNAO, 2015).

Parallel to the CoF efforts, the CNA launched its first National Expert Commission. In its 2012 report titled *A Nursing Call to Action*, it affirmed that "nurses, through their sheer numbers and collective knowledge are a mighty force for change" (CNA, 2012a, p. 1). The report stated that "registered nurses are deeply engaged in system transformation because they care about human health and about delivering responsible health care. But more than caring, it is the professional and social responsibility of nurses to take a strong leadership stand on behalf of Canadians" (CNA, 2012a, p. 1). This deep sense of duty is echoed by many organizations across the nation, and RNAO is among those strongly committed to shaping the future of health and health care in Ontario.

CoF estimated, when looking specifically, that Ontario will lose in excess of $13 billion over 10 years under the new fiscal arrangement with the federal government (CoF, 2012). This reality spurred the provincial government's determination to act on several fronts, starting with a full review of all public services led by economist Don Drummond. The Commission on the Reform of Ontario's Public Services report outlines 362 recommenda-tions, with over 100 for health care. RNAO, who had met with Mr. Drummond on several occasions during the consultations, gave mixed reviews. On the one hand, RNAO was highly critical about recommendations that suggested the private sector could deliver more efficient and cost-effective health services. It also opposed recommendations that proposed freezes in social spending, which would have translated into real per capita cuts. So far, the Ontario government has also rejected such recommendations.

On the other hand, RNAO was highly influential and fully endorsed recommendations to bring primary care under the control of Local Health Integration Networks (LHIN) to foster higher integration, as well as to expand scope of practice for all regulated health providers. RNAO also applauded the report's specific acknowledgement of the central role nurses play in the health system, and its potential for improved health outcomes and cost savings. Equally important was the report's recommendation to ensure that evidence-based care becomes the norm, a recommendation that resonated with RNAO's long-established leadership in developing and actively supporting implementation of best practice guidelines (BPGs) (Grinspun, Melnyk, & Fineout-Overholt, 2014; RNAO, 2015).

Soon after the release of the Drummond Report, RNAO issued two groundbreaking reports that were poised to shape health and nursing policy provincially, nationally, and internationally. The first, *Primary Solutions for Primary Care* (RNAO, 2012b), outlines a two-phased blueprint to maximize and expand the role of nurses in primary care that includes RN prescribing. RNAO recommends that the move to RN prescribing be based on an enabling framework that improves access to care by recognizing the broad depth of RN expertise. This report has already shaped health policy in Ontario. In her address to nurses attending RNAO's 88th Annual General Meeting in 2013, Ontario's Premier Kathleen Wynne said she recognized that nurses want their scope of practice to match their expertise. The changes announced by the Premier included allowing RNs to prescribe medi-cations. This was followed by a formal commitment to RN prescribing from the Ontario Liberal Party during the elections campaign in May 2014. Most recently, at RNAO's 15th Annual Queen's Park event in February 2015, the Minister of Health and Long-Term Care, alongside the Premier, announced that the province is proceeding with RN prescribing. RNAO's report has also served to shape national nursing positions and this is reflected in CNA's National Expert Commission Report (2012a), which recommended that the scope of practice of RNs be expanded to include prescribing in an effort to support patient care and health system sustainability.

The second report, *Enhancing Community Care for Ontarians (ECCO)*, (RNAO, 2012c) released first in 2012 and then updated in 2014, proposes shifting health care from an illness model to a health-oriented one by urging substantive investments in upstream programs in social and environmental programs, and by repositioning the system to be anchored in primary and community care as opposed to the current focus on illness and hospital care. This, RNAO argues, will strengthen our publicly-funded, not-for-profit health system and make it more responsive to the public's needs, better coordinated, easier to navigate, more efficient, and cost-effective.

Figure 19.3 depicts the ECCO model. Critical areas of focus are health promotion, disease prevention, mental health, and chronic disease prevention and management. These

FIGURE 19.3:   RNAO ECCO Model Overview

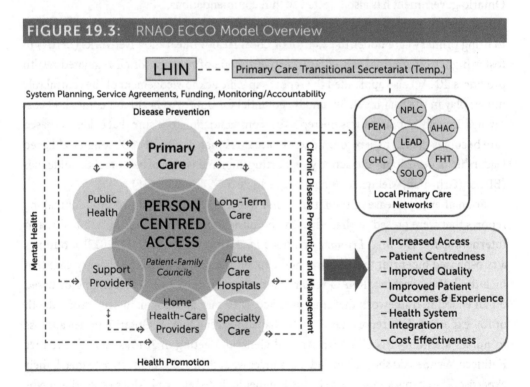

Note: LHIN = Local Integration Networks for Ontario; AHAC = Aboriginal Health Access Centres; CHC = Community Health Centres; FHT = Family Health Teams; NPLC = Nurse Practitioner-Led Clinics; PEM = Primary Care Enrolment Model; Solo = Solo Practitioner Practice.

Source: Registered Nurses' Association of Ontario (RNAO), 2012a. Reprinted with permission.

changes must be accompanied by enabling nurses and all other regulated health profession-als to work to their full scopes of practice in interprofessional teams, and using evidence to guide clinical- and work-environment practices.

The report has already influenced action. The views of Deb Matthews, then Ontario's Minister of Health, were reflected in *Ontario's Action Plan for Health Care* (Ontario Ministry of Health and Long Term Care [MOHLTC], 2012), which supported a continued shift of care delivery to the home and community settings to improve patient outcomes and system cost-effectiveness. Similarly, Ontario's current Minister of Health Dr. Eric Hoskins' *Patients First: Action Plan for Health Care* (Ontario MOHLTC, 2015) reflects a similar view, based on a person-centred agenda like ECCO. Most recently, ECCO's priorities are well reflected in the Report of the Expert Group on Home and Community Care, chaired by nurse leader Dr. Gail Donner, which was released by the Ontario government in March 2015. The next provincial report to be soon released by the Ontario government, and perhaps the most important, focuses on primary care.

Alongside the flurry of reports, we must juxtapose a dose of reality-based action. No substantial improvement in timely access, efficiency, and cost-effectiveness can be achieved without a fulsome participation of nurses, and any barriers that limit such participation must be torn down. This axiom is as true for Ontario as it is for Canada, or any other country where nursing is its largest workforce. Turning the tide from Canada being a lower performer to top performer is within reach; nurses' practice-power must be unleashed to its full and expanded potential, APNs must move to the driver's seat, and all must work in high-functioning inter-professional teams that deliver person-centred and evidence-informed practices.

Figure 19.4 shows the three pillars that are essential to improve timely access to person-centred care, optimize health outcomes, and achieve health system effectiveness. These include full scope of practice, interprofessional care, and evidence-based practice. Simply put, timely access to health care services can significantly improve if all health profession-als are working to their optimal scopes and in high-functioning interprofessional teams (Grinspun, 2007; Grinspun & Aninyam, 2014; RNAO, 2013).

The facts speak for themselves. In 2014, there were 293,205 RNs working in nursing (including NPs) in Canada, and a further 12,901 not working in nursing (or not specified), for a total of 306,106 RNs (Canadian Institute for Health Information [CIHI], 2015). Of these, there were 3,966 NPs working in nursing, and a further 178 not working in nursing (or not specified), for a total of 4,144 NPs (CIHI, 2015). Although there is no agreed-upon number of CNSs in Canada, estimates, based on self-declared statements, were around 2,200 in 2010, and of these only 800 nurses reporting to be CNSs had a graduate degree (CNA, 2012b). Just imagine, if this robust workforce were utilized to their optimal practice scopes, what that would do for timely health care access!

Let's look as an example at primary care in the province of Ontario. In 2014, there were 1,144 working NPs and 4,158 RNs in the general class working in primary care in Ontario

FIGURE 19.4:   Pillars for Health System Effectiveness

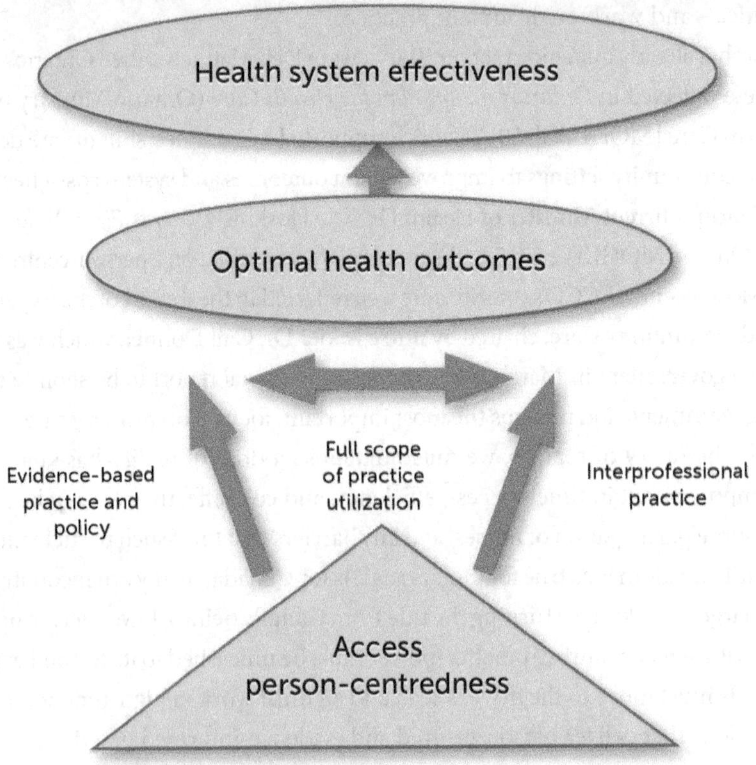

Source: Grinspun, 2012. Reprinted with permission.

(special data request to the College of Nurses of Ontario). As discussed in previous chapters, a good percentage of these NPs work below their full practice scope, despite having the legislative authority to do otherwise. The same holds true for CNSs. The situation is no better for RNs. Allard, Frego, Katz, & Halas (2010) found in a survey of primary care RNs from across Canada that only 61% of those who responded felt they were practicing to their full scope. Likely, the percentage of RNs in primary care who are underutilized is even higher given that the nature of the survey—self-reported—may have introduced social desirability bias where respondents answer in a way that will be seen favourably by others and not undermine their roles.

The scope of practice underutilization of APNs and RNs poses a substantive cost to Canadians and the health system, both in terms of timely access and value for service return on taxpayers' investments. On the first (timely access), if the majority of NPs, CNSs, and RNs practice scope were optimized, it is entirely foreseeable that people would have same-day access to primary care. Meanwhile, only 43.1% of Ontarians are able to see their family physician on the same or next day when ill (Health Quality Ontario, 2013). On the second (return on investment), total payments to Ontario's family physicians increased by $1.3 billion or 54% (after inflation) over a period of five years between 2003–04 and 2009–10. In 2009–10, the mean payment per full-time equivalent of family physicians was $300,100, which equates to anywhere between two-and-a-half to three times the salary of an NP and five times the current salary of an RN in primary care.

Consumer preferences, combined with financially strapped governments, have led to greater consideration of community care as a means to curb costs. Primary care and home health care are the two sectors increasingly receiving attention. While primary care can help people stay healthy, and delay as well as manage chronic conditions, high-quality home care can support them to remain active members of their communities. Nurses have always played a central role in community care, and NPs and CNSs must assert their clinical and advocacy roles in leading primary care and home health care.

In Ontario, significant gains have been made in cementing the role of primary care NPs in Community Health Centres (CHC), Aboriginal Health Access Centres (AHAC), Family Health Teams (FHT), and NP-led clinics, with 26 of the latter being fully operational and providing same-day access to thousands of Ontarians. Ontario also enables NPs, through legislative changes, to treat, transfer, and discharge hospital in-patients. Since 2012, legislation has also allowed NPs to admit hospitals' in-patients, a function that has yet to fully mature. NPs are also taking a lead in long-term care homes, and their numbers and roles are being expanded to primary attending provider. What will it take to scale-up even further the NP as a leading role, both within Ontario and across the country? Equally important, how can it be ensured the same happens with the invaluable role of the CNS?

Understanding Whole System Change to Spur Innovations and Improve Health Outcomes

It took almost 40 years for NPs to have legislated authority. It will likely take four to five years for RNs to achieve the same. Determining the potential speed of scope expansion adoption lies in understanding the factors that influence the uptake of innovations and the mechanisms that come into play that either accelerate or hinder adoption. The case of NPs in Canada can help illustrate this best.

In a seminal paper on understanding WSC, Edwards, Rowan, Marck, and Grinspun (2011) asked if the vast evidence pointing to the effectiveness of NPs was insufficient to trigger rapid adoption and growth; what else was needed? The authors then mapped out all the factors that influenced on the progress of NP adoption. These are summarized in Figure 19.5.

The following five lessons were learned:

FIGURE 19.5: Whole Systems Change in Health Care: Basic Elements

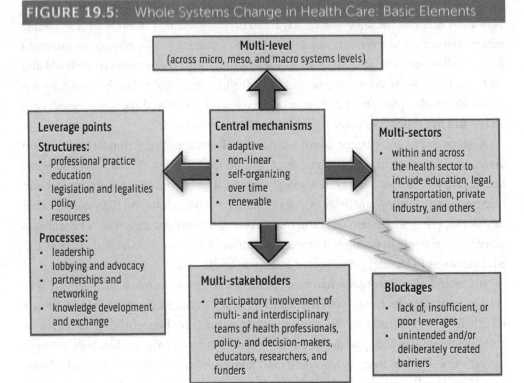

Source: Edwards, Rowan, Marck, & Grinspun, 2011. Reprinted with permission.

1. WSC is a complex, social, and ecological phenomenon, characterized by dynamic interactions among institutional, political, educational, and at times legislative forces involving multiple stakeholders and multiple sectors within micro, meso, and macro system levels over time (Edwards et al., 2011).

2. Program developers and change agents need to consider potential leverage points and blockages to capitalize on and/or mitigate their interrelated potential to either accelerate or decelerate WSC at varying points in time (Edwards et al., 2011).

3. When introducing health systems innovations, it is important to assess not only the outcomes of the innovation but also the context of uptake (Edwards et al., 2011).

4. WSC is nonlinear and cross-scale, which means that sustainable system changes occur across a panarchy of slower- and faster-moving adaptive cycles that transect system hierarchies over time (Edwards, Davies, Ploeg, Virani, & Skelly, 2007; Gunderson & Holling, 2002; Gunderson, Light, & Holling, 1995).

5. Diverse, multi-level, and multisectoral forms of leadership are essential to foster whole systems change (Edwards et al., 2011).

These important lessons help us understand the vital importance of active professional organizations. A revitalized RNAO took it upon itself to organize the nursing community with a laser-like focus from 1996 until the proclamation of the NP legislation in 1998. Part of the multi-pronged strategy involved meeting strategically with the Minister of Health to discuss NP initiatives, while also orchestrating: (a) a letter writing campaign to Ontario's Minister of Health, the Premier, and opposition leaders to influence their decision regarding the urgent need for NP legislation; (b) a multi-organizational press conference; (c) visits by NPs and RNs with local politicians in their ridings; and (d) media engagement to help the media and public understand NPs as a health system solution.

Improving the health system and health outcomes of Canadians requires the ongoing and persistent engagement of nursing as a collective in the political process. This engagement must be multi-partisan to enrich our democracy and grow the respect achieved from the public, politicians, and the media. By targeting specific policies aimed at closing the gap between what Canadians need and what nursing can offer, contributions to the health of Canadians, along with the health and health care performance of the country, can be improved. Accepting the duty of nursing as a body politic to advance WSC is central to ensuring that Canadians will fully benefit from the APNs' roles and from nurses as a whole. The role of professional associations and labour unions is paramount for this to happen.

In another seminal article, Cohen et al. (1996) delineated four stages of nursing's political development, and recommended strategies for implementing the fourth and most complex stage. Nursing in Canada has long evolved from the first stage—the "buy-in" stage where the profession recognizes the importance of political activism, but the nature of action is reactive and inward-focused, driven mainly by the interests of nursing. However, it is towards a much more sophisticated stage that nursing must evolve in order to fundamentally affect change. Nursing as a body politic in Canada must deliberately and skillfully attain what Cohen and colleagues deem as stage four, where nursing "leads the way." This is a stage in which the profession is envisioned as providing true political leadership on broader policy issues that speak to the public's interests. The profession is proactive on leadership and agenda-setting for a broad range of health and social policy issues, introducing terms that reorder the debate, and initiating coalitions beyond nursing for broad policy concerns. At this stage, many nurses are sought to fill nursing and health policy positions because of the value of nursing expertise and knowledge. The authors argue that the further the profession is able to move into this stage, the more the public will benefit from nursing's expertise and the advocacy on behalf of the public (Cohen et al., 1996).

Activism on broader health and social issues does not preclude continued vigilance on professional issues related to nursing practice. Indeed, the fourth stage does not rule out pursuit of self-interests; it merely does so within a context that emphasizes the larger public good. Pursuit of stage four can be enhanced by building coalitions and constituencies around health and social issues, leadership development and supporting visionaries and risk-takers, mobilizing nursing for campaigns, integrating health policy into curricula, developing public media expertise, and gaining increased sophistication in policy analysis and related research (Cohen et al., 1996).

Ennen (2001) defines four spheres for political action that deserve close attention. Government (the first sphere for political action) plays a critical, far-reaching role in nursing and health care. It defines and regulates nursing practice, sets and influences reimbursement systems for health care and nursing services, and sets the policy agenda related to health care provision. Here the ambit of regulation of professional nursing practice is central. Public law defines for whom nurses care, as well as when, where, and how care is delivered. It also regulates APN educational requirements and certification processes, as well as how they practice within the health care system.

Licensure, a prerogative of the state (in Canada, the provinces and territories), is deter-mined by a legislative process that sets rules and regulations governing licensure and desig-nates an agency responsible for law enforcement (in Canada, the regulatory colleges). The current licensure laws have raised the standards of education and established codes for the ethical behaviour of RNs and NPs, and created a state registry of persons meeting these criteria. Workplace is the second sphere for action. The policy and political nuances of the workplace can have a profound impact on the quality of nurses' professional lives. Professional organizations constitute the third sphere; they shape the practice of nursing through political influence and policy-making.

Developing standards of practice, lobbying for changes in the scope of practice, and playing a role in collective action are three services that professional organizations provide their members and the nursing profession as a whole. Strong professional organizations identify issues of concern to nursing and health care, and bring them to the attention of the public. Community, the fourth sphere of political action, is more than a practice arena for nursing. Rather, it is a social unit involving a variety of special interest groups, community activities, health and social problems, and available resources to solve identified problems.

Advocacy is also essential for nurses at the point of care to impact practice and the well-being of patients. Tomajan (2012) describes advocacy skills every nurse can employ to advocate for a safe and healthy work environment, and explains how nurses can advocate for nursing as part of their daily activity whether they are point-of-care nurses, nurse man-agers, or nurse educators. These advocacy practices are applicable, whether in advocating on one's own behalf, for colleagues at the unit level, or for issues at the organizational or system level. It is argued that advocacy requires a set of skills that includes problem solv-ing, communication, influence, and collaboration, skills akin to those that nurses use to deliver clinical care. Point-of-care nurses build on their public image of being the most trusted profession by communicating and advocating for a more accurate view of their contributions to health care and society. Managers and administrators advocate in their daily work to obtain required resources for their nursing staff and promote healthy work environments. Nurse educators play a critical role in preparing nurses to strengthen the profession through advocacy. Finally, nurses themselves must be involved in shaping public policy directly or indirectly affecting practice.

Conclusion

Canada's fiscal realities bring challenges and opportunities to the APN role. To thrive, APN roles must be understood and positioned as a key solution to the health and health care imperatives facing the public, both as funders and users of health services. Augmenting the narrative of NPs and CNSs (which already contains remarkable clinical expertise and proven health and system outcomes) with a nursing collective that is leading the way sets the agenda purposefully to benefit the public.

Critical Thinking Questions

1. What is Canada's health and health care performance compared to other OECD countries?
2. How can a health system redesign help improve Canada's performance?
3. How can APNs (NPs and CNSs) be positioned as a response to solve Canada's challenges?
4. What does it take to create whole system change (WSC)?

Note

1.   I would like to thank Josephine Mo, my Executive Assistant at RNAO, for her ready assistance in preparing the references and reviewing the draft. Also, my gratitude to Tim Lenartowych, RNAO's Director of Nursing and Health Policy, and Kim Jarvi, Senior Economist, for some of the statistical data and for our ongoing collaboration.

References

Allard, M., Frego, A., Katz, A., & Halas, G. (2010). Exploring the role of RNs in family practice residency training programs. *Canadian Nurse, 106*(3), 20–24.

Canadian Institute for Health Information. (2015). *Regulated nurses, 2014*. Ottawa, ON: CIHI. Retrieved from https://secure.cihi.ca/free_products/RegulatedNurses2014_Report_EN.pdf

Canadian Nurses Association (CNA). (2012a). *A nursing call to action: Expert Commission report*. Retrieved from http://www.cna-aiic.ca/~/media/cna/files/en/nec_report_e.pdf

CNA. (2012b). *Strengthening the role of the clinical nurse specialist in Canada: Background paper.* Ottawa, ON: CNA. Retrieved from https://www.cna-aiic.ca/~/media/cna/page-content/pdf-fr/strengthening_the_cns_role_background_paper_e.pdf?la=en

Cohen, S.S., Mason, D.J., Kovner, C., Leavitt, J.K., Pulcini, J., & Sochalski, J. (1996). Stages of nursing's political involvement: Where we've and where we ought to go. *Nursing Outlook, 44*(6), 259–266.

Council of the Federation (CoF) Working Group on Fiscal Arrangements. (2012). *Assessment of the fiscal impact of the current Federal Fiscal Proposals.* Retrieved from http://www.pmprovincesterritoires.ca/phocadownload/publications/cof_working_group_on_fiscal_arrangements_report_and_appendices_july.pdf

Davis, K., Stremikis, K., Squires, D., & Schoen, C. (2014). *Mirror, mirror on the wall: How the performance of the U.S. health care system compares internationally* (2014 update). Retrieved from http://www.commonwealthfund.org/publications/fund-reports/2014/jun/mirror-mirror

Edwards, N., Davies, B., Ploeg, J., Virani, T., & Skelly, J. (2007). Implementing nursing best practice guidelines: Impact on patient referrals. *BioMed Central Nursing, 6*(4), 1–9.

Edwards, N., Rowan, M., Marck, P., & Grinspun, D. (2011). Understanding whole systems change in health care: The case of nurse practitioners in Canada. *Policy, Politics & Nursing Practice, 12*(1), 4–17. doi: 10.1177/1527154411403816

Ennen, K. (2001). Shaping the future of practice through political activity: How nurses can influence health care policy. *American Association of Occupational Health Nurses (AAOH) Journal, 49*(12), 557–571.

Expert Group on Home and Community Care. (2015). *Bringing care home.* Toronto: Ministry of Health and Long-Term Care.

Grinspun, D. (2007). Healthy workplaces: The case for shared clinical decision making and increased full-time employment. *Healthcare Papers, 7*(Spec No: 85–91), 109–19.

Grinspun, D. (2012). *Healthcare in a time of fiscal restraint: Collaborating for system sustainability.* Keynote Address, McMaster University, 2012.

Grinspun, D., & Anyinam, C. (2014). Leadership. In S. Coffey & C. Anyinam (Eds.). *Interprofessional health care practice* (1st ed., pp. 131–158). Toronto, ON: Pearson.

Grinspun, D., Melnyk, B.M., & Fineout-Overholt, E. (2014) Advancing optimal care with rigorously developed clinical practice guidelines and evidence-based recommendations. In B.M. Melynk & E. Fineout-Overholt (Eds). *Evidence-based practice in nursing and healthcare. A guide to best practice* (3rd ed., pp. 182–201). Philadelphia, PA: Lippincott Williams & Wilkins.

Gunderson, L.H., & Holling, C.S. (Eds.). (2002). *Panarchy: Understanding transformations in human and natural systems.* Washington, DC: Island Press.

Gunderson, L.H., Light, S.S., & Holling, C.S. (Eds.). (1995). *Barriers and bridges to the renewal of ecosystems and institutions.* New York, NY: Columbia University Press.

Health Quality Ontario (2013). *Yearly report on Ontario's health system.* Retrieved from http://www.hqontario.ca/portals/0/Documents/pr/hqo-yearly-report-2013-en.pdf

National Expert Commission. (2012). *A nursing call to action: The health of our nation, the future of our health system.* Ottawa, ON: CNA. Retrieved from https://www.cna-aiic.ca/~/media/cna/files/en/nec_report_e.pdf

Organisation for Economic Co-operation and Development (OECD). (2014a). *Social expenditure database (SOCX)*. Retrieved from http://www.oecd.org/social/expenditure.htm

OECD. (2014b). *Social expenditure update: Social spending is falling in some countries, but in many others it remains at historically high levels*. Retrieved from http://www.oecd.org/els/soc/OECD2014-Social-Expenditure-Update-Nov2014-8pages.pdf

OECD. (2015). *Social expenditure – Detailed data*. Retrieved from http://stats.oecd.org/Index.aspx?DataSetCode=SOCX_DET

Ontario Ministry of Health and Long-Term Care (MOHLTC). (2012). *Ontario's action plan for health care*. Toronto, ON: MOHLTC. Retrieved from http://health.gov.on.ca/en/ms/ecfa/healthy_change/docs/rep_healthychange.pdf

Ontario MOHLTC. (2015). *Patients first: Action plan for health care*. Toronto, ON: MOHLTC. Retrieved from http://health.gov.on.ca/en/ms/ecfa/healthy_change/docs/rep_patientsfirst.pdf

Registered Nurses' Association of Ontario (RNAO). (2012a). *Primary solutions for primary care: Maximizing and expanding the role of the primary care nurse in Ontario*. Retrieved from http://rnao.ca/sites/rnao-ca/files/Primary_Care_Report_2012_0.pdf

RNAO. (2012b). *Primary solutions for primary care: Stakeholders' voices*. Retrieved from http://rnao.ca/news/media-releases/2012/06/28/provincial-task-force-action-plan-will-ensure-same-day-access-patient/stakeholders

RNAO. (2012c). *Enhancing Community Care for Ontarians (ECCO 1.0)*. Retrieved from http://rnao.ca/sites/rnao-ca/files/RNAO_ECCO_WHITE_PAPER_FINAL_2.pdf

RNAO. (2013). *Developing and sustaining interprofessional health care*. Retrieved from http://rnao.ca/bpg/guidelines/interprofessional-team-work-healthcare

RNAO. (2014). *Queen's Park day 2014 briefing notes: Renewal of federal health accord*. Retrieved from http://rnao.ca/policy/briefing-notes/queens-park-day-2014-briefing-notes

RNAO. (2015). *Best practice guidelines program*. Retrieved from http://rnao.ca/bpg

Tomajan, K., (2012). Advocating for nurses and nursing. *Online Journal of Issues in Nursing*, *17*(1), 4. doi: 10.3912/OJIN.Vol17No01Man04

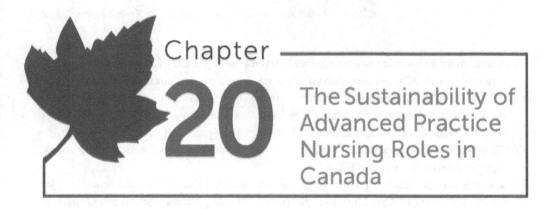

Chapter 20

The Sustainability of Advanced Practice Nursing Roles in Canada

Esther Sangster-Gormley

Esther Sangster-Gormley is an Associate Professor and Nurse Practitioner Program Coordinator, and teaches in the NP program at the University of Victoria, School of Nursing in British Columbia. She has spent much of her career as an NP, practicing in Florida until relocating to the University of New Brunswick, where she taught in the NP program. Esther has been involved in efforts that contribute to NP role sustainability both provincially and nationally. Over the last 10 years, Esther's research focus has been on the implementation and integration of NPs.

KEY TERMS

advanced practice nurse
  (APN)
primary health care
  (PHC)
sustainability

OBJECTIVES

1. Develop strategies to sustain the advanced practice nursing (APN) role within an organization.
2. Discuss ways of advocating for APN role sustainability.
3. Discuss contextual factors influencing APN role sustainability.

Introduction

The combined high cost of health care, aging demographics, and a global shortage of health care professionals is pressuring governments in Canada and worldwide to look for ways to change how health care is delivered. Advanced practice nursing (APN) roles are gaining more international attention as an option for meeting health care demands. Currently, approximately 50 countries have created or are in the process of creating APN roles (Kleinpell et al., 2014). As APN roles continue to evolve, it is important to consider the challenges that exist and the support necessary to ensure CNSs, NPs, and other advanced practice nurses are fully utilized and their roles are integrated and sustained within the health care system. In this chapter, sustainability of advanced nursing roles means that they are essential to the health care system and will continue to be supported in the future.

Global Emergence of Advanced Practice Nursing Roles

Multiple factors are contributing to the willingness of international governments to recognize the contributions nurses in advanced roles have made, and consider creating further opportunities to utilize nursing's potential more fully. A shortage of physicians and other health care workers, increasing emphasis on primary health care, and the complexity of hospitalized patients are drivers that are influencing the willingness to extend nursing's capacity within health care. Likewise, nurses' demands for more career choices, along with opportunities to remain in clinical practice, have prompted decision-makers to consider advanced nursing roles with increasing responsibility and autonomy (Schober & Affara, 2006). However, and for a variety of reasons, there is variation in how APN roles are emerging globally.

A global definition of APN is a starting point toward consistency in how APN roles are described. The International Council of Nursing (ICN) consulted extensively to establish the definition, characteristics, and scope of practice of nurses in advanced roles. ICN defines an advanced practice nurse as a registered nurse with expert knowledge, complex decision-making skills, and the clinical competence for practice beyond that of an RN. While a master's degree is recommended for entry to practice, the country and context within which the advanced practice nurse is credentialed influences how their practice is enacted (ICN, 2013). This definition allows countries the latitude to adjust APN roles to meet their economic, social, and political context. Consistency in defining the role, regardless of country of origin, contributes to a better understanding of the roles.

Global Challenges to Advanced Practice Nursing Roles

The global emergence of new nursing roles is not without challenges. Most often, differences in educational requirements, variation in scopes of practice and titles, and the nursing profession's strength and readiness to advance nursing to a higher level within the health care system impacts the uptake of APN roles (Kleinpell et al., 2014; Pulcini, 2014). Nursing leaders within organizations are vital to the introduction and sustainability of APN roles. At the same time, it must be acknowledged that the nursing profession's power base is stronger in some countries than in others. Consequently, the power differences between nursing and medicine will impact nursing leaders' capacity to launch and sustain APN roles.

Equally important is the fact that remuneration for health care services affects APN roles, particularly NPs. The ability to practice to full scope is limited in countries where regulatory and reimbursement structures restrict APNs from being directly reimbursed for the care they deliver. For example, in countries like Canada with universal government-sponsored health care, legislation may limit reimbursement for primary health care services to physicians on a fee-for-service basis. Box 20.1 is a summary of global challenges to APN sustainability.

BOX 20.1

Global Challenges to APN Sustainability

- Lack of uniform scope and standards of practice
- Variation in country-specific regulations and legislation enabling the role
- Differences in prescribing privileges
- Inconsistent educational standards and certification/registration requirements
- Inconsistent requirements for physician supervision
- Issues with reimbursement/remuneration for care
- Variance in role recognition and title protection
- Independent practice authority not existing in some countries

Source: Adapted from Kleinpell et al., 2014; Sheer & Wong, 2008.

It is important for Canadian APNs to be aware of global challenges to sustainability, as those challenges may often be the same ones directly impacting Canadian NP and CNS practice.

Motivators for Advanced Practice Nursing Roles in Canada

Reforming the Canadian health care system has been advocated for years (Health Council of Canada [HCC], 2005), and can be traced back to 1978 and the World Health Organization's (WHO) meeting in Alma-Ata. The Declaration of Alma-Ata recognized that **primary health care (PHC)** should be essential care that is universally available to individuals, families, and communities and fosters self-reliance and self-determination (WHO, 1978). Over the years, numerous Canadian reports have highlighted the need for changes to the way PHC is delivered (HCC, 2005; Lewis, 2004). National concerns previously identified included inadequate attention to health promotion and disease prevention, lack of continuity of patient care between providers and institutions, patients experiencing difficulty in obtaining access to care, and barriers to integrating primary care providers (such as NPs) into the health care system (Health Canada, 2006; HCC, 2005).

As nursing's nationally recognized professional organization, the Canadian Nurses Association (CNA) has viewed the need to address PHC reform as an opportunity to strengthen nursing's position in the health care system and promote advanced nursing roles (CNA, 2007). CNA's vision for nursing includes leaders who actively use advanced technology to redesign care processes in both acute and community care, and establishing nurse-led models of care that focus on health promotion and prevention resulting in engaged patients and families. The CNA exerts influence on policy-makers through published reports and position statements articulating the contributions all nurses, including NPs and CNSs, make to the health care system (CNA, 2013). Admittedly, increasing public and policy-makers' awareness of nursing's contributions is critically important; regrettably there are other issues that influence role sustainability.

Factors Affecting NP Role Sustainability

Sustaining APN roles is a complex process influenced by socio-political (macro-level), organizational (meso-level), and individual (micro-level) factors that are interconnected and work synergistically to facilitate or hinder sustainability (Champagne, 2002). Ongoing sustainability requires all sectors to work continuously and collaboratively over the long term. NPs provide an illustration of the complex process of implementing and sustaining an APN role.

NPs were introduced into the Canadian health care system almost 50 years ago, yet in 2013 less than 4,000 were registered (Canadian Institute for Health Information [CIHI], 2014). Initially, in the 1980s and 1990s, NP sustainability was influenced by an oversupply of family physicians, limited public awareness and understanding of the role, and an absence of legitimizing legislation and regulation. Other factors included the lack of government funding for educational programs, ambiguous support from organized medicine and nursing, and no identified funding models to support NP practice (Calnan & Fahey-Walsh, 2005; deWitt & Ploeg, 2005; Haines, 1993). Fortunately, the Canadian landscape has been changing over the years and many of these impediments have been remedied.

Since the mid-1990s, there has been a resurgence of interest in the NP role by federal and provincial governments as a way to influence change in Canada's health care system (Hutchison, Abelson, & Lavis, 2001; Lewis, 2004; Romanow, 2002). Early expectations were that NPs would reduce the costs of health care, provide high-quality care, and increase access to health care services (DiCenso, Paech, & IBM Corporation, 2003; Sidani & Irvine, 1999). The ability of NPs to meet these expectations and thrive in our health care system continues to be influenced by the degree of administrative and physician support, acceptance by other practitioners, a clear rationale for the position, and legislation and regulation to support the role (van Soeren & Micevski, 2001).

Legislative and regulatory changes have occurred incrementally. Alberta led the way by enacting legislation for NP practice in 1996 and Ontario in 1998 (Kaasalainen et al., 2010). The last territory to enact legislation was the Yukon in 2009, 13 years after Alberta. However, the early efforts to regulate NP practice were significant because it was the absence of legislation and regulation that, in part, was a major threat to sustainability. These changes have had a favourable influence on sustainable NP roles, but NP remuneration and lack of a legislated funding model continues to be a threat to NP sustainability.

Funding models for NP practice have consistently been identified as a barrier to role sustainability (DiCenso et al., 2010). A brief review of the Canada Health Act might help to illuminate the NP remuneration issue. The Canada Health Act ensures that eligible residents in all provinces and territories have reasonable access to necessary hospital, physician, and extended-care services. Extended care includes long-term residential and home care (Health Canada, 2013). Within provincial and territorial governments, ministries of health are responsible for administering health care financial resources. At the federal level, payment for acute and primary health care is limited to services provided through hospitals, and by physicians and dentists. However, provincial and territorial governments have expanded the list of providers to include, for example, midwives, optometrists, and acupuncturists.

Currently, no provincial or territorial legislation includes NPs as service providers eligible for payment through their medical services plan. In all Canadian jurisdictions, NPs and CNSs are salaried employees of health authorities. This funding model relies on ministries of health to allocate additional money to health authorities to fund NP positions. In the case of the CNS, the health authority's global nursing budget funds CNS positions (DiCenso et al., 2010). Changes to the current funding model to allow NPs to be recognized and reimbursed are possible, but will require provinces and territories to enact legislative changes to their health acts, along with the political will to do so.

The Shifting Landscape

For more than a decade, governments, regulators, educators, employers, and prospective NPs across Canada have expended substantial resources to implement or expand the NP role. For instance, in 2000 the Government of Canada funded the $800-million Primary Health Care Transition Fund (PHCTF) (Health Canada, 2004) to support provincial and territorial initiatives to introduce new approaches to PHC delivery, including expanded efforts to integrate NPs in the health care system. One pan-Canadian project that was funded through the PHCTF was the Canadian Nurse Practitioner Initiative (CNPI); Health Canada provided $8.9 million to the CNA. The initiative began in 2003 and was completed in 2006. Consultation with representatives of governments, nursing organizations, regulators, employers, educators, and other health professionals across Canada resulted in a framework for integration and sustainability of the NP role (CNPI, 2006). As a result of the CNPI, efforts to standardize educational programs and consistent NP legislation and regulation across the country have been ongoing (CNPI, 2006; DiCenso et al., 2010). The 2006 recommendations resulting from the CNPI are listed in Box 20.2.

BOX 20.2

2006 CNPI Recommendations

- Develop consistency in federal, provincial, and territorial legislation and regulation pertaining to NPs
- Implement consistent approaches to NP practice
- Conduct a pan-Canadian, needs-based human resource plan for NPs
- Implement a pan-Canadian approach to NP education
- Adopt the Implementation and Evaluation Toolkit as a guide to support ongoing implementation of the NP role
- Devise a five-year, pan-Canadian social marketing campaign to promote the NP role

Source: Adapted from CNPI, 2006.

Since 2006, the CNA has continued to collaborate with other professional associations; regulators; federal, provincial, and territorial governments; and health care organizations to implement the CNPI's recommendations. In 2009, CNA published a progress report on the status of which CNPI recommendations had been achieved. The NP title is now protected in all jurisdictions, meaning only those registered as NPs can use the title. At the time of the report, a master's degree was not required in all provinces and inconsistency in scope of practice and registration requirements continued to exist (CNA, 2009b). In 2012, the Canadian Association of Schools of Nursing (CASN) created a national framework and guiding principles for NP education (CASN, 2012b). The education framework came about in response to concerns raised by educators, NPs, and nursing associations for national standards to guide NP education. The framework contributes to national consistency in preparation of NPs in Canada, and sets graduate education as a requirement for entry to practice (CASN, 2012b).

Similarly, nursing regulators, working through the CNA, collaborated to develop core entry-level competencies for NP practice (CNA, 2010). The core competencies were used by CNA to develop the national NP registration examination. The landscape for NPs continues to shift toward more harmonization than differences, but the same cannot be said for CNSs.

Factors Affecting CNS Role Sustainability

While the CNS role has existed in Canada for 40 years, the number of CNSs has fluctuated, largely as a result of economic variables. In times of economic constraint positions were eliminated, only to be reinstated or created when monies were available for reinvestment in health care. It is difficult to determine the number of CNSs currently employed in Canada. The CIHI's regulated nurses database includes the CNS role under "other positions," thus rendering the role invisible and difficult to track. According to Bryant-Lukosius (2010), from 2000 to 2008 the numbers of CNSs decreased from 2,624 to 2,222; the numbers continue to decline (CNA, 2012). Reversing the decline will require policy- and decision-makers to allocate funding for new positions. However, the role continues to lack support from policy-makers who do not understand CNSs' contributions in the health care system (Bryant-Lukosius, 2010). Without the reallocation of funds for CNS positions, the sustainability of the role in Canada is questionable (CNA, 2012). Other factors are also influencing sustainability of the CNS role.

CNSs were introduced to promote nursing excellence in acute and community care. A primary function of CNSs was to educate and mentor nursing staff in the delivery of high-quality, evidence-informed care. They were expected to be a conduit for the uptake of knowledge generated through research, as well as nursing staff's utilization of evidence to inform their practice (CNA, 2008). There are five key components of the CNS role: clinician, consultant, educator, researcher, and leader (CNA, 2009a). Given the declining numbers of CNSs in Canada, the initial intent for the role has not been fully realized for a variety of reasons.

According to the CNA's advanced nursing practice framework, CNSs are expected hold a master's or doctorate degree and demonstrate advanced nursing competencies (2008). The CNS role is within the scope of practice of an RN, and therefore regulators do not require additional registration or credentialing. In Canada, the CNS title is not protected and an RN can assume the title without a graduate education. This is also occurring as employers have created CNS positions and hired baccalaureate-prepared RNs to fill them. The mismatch of professional expectations and employer implementation of the role is due to misunderstanding of the role and minimum requirements for its occupants (Kilpatrick et al., 2013). Lack of role clarity is symptomatic of the current Canadian landscape in which there are no standards for CNS education, and only 33% of universities offer CNS-specific programs (CASN, 2012a). What's more, there is very little Canadian research demonstrating the benefit of the CNS role or best practices to inform role implementation (Bryant-Lukosius et al., 2010).

In spite what seems to a bleak outlook for the CNS role in Canada, there are changes occurring that will contribute to improving how the role is understood. In 2014, the CNA began a pan-Canadian initiative to develop a common vision for the CNS role and determine core competencies (Sutherland Boal, 2014). This work is vital to sustainability of CNSs and will provide guidance and support for regulators, educators, employers, and CNSs themselves. Establishing core competencies is a major step in better identifying the CNS role. However, without title protection, national standards for CNS education, and mechanisms for credentialing, sustainability of the role will continue to be in question.

BOX 20.3

Strategies to Promote APN Role Sustainability

- Clearly define APN roles
- Standardize regulation and education of APNs
- Use a systematic process to implement new roles based on patient needs and stakeholder involvement
- Incorporate APN roles into federal and jurisdictional health and human resource planning
- Increase public awareness of the value APN roles through media campaigns
- Establish innovative collaborative models to leverage APN knowledge, skills, and abilities
- Fund research into the value-added benefit of APNs
- Educate health ministries, administrative entities, credentialing committees, and medical staff on how APNs assist in updating hospital bylaws
- Encourage patients to advocate for APNs as competent providers

---

Source: Adapted from DiCenso et al., 2010; Kleinpell et al., 2014.

Conclusion

In reviewing the context of APN roles it is clear that the future of these roles in the Canadian health care system will continue to be influenced by political and organizational contexts. APNs will be asked to provide evidence that demonstrates their value and cost-effectiveness to patients and the health care system. Box 20.3 outlines strategies that can be undertaken by APNs, regulators, and educators to ensure these roles are sustained and thrive in the changing health care environment. Further strategies to promote APN roles highlight work all APNs can undertake to become positive agents of change by advocating for the good of the public and professional growth. As leaders in the nursing profession, APNs cannot afford to passively wait for others to advance their roles. Sustainable roles will require APNs to take every opportunity to actively participate in policy discussions within their organizations, as well as at the provincial and federal levels, that determine or affect their professional practice.

Critical Thinking Questions

1. How has political context influenced APN role sustainability in Canada?
2. What might have happened if APN roles were introduced after a pan-Canadian approach to education, regulation, and legislation had been established?
3. What would you recommended if you were involved in introducing a new APN role to ensure its sustainability?

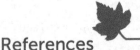

References

Bryant-Lukosius, D. (2010). The clinical nurse specialist role in Canada: Forecasting the future through research. *Canadian Journal of Nursing Research, 42*(2), 19–25.

Bryant-Lukosius, D., Carter, N., Kilpatrick, K., Martin-Misener, R., Donald, F., Kaasalainen, S., … DiCenso, A. (2010). The clinical nurse specialist role in Canada. *Nursing Leadership, 23*(Special Issue December), 140–166.

Calnan, R., & Fahey-Walsh, J. (2005). *Practice consultation initial report.* Ottawa, ON: CNPI. Retrieved from http://www.npnow.ca/docs/tech-report/section3/02_Practice_AppendixA.pdf

Canadian Association of Schools of Nursing (CASN). (2012a). *Nursing masters education in Canada final report.* Ottawa, ON: CASN. Retrieved from http://www.casn.ca/vm/newvisual/attachments/856/Media/20121213ENMNescanFinalReport2.pdf

CASN. (2012b). *Nurse practitioner education in Canada: National framework of guiding principles and essential components.* Ottawa, ON: CASN. Retrieved from http://www.casn.ca/en/Competencies_and_Indicators_168/items/4.html

Canadian Nurses Association (CNA). (2007). *Advanced nursing practice: Position statement.* Ottawa, ON: CNA. Retrieved from http://www.cna-aiic.ca/en/download-buy/nurse-practitioners-clinical-nurse-specialists

CNA. (2008). *Advanced nursing practice: A national framework.* Ottawa, ON: CNA.

CNA. (2009a). *Position statement: Clinical nurse specialist.* Ottawa, ON: CNA. Retrieved from https://www.cna-aiic.ca/~/media/cna/page-content/pdf-en/clinical-nurse-specialist_position-statement.pdf?la=en

CNA. (2009b). *Recommendations of the Canadian nurse practitioner initiative: Progress report.* Ottawa, ON: CNA. Retrieved from http://www.cna-aiic.ca/~/media/cna/files/en/cnpi_report_2009_e.pdf

CNA. (2010). *Canadian nurse practitioner core competency framework.* Ottawa, ON: CNA. Retrieved from https://www.cna-aiic.ca/~/media/cna/files/en/competency_framework_2010_e.pdf

CNA. (2012). *Strengthening the role of the clinical nurse specialist in Canada: Background paper.* Ottawa, ON: CNA. Retrieved from http://cna-aiic.ca/~/media/cna/page-content/pdf-fr/ strengthening_the_cns_role_background_paper_e.pdf?la=en

CNA. (2013). *Registered nurses: Stepping up to transform health care.* Ottawa, ON: CNA. Retrieved from http://www.cna-aiic.ca/~/media/cna/files/en/registered_nurses_stepping_ up_to_transform_health_care_e.pdf

Canadian Institute for Health Information (CIHI). (2014). *Regulated nurses, 2013.* Ottawa, ON: CIHI. Retrieved from https://secure.cihi.ca/free_products/Nursing-Workforce-2013_EN.pdf

Canadian Nurse Practitioner Initiative (CNPI). (2006). *Nurse practitioners: The time is now: A solution to improving access and reducing wait times in Canada.* Ottawa, ON: CNA. Retrieved from http://www.npnow.ca/docs/tech-report/section1/01_Integrated_Report.pdf

Champagne, F. (2002). *The ability to manage change in health care organizations.* (Discussion paper No. 39). Ottawa, ON: Commission on the Future of Health Care in Canada. Retrieved from http://publications.gc.ca/collections/Collection/CP32-79-39-2002E.pdf

deWitt, L., & Ploeg, J. (2005). Critical analysis of the evolution of a Canadian nurse practitioner role. *Canadian Journal of Nursing Research, 37*(4), 116–137.

DiCenso, A., Bryant-Lukosius, D., Martin-Misener, R., Donald, F., Abelson, J., Bourgeault, I., ... Harbman, P. (2010). Factors enabling advanced practice nursing role integration in Canada. *Nursing Leadership, 23*(Special Issue December), 211–238.

DiCenso, A., Paech, G., & IBM Corporation. (2003). *Report on the integration of primary health care nurse practitioners into the province of Ontario.* Toronto, ON: MOHLTC. Retrieved from http://www.health.gov.on.ca/en/common/ministry/publications/reports/nurseprac03/ nurseprac03_mn.aspx

Haines, J. (1993). *The nurse practitioner: A discussion paper.* Ottawa, ON: Canadian Nurses Association.

Health Canada. (2004). *Archived information: Primary health care.* Ottawa, ON: Health Canada. Retrieved from http://publications.gc.ca/collections/Collection/CP32-79-39-2002E.pdf

Health Canada. (2006). *About primary health care.* Ottawa, ON: Health Canada. Retrieved from http://www.hc-sc.gc.ca/hcs-sss/prim/about-apropos-eng.php

Health Canada. (2013). *Canada health act annual report, 2012–2013.* Ottawa, ON: Health Canada. Retrieved from http://www.hc-sc.gc.ca/hcs-sss/pubs/cha-lcs/2013-cha-lcs-ar-ra/ index-eng.php

Health Council of Canada (HCC). (2005). *Health care renewal in Canada: Accelerating change.* Ottawa, ON: Carleton University. Retrieved from http://www.healthcouncilcanada.ca/

Hutchison, B., Abelson, J., & Lavis, J. (2001). Primary care in Canada: So much innovation, so little change. *Health Affairs, 20*(3), 116–131.

International Council of Nurses (ICN). (2013). *Definition and characteristics of the role.* Retrieved from http://international.aanp.org/Practice/APNRoles

Kaasalainen, S., Martin-Misener, R., Kilpatrick, K., Harbman, P., Bryant-Lukosius, D., Donald, F., ... DiCenso, A. (2010). A historical overview of the development of advanced practice nursing roles in Canada. *Nursing Leadership, 23*(Special Issue December), 35–68.

Kilpatrick, K., DiCenso, A., Bryant-Lukosius, D., Ritchie, J., Martin-Misener, R., & Carter, N. (2013). Practice patterns and perceived impact of clinical nurse specialist roles in Canada: Results of a national survey. *International Journal of Nursing Studies, 50*(11), 1524–1536.

Kleinpell, R., Scanlon, A., Hibbert, D., Ganz, F., East, L., Fraser, D., ... Beauchesne, M. (2014). Addressing issues impacting advanced nursing practice worldwide. *OJIN: The Online Journal of Issues in Nursing, 19*(2), Manuscript 5. doi: 10.3912/OJIN.Vol19NO02Man05

Lewis, S. (2004). *A thousand points of light? Moving forward in primary health care.* Winnipeg, MB: Primary Care Framework.

Pulcini, J. (2014). Chapter 6: International development of advanced practice nursing. In A.B. Hamric, C.M. Hanson, M.R. Tracey, & E.T. O'Grady. *Advanced practice nursing: An integrative approach* (5th ed.), (pp. 133–146). St. Louis, MO: Elsevier.

Romanow, R. (2002). *Building on values: The future of health care in Canada: Final report.* Saskatoon, SK: Commission on the Future of Health Care in Canada.

Schober, M., & Affara, F. (2006). *International council of nurses: Advanced nursing practice.* Malden, MA: Blackwell Publishing.

Sheer, B., & Wong, F. (2008). The development of advanced nursing practice globally. *Journal of Nursing Scholarship, 40*(3), 204–211.

Sidani, S., & Irvine, D. (1999). A conceptual framework for evaluating the nurse practitioner role in acute care settings. *Journal of Advanced Nursing, 30*(1), 58–66.

Sutherland Boal, A. (2014). Strengthening the CNS role. *Canadian Nurse, 110*(6), 19.

van Soeren, M., & Micevski, V. (2001). Success indicators and barriers to acute nurse practitioner role implementation in four Ontario hospitals. *American Association of Critical Care Nursing, 12*(3), 424–437.

World Health Organization. (1978). *Declaration of Alma-Ata: International conference on primary health care, Alma-Ata, USSR, 6–12, September, 1978.* Retrieved from http://www.who.int/publications/almaata_declaration_en.pdf

Chapter 21

Advanced Practice Nursing from a Global Perspective

Roberta Heale

Roberta Heale is an Associate Professor at Laurentian University, School of Nursing, and NP–Family/All Ages in Sudbury, Ontario. In 2006, Roberta and her colleague, Marilyn Butcher, were awarded the development of Canada's first NP-led clinic in Sudbury. Roberta's commitment to her profession is evident in her research related to her NP role and her ongoing practice as an NP. She is an active member with the International NP/APN Network as the Chair of the Communications Subgroup.

KEY TERMS

advanced practice
  nursing (APN)
jurisdiction
nursing regulation
title protection

OBJECTIVES

1. Develop an understanding of advanced practice nursing (APN) roles across the globe.
2. Reflect on variations in educational, regulatory, and credentialing requirements for APNs.
3. Review various facilitators and barriers to the development and implementation of APN roles internationally.
4. Understand variation in scopes of practice of APNs.

Introduction

The first **advanced practice nursing (APN)** roles to be recognized were in the United States in the mid-1960s, which arose as a result of a shortage of physicians. During this time, registered nurses became authorized to perform some medical tasks (Duffield, Gardner, Chang, & Catling-Paull, 2009). Since then, APN roles have evolved in various forms across the globe (Duffield et al., 2009). *APN* is an umbrella term, meant to denote registered nurses who work at a higher level than basic nursing (Sheer & Wong, 2008). The International Council of Nurses (ICN) defines APN as

> a registered nurse with the expert knowledge, complex decision making skills and clinical competency for advanced practice. Each country or **jurisdiction** [emphasis added] determines how the APN will be credentialed to practice. In addition, a master's degree is recommended for entry level. (2010, p. 1)

Where they exist, each APN role is operationalized in a unique manner. Unfortunately, the wide range of titles, educational and credentialing requirements, and scopes of practice has made it difficult to determine if a role is in fact representative of advanced practice (Bryant-Lukosius, DiCenso, Browne, & Pinelli, 2004). The result is extensive variations of, and in many cases confusion about, the understanding of the APN role across jurisdictions (Bryant-Lukosius et al., 2004).

Evolution of APN Roles

APN roles evolved for a variety of reasons. In most countries, improved access to care was the catalyst for development of APN roles (Delamaire & Lafortune, 2010). The need for enhanced delivery of care to rural and remote locations promoted the initiation of APN roles in both Australia and Canada (Delamaire & Lafortune, 2010). Similarly, although Nicaragua doesn't have a recognized APN role, severe health care shortages in rural areas have resulted in nurses working in an advanced practice capacity (Sequeira et al., 2011).

Unmet health needs have also been a catalyst for APN role development (Bryant-Lukosius et al., 2004; Furlong & Smith, 2005). In Thailand, there were gaps in maternity services, so all APNs are now trained as midwives (Ketefian, Redman, Hanucharurnkul, Masterson, & Neves, 2001). Aging populations and related increases in chronic diseases promoted the development of APNs in primary health care in several countries, such as Australia and Finland (Delamaire & Lafortune, 2010).

Many worldwide health care systems have seen rapid expansions in both knowledge and technology. The associated costs of these system changes are high, as are costs in specific areas such as physician remuneration (Bryant-Lukosius et al., 2004; Furlong & Smith, 2005). Ultimately, delegation of medical tasks to less expensive APNs has been seen as a viable cost-containment mechanism (Bryant-Lukosius et al., 2004; Delamaire & Lafortune, 2010). In Cyprus, keeping the growth in health care costs in check was a main driver for their development of APN roles (Delamaire & Lafortune, 2010). In many countries, including Canada, improving quality of care is an expected outcome of the introduction of APNs with the belief that improved quality of care may also result in cost savings to the health system as a whole (Delamaire & Lafortune, 2010).

Titles and Roles

There is a plethora of titles and job descriptions for APNs across the globe, and even within certain jurisdictions (Furlong & Smith, 2005). Table 21.1 provides a compilation of existing APN roles in variety of countries. You will notice that the status of APN role development also varies.

TABLE 21.1: Country and APN Titles	
Country	**Roles**
Angola	NP, CNS
Argentina	none
Australia	NP, APN, CNS, clinical nurse consultant
Austria	APN, NS
Bahamas	NP, APN, nurse midwife
Belgium	*
Belize	Psychiatric NP
Bolivia	NP
Botswana	NP, NS
Canada	NP (Family/all ages or acute care (adult, pediatric, neonatal)), CNS, nurse anesthetist
China	NP, CNS, APN
Columbia	*
Congo	none
Costa Rica	*
Cyprus	APNs (diabetic nurses, community mental health nurses, mental health nurses for drug and alcohol addiction, or community nurses)
Czech Republic	NS *
Finland	CNS, APN
France	NS
Gambia	none
Germany	*
Greece	NS*
Hong Kong	NS, APN
Islamic Republic of Iran	NP, APN, CNS, NS
India	NP*
Italy	CNS, NS
Japan	Certified nurse specialist
Korea	APN

continued

TABLE 21.1: Country and APN Titles *(cont.)*

Country	Roles
Malaysia	CNS
Mexico	*
Mongolia	NP
Namibia	Midwifery and neonatology specialist midwife, NS (critical care and psychiatry)
Netherlands	NP, CNS
New Zealand	NP, CNS, APN
Nicaragua	*
Paraguay	*
Poland	CNS*, NS*, nurse midwife
Republic of Ireland	APN, CNS
Russia	*
Sierra Leone	NS, nurse midwife
Singapore	APN
South Korea	APN
Spain	APN
Sri Lanka	none
Suriname	none
Swaziland	NP, nurse midwife
Sweden	Advanced clinical nurse specialist
Taiwan	NP
Thailand	NP, APN, CNS, NS
Togo	NP, APN, CNS
United Kingdom	CNS, APN, nurse consultants, matrons
United States	NP, CNS, nurse midwife, nurse anesthetist

NP = nurse practitioner; CNS = clinical nurse specialist; APN = advanced practice nurse; NS = nurse specialist; * = under development

Source: Adapted from Delamaire & Lafortune, 2010; Heale & Rieck-Buckley, 2015; Lindblad, Hallman, Gillsjö, Lindblad, & Fagerstrom, 2010; Sequeira et al., 2011; Sheer & Wong, 2008.

Along with the variation in role titles, there is also wide variation in APN practice. The scope of practice of the APN is typically understood to include such things as communicating a diagnosis, prescribing medication, ordering diagnostic testing, admitting to hospital, performing controlled medical acts such as intubation, and practicing independently or autonomously. However, the tasks associated with advanced practice differ considerably across jurisdictions. For example, clinical nurse specialists (CNS) in Canada do not have separate regulation from the RN. They do not have the authority to autonomously order tests, diagnose, or prescribe. This is in contrast with CNSs in other countries, such as the US, where many states have regulations that authorize them to perform many of these tasks independently (Delamaire & Lafortune, 2010). Not only are there differences in the scope of practice of APNs between countries, there are often differences in the authorized scope of practice for the same APN title in different jurisdictions within an individual country. Regulation for APN roles is developed for each state in the US. Legislation across the country has gone through many changes since the 1970s, and only in recent years have most states allowed APNs independent broader prescribing authority. However, in most states, NPs must still collaborate with a physician in order to prescribe (Delamaire & Lafortune, 2010). For example, a law that took effect January 1, 2015, through collaborative agreement, finally allowed NPs in New York State with 3,600 hours of practice experience to work without physician supervision. To date, there are over 20 states where NPs are able to practice with this wider autonomy (American Association of Nurse Practitioners [AANP], 2016; Rubenfire, 2014).

In countries where the APN role is in the developmental stage, nurses are often authorized to perform some, but not all, tasks associated with advanced practice. The recognition of APNs in Belgium, for example, hasn't officially occurred; however, some nursing programs at the graduate level are supporting the development of APN streams and nurses can perform some advanced tasks in hospital or primary health care such as consultation and referral to specialists and management of chronic diseases (Delamaire & Lafortune, 2010).

Roles and responsibilities of APNs vary within a jurisdiction. In the United Kingdom, being a CNS does not necessarily mean that the nurse is able to diagnose, treat autonomously, or use advanced decision-making and judgment in practice (Delamaire & Lafortune, 2010). In addition, all basic nurses in the UK are able to prescribe medications as long as they have a baccalaureate degree, three years' experience, and have successfully completed a program that includes 26 days of theory and 12 days in practice (Delamaire & Lafortune, 2010). Table 21.2 provides a snapshot of the scope of practice of APNs in nine countries.

Regulation

There are several methods of regulating health care providers. Two main types of **nursing regulation** are state- and profession-based (ICN, 2009). Regulation of health care providers may occur by statute or government decree, or through a professional body (Bryant, 2005). In some cases, there is separate legislation for both basic nursing as well as APN roles. In other situations, APN roles are legitimized through credentialing processes but do not require a separate legislation or license beyond the basic nursing criteria (DiCenso & Bryant-Lukosius, 2010). Employers, through their organizational objectives and policies, may restrict the APN role and impose a form of regulation (Bryant, 2005). In many cases,

TABLE 21.2: APN Scope of Practice

Country	APN Role	Diagnose	Prescribe	Order Diagnostic Tests	Admit to Hospital	Perform Controlled Medical Acts	Practice Independently/ Autonomously
Angola	NP	Yes	Yes	–	Yes	Yes	Yes
	CNS	Yes	Yes	–	Yes	Yes	Yes
	NS	–	–	–	–	–	–
Bahamas	NP	–	–	–	–	–	–
	APN	Yes	Yes	Yes	Yes	Yes	Yes
	NS	–	–	–	–	–	–
	Nurse-Midwife	Yes	Yes	Yes	Yes	Yes	–
Canada	CNS	–	–	–	–	–	–
	NP*	Yes	Yes	Yes	Yes	Yes	Yes
Finland	APN	Yes	Yes	Yes	–	–	Yes
	CNS	–	–	–	–	–	–
Iran	NP	Yes	–	–	Yes	Yes	–
	APN	Yes	–	–	Yes	Yes	–
	CNS	Yes	–	Yes	Yes	Yes	Yes
	NS	Yes	–	–	–	–	–
New Zealand	NP	Yes	Yes	Yes	Yes	Yes	Yes
Norway	CNS	–	–	–	–	–	–
Republic of Ireland	APN	Yes	Yes	Yes	Yes	Yes	Yes
	CNS	–	–	–	–	–	–
United States	CNS*	Yes	Yes	Yes	Yes	Yes	Yes
	NP*	Yes	Yes	Yes	Yes	Yes	Yes

Note: *varies by jurisdiction

Source: Adapted from Heale & Rieck-Buckley, 2015.

changes to existing regulation in a jurisdiction are required to eliminate barriers to the expanded scope of practice of the APN (Delamaire & Lafortune, 2010).

Control over the nursing profession varies. While across Canada nursing colleges have an important role in the governance of nursing through self-regulation, in many countries powerful governmental influence and political priorities have a strong impact on APN roles both through funding and policy development (Bryant-Lukosius et al., 2004). The result is that in some countries the nursing profession is "managed" by a branch of government rather than by an independent nursing college. Thus, while it is within the mandate of the nursing profession to ensure the development of appropriate competencies and standards for APN practice related to legislation, at times this is not the case.

Where regulation for APNs exists, it typically outlines the specific authority that is granted to the APN. This is often the basis for the scope of practice, or practice standards. Some regulation is very specific and restrictive, while other regulation provides more flexibility in the manner in which the APN role is implemented. The UK has the least restrictive regulation while the US has the most restrictive (Ketefian et al., 2001). In the UK, there is only the basic nursing license. Nurses are given APN status through training programs that prepare them for expanded scope of practice. In the US, legislation beyond that required for basic RN licensure specifically outlines the tasks that the APN is authorized to perform (Delamaire & Lafortune, 2010).

The existence and type of APN regulation may also include **title protection** for the APN role. Title protection ensures that only those officially authorized to do so are able to practice under an APN title. Although this is the ideal, the reality is that many countries do not have protected titles for APN roles (Bryant-Lukosius et al., 2004). Regulation of the APN role may also be centralized or decentralized. Decentralized regulation often results in different legislation and scope of practice of APNs in different jurisdictions within a specific country. This is the case in both Canada and in the US. An APN in one province, or state, may have difficulty with portability of their license across jurisdictions. In order to avoid this situation, Australia passed legislation in 2010 that harmonized APN legislation in that country (Delamaire & Lafortune, 2010). Regulation, or at least official authorization of APN roles, is essential for their successful implementation. This is a difficult objective given that some countries are in the early stages of registering basic nursing and will not be in a position to develop APN roles for some time. Argentina, for example, started the process of a national licensing registry for nurses in 2008 (Ministerio de Salud, n.d).

Inconsistencies in the regulation of APN roles across countries result in differences in terms of the clinical practice of the same roles in different jurisdictions. For example, CNSs do not have separate regulation from that of the registered nurse in Canada (DiCenso & Bryant-Lukosius, 2010), while many states in the US have regulated the CNS role including such things as title protection, diagnosing, and prescribing authority (Delamaire & Lafortune, 2010). Although the focus of practice is similar in both countries whereby the

CNS manages disease and promotes health among clients, families, and communities, the regulation of the CNS role in the US offers those practitioners an expanded practice framework and some protection that is not available to their Canadian counterparts.

Educational Requirements

In many circumstances, regulation and/or registration boards determine the practice criteria for APN roles. These boards must ensure that nurses are able to safely and effectively meet the competencies of the role, which points to the need for appropriate educational programs. Also required are processes for review of the quality of education, the development of continuing education opportunities, and procedures for re-licensing and measurement of ongoing competencies (Bryant, 2005).

Educational institutions and nursing organizations that support APN roles have a responsibility to deliver APN programs that will ensure that graduates are able to meet competencies required for safe and effective practice (Furlong & Smith, 2005). Policy and documentation related to the competencies of the APN should precede the development of educational programs, however, this has often not been the case. One example is the consortium NP educational program in Ontario, Canada, which was developed and delivered for several years prior to the enactment of legislation to support nurse practitioner practice (NPAO, 2011).

Many countries and/or jurisdictions do not have graduate preparation for entry to practice as an APN (Delamaire & Lafortune, 2010; Sheer & Wong, 2008). Despite the development of graduate nursing education programs, in some countries (such as Brazil), these are designed for faculty roles or for those who will conduct research rather than for advanced practice training (Ketefian et al., 2001).

Barriers to the Development of APN Roles and APN Practice Internationally

There are many obstacles to the successful development and implementation of APN roles (Bryant-Lukosius et al., 2004). Specific barriers to the development of APN roles and growth of APN practice vary considerably, however, some common themes have emerged. Physician opposition, and opposition from other health care providers, is a barrier (Delamaire & Lafortune, 2010; Heale & Rieck-Buckley, 2015). In Thailand, physician opposition to NP initiatives squelched the development of this APN role (Ketefian et al., 2001).

Nursing leadership is essential in influencing health care policy, as well as APN role development and implementation. However, skill level and motivation of nursing organizations to evoke change can be an obstacle to the development and implementation of

TABLE 21.3: Reported Number of APNs in Selected Countries (as of December 2011)

Country	APN Role	Reported Numbers
Bahamas	NP	12
	APN	300
	Nurse midwife	800
Bolivia	NP	2,995
Canada	CNS	2,288*
	NP	3,000
Finland	APN	50
	CNS	unknown
Greece	CNS	unknown
	NS	1,600
Iran	NP	2,500
	APN	400
	CNS	300
	NS	unknown
Malaysia	CNS	6
Poland	CNS	15–20,000
	NS	60,000
Thailand	NP	16,000
	APN	1,187
	CNS	900
	NS	>10,000
United States	CNS	59,242**
	NP	205,000***

Notes: *from DiCenso & Bryant-Lukosius, 2010; **from Delamaire & Lafortune, 2010; ***from PR Newswire, 2015

Source: Adapted from Heale & Rieck-Buckley, 2015.

these roles (Delamaire & Lafortune, 2010; Heale & Rieck-Buckley, 2015). This is the case in Mexico where, although nurses are able to specialize in intensive or critical care, as of 2013 there was no specific APN role in that country; this is largely due to the lack of nursing leadership in health care (Kruth, 2013).

The development and progress of APN roles are impeded by such things as lack of recognition of the APN contribution by health policy- and decision-makers (Villegas & Allen, 2012). Restrictive legislation and regulation continues to be an issue in many countries (Delamaire & Lafortune, 2010; Villegas & Allen, 2012). Also, cultural considerations including the value and role of women in a society help to shape the expectations for nursing roles (Bryant-Lukosius et al., 2004).

Ongoing evaluation of APN roles and research evidence to support the value and quality of APN care is required (Pulcini & Hart, 2007). Although there is considerable evidence about well-established APN roles there is little or no evidence about emerging ones. In addition, it is difficult to make comparisons of APN evaluation from other countries given the wide variation in context among APN roles across jurisdictions (Brooten, Youngblut, Deosires, Singhala, & Guido-Sanz, 2012).

In many countries, the numbers of APNs compared to the numbers of nurses is small. In Canada in 2008, NPs represented 0.6% and CNSs 0.9% of all registered nurses (Delamaire & Lafortune, 2010). Where regulation for an APN role does not exist, the numbers practicing in the role may not be monitored. Table 21.3 provides a snapshot of the reported number of APNs in a variety of countries. It is often difficult for APN concerns to be heard and addressed given the low numbers, and even more difficult if there is no tracking system. In the Bahamas, "nurse midwife" is considered an APN role. In other countries, such as Canada, midwifery is not a nursing role but rather a separate health care provider category altogether.

A poor understanding about the scope of practice of an APN is a barrier in role realization. Organizational propensity to view APNs as a physician replacement and to limit APN practice inhibits the potential of an APN (Bryant-Lukosius et al., 2004; Delamaire & Lafortune, 2010). Role conflict, role overload, and variable stakeholder acceptance are further examples of barriers to the implementation of APN in health care (Bryant-Lukosius et al., 2004).

Globally, reimbursement and remuneration of health care providers, including APNs, is another barrier (Palumbo, Marth, & Rambur, 2011; Villega & Allen, 2012). An example is fee-for-service in primary health care, where the introduction of an APN could result in reduced income for the physician, whereas capitation, performance-based, and salaried physician remuneration models are more likely to encourage the development of APN roles (Delamaire & Lafortune, 2010).

Many countries deal with multiple levels of barriers to APN practice. In some US states, remuneration of the APN at less than physicians for similar work, professional liability insurance, staff privilege issues, designation as a primary care provider, and prescriptive authority are simultaneously issues affecting APN practice (Ketefian et al., 2001).

International Focus

The varied nomenclature used to describe APN roles, variation in regulation, educational standards, and scope of practice speaks to the need for a common understanding of APN roles, including consensus on competencies (Bryant-Lukosius et al., 2004). The need for a consistent approach to the development and implementation of APN roles has been widely acknowledged. Countries across the globe recognize the need for APN roles to have international standards for regulation, education, titles, and an identified scope of practice and core components of practice (Currie, Edwards, Colligan, & Crouch, 2007; Duffield et al., 2009; Furlong & Smith, 2005). At the same time the ICN (2009) identified the importance for every nurse to enter into policy debates that influence their profession, rather than remaining passive and allowing others to determine nursing practice in their country. This will ensure that nurses become constructive change agents for the benefit of the public, as well as for professional growth.

There are numerous strategies for the nursing profession to ensure relevance and promote APN roles. Nursing organizations have an opportunity to determine trends and unmet health care needs in their country and mobilize to address these needs through specialized APN services. Examples of these include Japan, in recognizing the population was aging and implementing an aging strategy; care of AIDS patients in the US; or Brazil targeting the younger population and their needs, such as smoking cessation (Ketefian et al., 2001).

Nurses and nursing organizations may lack the knowledge and skills to advocate, develop, and implement APN roles. To address this concern, in 2000 the International Nurse Practitioner (INP)/Advanced Practice Nursing Network (APNN) was established for the purpose of facilitating communication among representatives of countries with existing APN roles with representatives of those in development (Sheer & Wong, 2008). INP/APNN has additional objectives, which include to serve as a vehicle for the ICN to harness specialist expertise, to help the ICN more effectively meet its mandate as a global voice of the profession, to provide a mechanism to promote and disseminate information from any of the network members and the ICN, and to act as a base for future international collaboration around advanced practice and the NP role (Cross, 2014).

Conclusion

APN roles are recognized in many countries across the globe. Their development and implementation arose for a variety of reasons, most notably to increase access to care in areas with gaps in health care and physician services. These roles vary widely with respect to educational requirements, regulation, and scope of practice. Although many barriers continue to exist in the development and implementation of APN roles, INP/APNN provides a forum for nurses and nursing organizations to learn from and support one another in the success of APNs across the globe.

Critical Thinking Questions

1. What factors impact the ability of APNs in other countries and jurisdictions to work to their full scope of practice?
2. Compare and contrast mechanisms that authorize practice for APNs in the UK with NP and CNS roles in Canada.
3. You are a nurse and interested in advocating for the development of an APN role in your jurisdiction. What strategies could you implement to assist in the development of the role? What organizations or institutions would you contact to facilitate your goal? Why?

References

American Association of Nurse Practitioners (AANP). (2016). *State practice environment.* Austin, TX: AANP. Retrieved from https://www.aanp.org/legislation-regulation/state-legislation/state-practice-environment/66-legislation-regulation/state-practice-environment/1380-state-practice-by-type

Brooten, D., Youngblut, J.M., Deosires, W., Singhala, K., & Guido-Sanz, F. (2012). Global considerations in measuring effectiveness of advanced practice nurses. *International Journal of Nursing Studies, 49*(7), 906–912. doi: 10.1016/j.ijnurstu.2011.10.022

Bryant, R. (2005). *Regulation, roles and competency development.* Geneva, CH: ICN.

Bryant-Lukosius, D., DiCenso, A., Browne, G., & Pinelli, J. (2004). Advanced practice nursing roles: Development, implementation and evaluation. *Journal of Advanced Nursing, 48*(5), 519–529. doi: 10.1111/j.1365-2648.2004.03234.x

Cross, S. (2014). *Network history 1992–2000.* Retrieved from http://international.aanp.org/About/History

Currie, J., Edwards, L., Colligan, M., & Crouch, R. (2007). A time for international standards? Comparing the emergency nurse practitioner role in the UK, Australia and New Zealand. *Accident and Emergency Nursing, 15*(4), 210–216. doi: 10.1016/j.aaen.2007.07.007

Delamaire, M-L., & Lafortune, G. (2010). *Nurses in advanced roles: A description and evaluation of experiences in 12 developed countries.* OECD Health Working Paper No. 54. Retrieved from http://www.oecd.org/officialdocuments/publicdisplaydocumentpdf/?cote=delsa/hea/wd/hwp(2010)5&doclanguage=en. doi: 10.1787/5kmbrcfms5g7-en

DiCenso, A., & Bryant-Lukosius, D. (2010). Clinical nurse specialists and nurse practitioners in Canada. Ottawa, ON: Canadian Health Services Research Foundation. Retrieved from http://www.cfhi-fcass.ca/Libraries/Commissioned_Research_Reports/Dicenso_EN_Finals.flb.ashx

Duffield, C., Gardner, G., Chang, A.M., & Catling-Paull, C. (2009). Advanced nursing practice: A global perspective. *Collegian Journal of the Royal College of Nursing Australia, 16*(2), 55–62. doi: 10.1016/j.colegn.2009.02.001

Furlong, E., & Smith, R. (2005). Advanced nursing practice: Policy, education and role development. *Journal of Clinical Nursing, 14*(9), 1059–1066. doi: 10.1111/j.1365-2702.2005.01220.x

Heale, R., & Rieck Buckley, C. (2015). An international perspective of advanced practice nursing regulation. *International Nursing Review, 62*(3), 421–429. doi: 10.1111/inr.12193

International Council of Nurses (ICN). (2009). *Regulation 2020: Exploration of the present; Vision for the future.* Geneva, CH: ICN.

ICN. (2010). *Nurse practitioner/advanced practice nurse: Definition and characteristics.* Retrieved from http://www.icn.ch/images/stories/documents/publications/fact_sheets/1b_FS-NP_APN.pdf

Ketefian, S., Redman, R.W., Hanucharurnkul, S., Masterson, A., & Neves, E.P. (2001). The development of advanced practice roles: Implications in the international nursing community. *International Nursing Review, 48*(3), 152–163.

Kruth, T. (2013). Advanced practice nursing in Mexico. *International Advanced Practice Nursing.* Retrieved from http://internationalapn.org/2013/08/15/mexico/

Lindblad, E., Hallman, E-B., Gillsjö, C., Lindblad, U., & Fagerström, L. (2010). Experiences of the new role of advanced practice nurses in Swedish primary health care: A qualitative study. *International Journal of Nursing Practice, 16*(1), 69–74. doi: 10.1111/j.1440-172X.2009.01810.x

Ministerio de Salud (n.d). *Registro unico de profesionales de la Salud.* Retrieved from http://rups.msal.gov.ar/turnos/

Nurse Practitioners' Association of Ontario (NPAO). (2011). *Nurse practitioner history in Ontario.* Retrieved from http://npao.org/nurse-practitioners/history/#.VIDTbyhql8M

Palumbo, M.V., Marth, N., & Rambur, B. (2011). Advanced practice registered nurse supply in a small state: Trends to inform policy. *Policy, Politics, & Nursing Practice, 12*(1), 27–35. doi: 10.1177/1527154411404244

PR Newswire. (2015). *2015 Nurse practitioner ranks surge to 205,0000, nearly doubling over past decade.* Retrieved from http://www.prnewswire.com/news-releases/2015-nurse-practitioner-ranks-surge-to-205000-nearly-doubling-over-past-decade-300023042.html

Pulcini, J., & Hart, M.A. (2007). Politics of advanced practice nursing. In D.J. Mason, J.K. Leavitt, & M.W. Chaffee (Eds.), *Policy & politics in nursing and health care* (5th ed., pp. 568–573). St. Louis, MO: Saunders Elsevier.

Rubenfire, A. (2014, December 30). *Some N.Y. nurse practitioners to be freed of doc supervision in 2015.* Retrieved from http://www.modernhealthcare.com/article/20141230/NEWS/312309974

Sequeira, M., Espinoza, H., Amador, J.J., Domingo, G., Quintanilla, M., & de los Santos, T. (2011). *The Nicaraguan health system: An overview of critical challenges and opportunities.* Seattle, WA: PATH.

Sheer, B., & Wong, F.K.Y. (2008). The development of advanced nursing practice globally. *Journal of Nursing Scholarship, 40*(3), 204–211. doi: 10.1111/j.1547-5069.2008.00242.x

Villegas, W.J., & Allen, P.E. (2012). Barriers to advanced practice registered nurse scope of practice: Issue analysis. *Journal of Continuing Education in Nursing, 43*(9), 403–409. doi: 10.3928/00220124-20120716-30

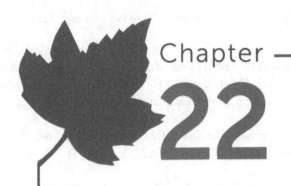

Chapter 22

Advanced Practice Nursing Roles, Education, and Future Trends

Cynthia Baker

Cynthia Baker is the Executive Director of the Canadian Association of Schools of Nursing (CASN) in Ottawa, Ontario. CASN is the national voice of nursing education in Canada. She is a Professor Emerita at Queen's University in Kingston, Ontario, where she was Director, School of Nursing and Associate Dean, Faculty of Health Sciences. Prior to Queen's University, she was Directrice, École des sciences infirmières at l'Université de Moncton in Moncton, New Brunswick.

KEY TERMS

advanced practice
   nursing (APN)
integration
interprofessional
   collaboration
trends

OBJECTIVES

1. Trace the evolution of education for advanced practice nursing (APN) in Canada in relation to trends in health care delivery.
2. Examine contextual factors influencing education programs for APNs and the role of graduates in the health care system over time.
3. Discuss future trends in APN in relation to historical and current challenges and opportunities.

Introduction

Future directions of a phenomenon are often best understood by examining historical forces that have shaped it in the past. The purpose of this chapter is to identify **trends** that are emerging in **advanced practice nursing (APN)** in Canada in light of the forces that have influenced its development. Health professional education has the mandate of preparing graduates for anticipated future health system realities. At any point of time, it reflects the actual and perceived trends of the day. The evolution of APN education in Canada is traced in this chapter, and the contextual forces driving this evolution examined in order to capture directions for the future.

Evolution of Advanced Practice Nursing Education

APN was launched in Canada nearly 50 years ago in 1967, when Dalhousie University opened a groundbreaking Outpost Nursing Program (Martin-Misener et al., 2010). In contrast with the United States, however, the subsequent growth of education for APN was slow and discontinuous for several decades (DiCenso & Bryant-Lukosius, 2010). Programs were often developed in response to time-limited, period-sensitive, contextual demands, and soon waned or disappeared as the particular contextual reality changed. Furthermore, until recently there have been considerable inconsistencies in the academic level of the completion qualifications and in the length of the programs.

In contrast, a renewed interest in nurse practitioner (NP) education emerged in the 1990s that led to a fairly steady growth in enrolments and graduates. This growth has been supported by an emerging professional infrastructure of policies and regulation for advanced nursing education and practice, creating an additional set of contextual factors influencing trends in APN in Canada.

Introduction of Education Programs for Advanced Practice

Canadian schools of nursing have introduced a succession of new educational options to prepare nurses for advanced practice roles as primary health care nurse practitioners (PHCNP), clinical nurse specialists (CNS), NPs in acute care settings, and most recently as nurse anesthetists. Each of these has encountered contextual challenges that affected their subsequent continuity.

Nurse Practitioners in Primary Health Care

Immediately after the Outpost Nursing Program was first launched at Dalhousie University, programs emerged across Canada. They focused on the clinical training of registered nurses to provide primary health care in isolated settings in the North (Martin-Misener et al., 2010). Programs to prepare NPs to work in urban settings also followed Dalhousie's Outpost Nursing Program, first at McMaster University and then at McGill University (Haines, 1993).

These early initiatives were introduced at a time when Canada was experiencing a shortage of family physicians. This stimulated interest in nurses who possessed greater medical skills (Donald et al., 2010). By 1972, however, this contextual factor changed, as Canada moved from a shortage to an oversupply of physicians. Despite positive evaluations of the role based on several randomized clinical trials, the interest in educating nurse practitioners evaporated except to prepare them to work in remote areas in the North (Martin-Misener et al., 2010).

Clinical Nurse Specialists

While the NP in primary health care role was vanishing in Canada during the 1970s, positions for clinical nurse specialists (CNS) emerged in urban hospitals in response to a different set of contextual factors. Advances in health care science and technology were rapidly increasing the complexity of nursing care during the decade, bringing a need for specialized nurses with greater knowledge and skills to support the bedside nurse in providing clinical care (Kaasalainen et al., 2010).

This new CNS role was understood to require deeper and more advanced nursing knowledge built on what nurses had learned in their entry-to-practice programs rather than on supplementary medical knowledge about the diagnosis and treatment of diseases. In contrast with NPs in primary health care, the CNS has typically required a graduate degree in nursing. In fact, definitions of the role often included the possession of a graduate degree in nursing among its defining attributes, and this is still the case. The Canadian Nurses Association (CNA) (2014), for example, recently stated that clinical nurse specialists are "registered nurses who have a graduate degree in nursing and expertise in a clinical nursing specialty" (p. 1).

CNSs were expected to have a high level of nursing expertise in a given clinical area along with abilities in leadership, education, and consultation. The nature of their clinical expertise, however, varied widely. It could be related to a specific population, practice setting, disease, subspecialty, or type of clinical problem (DiCenso & Bryant-Lukosius, 2010).

Although CNSs typically required a graduate degree in nursing, educational programs were not designated specifically for it. This may be because of the range and diversity in the clinical expertise associated with the role. It is worth noting, however, that the introduction of CNSs appears to have had an important impact on graduate programs in nursing in general, and on the later development of master's programs for nurse practitioners. Because the role required deeper nursing knowledge, it increased nurses' interest in graduate studies in the discipline and in advancing nursing-specific clinical knowledge. Moreover, the CNS role prompted the development of graduate programs in nursing that offer clinical nursing specializations (Alcock, 1996). The first such program was introduced at the University of Toronto in 1970, and many graduate programs developed since have had a clinical focus (Montemumo, 1987).

Despite the initial growth of positions for CNSs, fiscal efficiencies introduced in the early 1990s during a period of health care reform resulted in the elimination of many of these positions. The cutbacks were important in reducing the profile of the CNS during the decade and in a decline of interest in this role. The lack of role-specific graduate education has also been identified as a contributing factor (Martin-Misener et al., 2010). While there has been some renewed interest in the CNS role in recent years (CNA, 2014), this has not translated into the development of nursing education programs for it.

Nurse Practitioners in Acute Care

Although interest in the NP in primary health care roles had disappeared, universities began to introduce programs for a new type of nurse practitioner to work in acute care settings in the latter half of the 1980s. The first such program was opened at McMaster University in 1986 for neonatal nurse practitioners (NNP), and in 1993, the University of Toronto introduced a nurse practitioner program for acute care settings that was not focused on neonatology (Kaasalainen et al., 2010).

Schools of nursing delivered the acute care nurse practitioner programs at the graduate or post-graduate level, in line with education for the CNS role and in contrast with programs for the NP in primary health care. These programs represented something of a hybrid, educating nurses for a blended CNS and NP role. They were based on the premise that the graduate needed to learn components of the CNS role as well as the more medical components of the NP role (Kaasalainen et al., 2010). Graduates of these programs were unregulated, and were enabled through physician-approved medical directives and protocols (NPAO, n.d.).

Initially, NPs in acute care settings were called expanded role nurses, blended CNS/NPs, or APNs. Several years after their introduction, they became known as acute care nurse practitioners (ACNP), a term borrowed from the US, where it had been adopted initially to designate NPs working in critical care units (Simpson, 1997).

The initial contextual factors identified as the stimulus for the creation of ACNP education programs included a shortage of pediatric residents (Paes et al., 1989), a need to address the lack of continuity of care for seriously ill patients (Pringle, 2007), and the need to deliver increasingly complex care in acute care settings (Hravnak, Kleinpell, Magdic, & Guttendorf, 2009). While the neonatology programs were highly specialized, most acute care nurse practitioner (ACNP) programs were generic except for those in the province of Quebec. Students obtained the specialized knowledge and skills of a given specialty in the selection of their clinical placements, and in individualized learning activities.

Age-Based Nurse Practitioner Roles

In 2010, changes in nursing regulation had an impact on the ACNP designation and on ACNP education programs. The nursing regulatory bodies in Canada established the following streams for nurse practitioner registration: Family/All Ages (also referred to as Primary Health Care), Adult, and Pediatrics, organizing NP roles into age-based population categories being served, rather than on a specialization or setting. Despite this broad generalist approach, the more narrowly specialized NNP continues to be recognized. In addition, the Ordre des Infirmières et Infirmiers du Québec (OIIQ) retained a specialization focus rather than an age-based framework. NPs in Quebec sit one of four registration streams: First Line of Care (Primary Care), Neonatology, Cardiology, or Nephrology.

Nurse Anesthetist

In 2009, the University of Toronto introduced a post-graduate diploma for nurse anesthetists. This initiative was funded by the Government of Ontario as a potential solution to wait times for surgery resulting from a shortage of anesthetists. Although a small number of nurses graduated from the program, it has been discontinued because the nurse anesthetist role did not materialize in the Canadian health care system; this is in contrast with the US, where it is well established.

Renewal of the Nurse Practitioner Role

During the 1990s, interest in the NP in primary health care roles resurfaced within provincial governments. DiCenso et al. (2007) have attributed this to a combination of factors including cutbacks in medical residency positions, a need to offset rising costs with greater fiscal efficiency, and government interest in shifting care from hospitals to the community. Thus, some of the same factors that led to the elimination of CNS positions in acute care settings prompted a renewed attention to potential benefits of revitalizing the NP role.

In 1995, the Ontario provincial government funded a Council of Ontario University Programs in Nursing (COUPN) consortium of 10 nursing schools to develop and deliver a post-baccalaureate program for Primary Health Care Nurse Practitioners (PHCNP) in both English and French (Cragg, Doucette, & Humbert, 2003). The program was developed and offered conjointly by the 10 member schools of nursing, using distance delivered courses across consortium sites, and supported by face-to-face interactive learning activities and clinical practica carried out at each site. There has been some change in the membership of the COUPN consortium since its creation, and it now consists of nine schools. It continues to educate the majority of PHCNPs who graduate in Ontario.

The COUPN program was created as a one-year post-baccalaureate certificate program, in response to government requirements. It included course content related to roles, health promotion, and health system delivery. Because of the short time frame, however, the emphasis was on the additional medical knowledge and skills needed to diagnose and treat illness in primary health care. Advanced nursing knowledge was part of the education of CNSs and ACNPs. The COUPN consortium members decided it was essential to upgrade the PHCNP program to a graduate level despite government resistance, and to integrate APN competencies into the role. Curriculum work was carried out to bring all the NP certificate courses to a graduate level, and in 2008–09 each of the consortium member schools incorporated the revised and shared PHCNP courses with each school's core graduate courses into a two-year graduate nursing program. A one-year post-baccalaureate certificate, however, composed of the original but upgraded PHCNP courses, can still be obtained at some consortium sites.

Expansion of Nurse Practitioner Education

The introduction of the COUPN consortium program marked a revival of interest in educating NPs in primary health care throughout Canada. An environmental scan conducted by the Canadian Association of Schools of Nursing (CASN) in 2011 found that there had been a progressive increase in the number of programs for NPs in Canada between 2000 and 2009, and programs were being offered in all provincial/territorial jurisdictions except Prince Edward Island, Nunavut, and the Yukon. In 2013, the CASN National Faculty and Student Survey reported that 28 schools of nursing, representing a quarter of the schools in Canada, offered one or more NP program.

Overall, admissions into NP programs, along with the number of graduates, have been rising steadily. As Figure 22.1 demonstrates, although admissions dropped in 2011–2012, the number of students entering nurse practitioner programs across Canada rose in 2008–2009, 2009–2010, and 2012–2013. From 2011–2012 to 2012–2013, the numbers increased by 89.3% with 568 students entering nurse practitioner programs across the country.

This expansion of NP education is reflected in the growth of licensed NPs since 2007. The Canadian Institute for Health Information (CIHI) (2011) reported that between 2007 and 2011, the number of licensed NPs doubled from 1,344 to 2,777. By 2013, the number had risen to 3,655 (CIHI, 2013). Unfortunately, this data does not provide a full picture

FIGURE 22.1:   Admissions to Nurse Practitioner Programs, 2008–2009 to 2012–2013

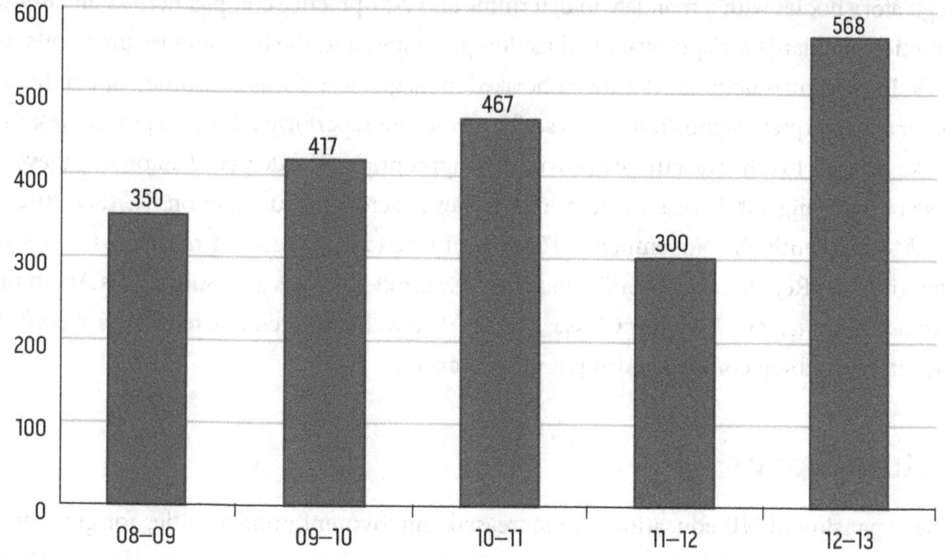

Source: Canadian Association of Schools of Nursing (CASN), 2014. Reprinted with permission.

of enrolment trends for APNs. There is no information on the education of CNSs because of the lack of role-specific programs to survey. Moreover, as they are not licensed there are no statistics on their numbers in the health care system (Bryant-Lukosius et al., 2010).

Emerging Infrastructure for Advanced Practice Nursing

A stronger infrastructure of national policies and provincial/territorial legislation emerged during the last decade, supporting the NP role in Canada. The Canadian Nurse Practitioner Initiative (CNPI), with broad representation from all major stakeholders, played a significant part in fostering this. A national consensus-based definition of the NP role was articulated by CNPI, and was widely accepted. It states that NPs are "registered nurses with additional educational preparation and experience who possess and demonstrate the competence to autonomously diagnose, order and interpret diagnostic tests, prescribe pharmaceuticals, and perform specific procedures within their legislated scope of practice" (CNPI, 2006, p. iii). The CNPI initiative also introduced a national core competency framework for NPs in 2005 that was reviewed and updated in 2010 through a consensus building approach (CNA, 2010). Another output of the CNPI initiative was the development of a national registration examination for the NP–Family/All Ages stream in both English and French. This exam was administered from 2005 until 2014.

Legislation was also developed supporting the NP role. Alberta was the first jurisdiction in Canada to introduce it in 1996, and, by 2009, all provinces and territories had followed suit. This increased the clarity of the extended scope of practice of the NP role, and provided nursing regulatory bodies with a mandate to determine entry-to-practice competencies, standards of practice, standards for approval of education programs, and the licensure requirements for NPs. In most jurisdictions NPs are authorized to diagnose a disease, disorder, or condition; order and interpret diagnostic tests; prescribe medications; perform advanced procedures; and make referrals to other health care providers as appropriate. The degree of autonomy they are given in carrying out these activities varies, however, across the jurisdictions (CASN, 2012).

More recently, in November 2012, Health Canada proclaimed the New Classes of Practitioners Regulations (NCPR) under the Controlled Drugs and Substances Act in the *Canada Gazette*, Part II ("New Classes," 2012). These changes remove federal barriers NPs face in prescribing controlled drugs and substances.

Future Trends

The expansion of NP education, the increased employment opportunities for graduates, and the policy and legislative infrastructure development have created forward momentum, and created a new set of challenges. There is a movement towards increased clarity in the educational expectations for APNs, and better **integration** of APNs in the interprofessional health care system. Given the historical vulnerability of advances in nursing practice to contextual changes, calls continue for further articulation and optimum alignment of roles with evolving health system realities.

Trends in Education

Despite external barriers, the trend has been to ground education for all types of NPs in an advanced nursing model at the graduate level. In 2011, CASN struck a Task Force on Nurse Practitioner Education, in response to nursing demands for further development of national educational standards. The resulting framework supported the growing consensus that NP programs be at the graduate level, and that this graduate education provide a broad-based nursing education that addresses core competencies for all APNs (clinical, research, leadership, and consultation and collaboration). Currently, as Table 22.1 demonstrates, although one post-baccalaureate program is still being offered in Canada, the majority of programs are at the graduate or post-graduate level.

NPs also appear to be integrating their extended scope of practice skills in an advanced nursing perspective. A recent research synthesis and study comparing NPs and physician

TABLE 22.1: Nurse Practitioner Program Levels by Province/Territory, 2014			
Province	Post-baccalaureate	Graduate	Post-graduate
Canada	1	25	7
NL	—	2	1
PE	—	1	—
NS	—	1	—
NB	—	2	—
QC	—	2	2
ON	1	9	3
MB	—	1	—
SK	—	1	—
AB	—	2	1
BC	—	3	—
NT	—	1	—
NU	—	—	—
YT	—	—	—

Source: Canadian Association of Schools of Nursing (CASN), 2014. Reprinted with permission.

assistants (PA) in Canada found both were appreciated by clients, but offered a different approach. The NPs utilized knowledge and autonomous decision-making skills in analytical activities associated with primary health care (Wong & Farrally, 2013). In addition, they incorporated an emphasis on population health and prevention, the social determinants of health, and the effects of illness on the lives of clients and families in their practice. The researchers attribute this to an education base embedded in a nursing model. The PAs, with an education grounded in a medical model, and trained to be assistants, were less focused on autonomous decision-making and analytical processes, and concentrated more on a technical orientation.

While the debate in Canada has been about a graduate-level requirement, in the US it has been about the Doctor of Nursing Practice (DNP) as the entry-to-practice degree level for NPs. The American Association of Colleges of Nursing (AACN) adopted this position in 2004, and recently reported that 243 DNP programs were enroling students at schools of nursing nationwide, and an additional 59 DNP programs were in the planning stages. In 2013, 14,688 students in the US were enroled in the DNP (AACN, 2014). There have been extensive discussions and debates about whether or not the DNP should be introduced in Canada at the annual CASN Graduate Study Forum, in 2010, 2011, and 2012.This forum is attended primarily by nursing faculty responsible for graduate studies in Canadian universities, and the Deans and Directors of CASN member schools. The consensus position that emerged concluded that, at the present time, the DNP is not supported by CASN, but with a recognition that it may be in the future.

Trends in Health System Integration

When the NP role was first introduced, a major driver was the lack of physicians. The role persisted in the remote North where the physician shortage continued, but dwindled in the South as soon as this was resolved. A shortage of physicians also played a role in the resurgence of interest in the NP role in the last decade, however, government efforts to shift care to the community and promote primary health care were also important. These additional contextual factors may account to some extent for the current increase of NPs in the health care system. Trends suggest, for instance, that graduates from NP programs are being integrated into new models of primary health care delivery. Many are working in community health centres, others in primary care services such as the family health team (FHT) or in NP-led clinics, and they remain the backbone of rural and remote primary health care services in Canada (Wong & Farrally, 2013).

Although employment in primary health care has been important, CIHI reported that 41% of NPs worked in acute care in 2011. Sectors identified include cardiology and cardiovascular surgery, geriatrics, medicine, pediatrics, nephrology, trauma, palliative care, oncology, and neonatology. NPs have also begun to be employed in emergency departments (ED), and are increasingly employed in ambulatory specialty areas in hospitals (Wong &

Farrally, 2013). Thus, the contextual factors that prompted the creation of the ACNP role, including the increased complexity of care, the need for long-term management of chronic conditions, and the aging of the population appear to be influencing a continued need for this type of NP. The data suggests that, in fact, many nurses educated to be primary health care providers are being employed in specialized areas of acute care.

The recent eligibility to prescribe controlled drugs and substances has brought a new set of challenges and opportunities for increasing optimum NP integration in both acute care and primary health care services. Currently practicing and future NPs need to learn about the specific complexities of controlled drugs and substance prescription, their potential for misuse and abuse, and the array of skills required for good prescribing practices (Kamarudin, Penm, Chaar, & Moles, 2013). Continuing education programs for practicing NPs, and curricular modifications to address these learning needs, are currently being examined and will be an important step in increasing NPs' ability to respond autonomously to client needs in the future.

Interprofessional collaboration is a key component of health system integration. Indeed, Martin-Misener et al. (2010) report that the need for interprofessional education for APNs has been consistently flagged in the literature. There has been a growing emphasis on interprofessional collaboration among other health professions in Canada in recent years. Team members' understanding, recognition, and acceptance of roles, however, is a necessary condition for interprofessional collaboration. This appears to be increasing for the NP. Wong and Farrally (2013) report, for example, that a key element of the NP role in the practice setting is to act as a liaison between the medical plan of care and the interprofessional plan of care. Thus, the trend appears to be an increasing integration of APNs in the interprofessional team.

Articulation of Education and Licensure Streams

Prior to the introduction of NP licensure, education programs were classified into primary health care and acute care streams. As noted earlier, except for Quebec, three licensure streams have been identified: the Family/All Ages, Adult, and Pediatrics. The highly specialized NNP, however, is also recognized. Moreover, as discussed, while many NPs in Canada are in primary health care services, 41% are employed in acute care and specialty settings (Wong & Farrally, 2013). Finally, the CNS role is not licensed, does not require a role-specific education, and tends to be less understood than the NP role.

The alignment of NP education with licensure requirements, health system service demands, client needs, and graduate employment patterns has created challenges in Canada. Issues revolve around designing program streams to fit an intersection of age-based care with an optimum set of acute and/or primary health care service competencies, and an optimum set of generalist and/or specialist competencies.

As the CNS role does not include components from the medical scope of practice, regulatory bodies do not license it. It is less well understood than the NP role and, as noted earlier, lacks a designated education program. Recently, however, the CNA (2014) has developed competencies for the role in order to facilitate a better understanding of it within the service delivery sector and as a guide to nursing education (see Chapter 5).

It is worth noting that articulation of APN streams created issues in the US, and resulted in a proliferation of categories and inconsistencies across jurisdictions. The Advanced Practice Registered Nurse (APRN) Consensus Model (2008) was developed over four years to tackle this problem. Known as LACE (legislation, accreditation, certification, education), it is endorsed by over 40 American nursing organizations and is being progressively implemented by individual states. The model defines four APRN roles: nurse anesthetist, nurse midwife, CNS, and NP. In each of these roles, the APRN must be educated in one of six population foci: family/individual across the lifespan, adult-gerontology, neonatal, pediatrics, women's health/gender related, and psychiatric/mental health. Further specialization within a foci and role is optional, but must be based on APRN role/population-based competencies. Specialties are recognized and represent a more focused area of education and practice within a role. Examples include oncology, nephrology, and palliative care.

Currently, US licensing examinations, for some of the NP foci, are used by Canadian regulating bodies and are approved for one or more of the three streams recognized in Canada. It is too early to know if other LACE foci or other APN roles, such as the nurse anesthetist, will be adopted in Canada.

Conclusion

Although APN was introduced in Canada a half a century ago, the roles, and the education programs for these roles, have been vulnerable to sudden contextual changes. While this vulnerability persists, the needs of an aging population, the associated disease burden, and the increasing complexity of care are likely to support the trend of a growing number of APNs in the health care system.

There have been tensions over the years between a generalized education and a specialized practice, as well as between a context-specific education program and a shifting environment. Although these issues are unresolved, considerable progress has been made in the last two decades in articulating APN roles, competencies, and educational requirements; this trend is likely to continue.

A solid body of evidence, spanning five decades, shows the value APNs bring to the health care system and this is increasingly being recognized. There appears to be contextual support for a continuation of the current trends of a fuller contribution, a greater integration of APNs in health care services, and membership in the interprofessional health care team.

Critical Thinking Questions

1. How are current contextual factors influencing the evolution of APN in Canada?
2. What factors have influenced the lack of education programs designated for CNSs in Canada, and has this had an impact on the role?
3. Is there a misalignment between the curricula of education programs for APNs and their employment settings in the health care system?
4. What has contributed positively to the evolution of APN in Canada and why?

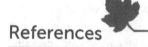

References

Advanced Practice Registered Nurse (APRN) Joint Dialogue Group (2008). *Consensus model for APRN regulation: Licensure, accreditation, certification & education.* Retrieved from http://www.aacn.nche.edu/education-resources/APRNReport.pdf

Alcock, D. (1996). The clinical nurse specialist, clinical nurse specialist/nurse practitioner and other titled nurse in Ontario. *Canadian Journal of Nursing Administration, 9*(1), 23–44.

American Association of Colleges of Nursing (AACN). (2014). *Fact sheet: The doctor of nursing practice (DNP).* Washington, DC: AACN.

Bryant-Lukosius, D., Carter, N., Kilpatrick, K., Martin-Misener, R., Kaasalainen, S., Harbman, P., … DiCenso, A. (2010). The clinical nurse specialist role in Canada. *Nursing Leadership, 23*(Special Issue December), 140–166.

Canadian Association of Schools of Nursing (CASN). (2011). *Nurse practitioner education in Canada.* Ottawa, ON: CASN. Retrieved from http://www.casn.ca

CASN. (2012). *Nursing masters education in Canada. Final Report 2012.* Ottawa, ON: CASN Retrieved from http://www.casn.ca

CASN. (2014). *Registered nursing education statistics 2012–2013.* Ottawa, ON: CASN. Retrieved from http://www.casn.ca

Canadian Nurses Association (CNA). (2010). *Canadian nurse practitioner core competency framework.* Ottawa, ON: CNA. Retrieved from http://mantnu.ca/Portals/o/Competency Framework 2010 e.pdf

CNA. (2014). *Pan-Canadian core competencies for the clinical nurse specialist.* Ottawa, ON: CNA. Retrieved from https://www.cna-aiic.ca/~/media/cna/files/en/clinical_nurse_specialists_convention_handout_e?la=en

Canadian Nurse Practitioner Initiative (CNPI). (2006). *Nurse practitioners: The time is now: A solution to improving access and reducing wait times in Canada.* Ottawa, ON: CNPI. Retrieved from http://www.npnow.ca/docs/tech-report/section1/01_Integrated_Report.pdf

Canadian Institute for Health Information (CIHI). (2011). *Regulated nurses: Canadian trends, 2007 to 2011.* Retrieved from https://secure.cihi.ca/estore/productFamily.htm?locale=en&pf=PFC2016&lang=en

CIHI. (2013). *Regulated nurses: 2013.* Retrieved from https://secure.cihi.ca/free_products/Nursing-Workforce-2013_EN.pdf

Cragg, C.E., Doucette, S., & Humbert, J. (2003). Ten universities, one program: Successful collaboration to educate nurse practitioners. *Nurse Educator, 28*(5), 227–231.

DiCenso, A., Auffrey, L., Bryant-Lukosius, D., Donald, F., Martin-Misener, R., Matthews, S., & Opsteen, J. (2007). Primary health care nurse practitioners in Canada. *Contemporary Nurse, 26*(1), 104–115.

DiCenso, A., & Bryant-Lukosius, D. (2010). The long and winding road: Integration of nurse practitioners and clinical nurse specialists into the Canadian health-care system. *Canadian Journal of Nursing Research, 42*(2), 3–8.

Donald, F., Martin-Misener, R., Bryant-Lukosius, D., Kilpatrick. K., Kaasalainen, S., Carter, N., … DiCenso, A. (2010). The primary health care nurse practitioner role in Canada. *Nursing Leadership, 23*(Special Issue December), 88–1013. doi: 10.12927/cjnl.2013.22271

Haines, J. (1993). *The nurse practitioner: A discussion paper.* Ottawa, ON: CNA.

Hravnak, M., Kleinpell, R., Magdic, K., & Guttendorf, J. (2009). The acute care nurse practitioner. In A. Hamric., J. Spross., and C. Hanson (Eds.). *Advanced practice nursing. An integrative approach,* (pp. 403–436). St. Louis, MO: Saunders.

Kaasalainen, S., Martin-Misener, R., Kilpatrick, K., Harbman, P., Bryant-Lukosius, D., Donald, F., & DiCenso, A., (2010). A historical overview of the development of advanced practice nursing in Canada. *Journal of Nursing Leadership, 23*(Special Issue December), 35–60.

Kamarudin, G., Penm, J., Chaar, B., & Moles, R. (2013). Educational interventions to improve prescribing competency: A systematic review. *British Medical Journal Open, 3*(8). doi: 10.1136/bmjopen-2013-003291

Martin-Misener, R., Bryant-Lukosius, D., Harbman, P., Donald, F., Kaasalainen, S., Carter, N., … Di Censo, A. (2010). Education of advanced practice nurses in Canada. *Journal of Nursing Leadership, 23*(Special Issue December), 61–87.

Montemuro, M. (1987). The evolution of the clinical nurse specialist: Response to the challenge of professional nursing practice. *Clinical Nurse Specialist 1*(3), 106–110.

New classes of practitioners regulations. (2012, May 5). *Canada Gazette, 146*(18). Government of Canada. Retrieved from http://www.gazette.gc.ca/rp-pr/p1/2012/2012-05-05/html/reg1-eng.html

Nurse Practitioners' Association of Ontario (NPAO). (n.d.). *Nurse practitioner history in Ontario.* Retrieved from http://npao.org/nurse-practitioners/history/#.VQHckI7F-84

Paes, B., Mitchell, A., Hunsberger, M., Blatz, S., Watts, J., Dent, P., … Southwell. D. (1989). Medical staffing in Ontario neonatal intensive care units. *Canadian Medical Association Journal, 140*(11), 1321–1326.

Pringle, D. (2007). Nurse practitioner role: Nursing needs it. *Nursing Leadership, 20*(2), 1–5.

Simpson, B. (1997). An educational partnership to develop acute care nurse practitioners. *Canadian Journal of Nursing Administration, 10*(1), 69–84.

Wong, S., & Farrally, V. (2013). *The utilization of nurse practitioners and physician assistants: A research synthesis.* Retrieved from http://www.msfhr.org/sites/default/files/Utilization_of_Nurse_Practitioners_and_Physician_Assistants.pdf

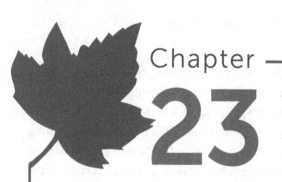

Chapter

23

The Future of Advanced Practice Nursing in Canada

Eric Staples

Eric Staples is an Independent Nursing Practice Consultant, who previously worked as an APN. He has served as an Assistant Professor at Dalhousie University in Halifax, Nova Scotia, where he was involved in implementing the Advanced Nursing Practice stream in 1998; at McMaster University, where he worked as NP coordinator in the Ontario Primary Health Care Nurse Practitioner Program; and at the University of Regina. He has served on a number of Canadian Association of Schools of Nursing (CASN) committees related to NP education, preceptorship, prescribing, and the development of the position statement on doctoral education in Canada.

KEY TERMS

advanced practice
  nursing (APN) roles
Doctor of Nursing
  Practice (DNP)
preceptorship
regulation
remuneration
role development and
  implementation

OBJECTIVES

1. Explore current, key issues impacting future APN practice.
2. Identify how APN roles and education are responding to health system changes across Canada.

Introduction

For the first time in Canada's history, there are more people aged 65 and older than children under the age of 15 (Statistics Canada, 2015). As of July 1, 2015, the federal agency reported that nearly one in six Canadians, approximately 5.78 million people, were at least 65 years old and the population under the age of 15 was 5.75 million. Based on these numbers, older adults are expected to account for 20.1% of the total population by 2024.

With an aging population, the demand for health care will grow exponentially, driven by increases in chronic diseases. Within a health system milieu that continues to see a shortage of both physician and nursing care providers, increasing complexity, and pressures to contain costs, **advanced practice nursing (APN) roles** can assist in meeting these growing needs. Where nursing shortages exist, the development of more APN roles may be seen, in response, to increase and retain nursing rates through the enhancement of nursing career prospects (MacDonald-Rencz & Bard, 2010) (see Chapter 20).

Within the last five years, the number of nurse practitioners (NPs), for example, has doubled, including a 25% increase over a one-year period (Picard, 2012). However, within this positive finding, APN roles must continue to be promoted, integrated, and sustained. New APN roles should only be introduced based on evidence of, or in response to, health care needs that have been identified for Canadians. To this extent, the Canadian Nurses Association (CNA) (2006a) purports that there should be a common framework that includes needs-based planning that anticipates health needs based on demographic, epidemiological, and cultural factors, and includes benchmarking for regional variation, and a review of specialty mix within and between disciplines. This points towards increasingly relying on interprofessional collaboration and practice.

Moving Towards the Future

Health care policy-makers and administrators are being required to seek new opportunities that enhance health care delivery. Many health care settings are moving away from traditional role boundaries to a mix of health professionals to provide care (MacDonald-Rencz & Bard, 2010). In Canada, the expansion of nursing roles (for example, registered nurse prescribing) is occurring in efforts to reorganize health service delivery and increase accessibility of health services, specifically community health services as a way to drive down overall health care costs.

The PEPPA framework, which is the "participatory, evidence-based, patient-centred process for APN role development, implementation, and evaluation" (Bryant-Lukosius & DiCenso, 2004, p. 532), is well accepted and supported in Canada for planning, preparing, and evaluating APN roles (see Chapter 4). Research data has identified key areas that will further the implementation of APN roles. Positive outcomes from NP practice (such as improved accessibility to health services and lowered wait times) have consistently been identified, but more research is required to identify the economic impact of NPs across all health care practice settings.

The impact of clinical nurse specialist (CNS) practice in Canada is even more obscure, partly due to lack of regulation and title protection of the role. With changes in the nursing workforce, CNSs are collaborating with and leading interprofessional teams. The role of the CNS is becoming even more critical for supporting nurses and providing clinical expertise. As the adoption of health care models based on interprofessional collaboration become more widespread, a unique opportunity exists to identify niches that are best filled by APNs.

Areas in Advanced Practice Nursing Requiring Further Development in Canada

The evolution of APN has paralleled a renewed focus in patient-centred care, as well as in demonstrating the expertise required to remain on the leading edge of clinical and technological health care advancements. Clinical leadership, support for nursing staff, and the advancement of research are uniting forces that can lead to improved patient outcomes and satisfaction. Indicators measuring patient outcomes and the cost benefits of APN will result in the development of more APN role opportunities. The variability in CNS specialties continues to make it more difficult to capture the same type of evaluative data for this role (MacDonald-Rencz & Bard, 2010).

Role Development

Successful **role development and implementation** is key to the full integration of APNs across Canada. A pan-Canadian approach has been suggested by the Canadian Nurses Association (CNA) (2008) and the Canadian Nurse Practitioner Initiative (CNPI) (2005) that would coordinate areas of recruitment; interprofessional collaboration and practice; education standards; and legislation and regulation that clarify APN roles, titles, and scopes of practice (DiCenso et al., 2010b). In relation to the CNS there is a call to establish funding not only for the role, but also for a research program to span over 10 years or more that will address implementation and outcomes of CNS practice (CNA, 2012b).

Financial investments, including stakeholder commitment required to create, support, and sustain NP roles, as well as those relating to remuneration, have been well described by Donald et al. (2010) and Kilpatrick et al. (2010). To address, for example, vacancy rates of NP positions in primary health care (PHC), and as a mechanism to increase the number of primary health care nurse practitioners (PHCNPs), Health Force Ontario in 2006 introduced the Grow Your Own NP program, which was updated in 2015 to reflect changes in today's health care environment. In this program, government funding, already allocated to organizations for PHCNP positions, could be used to sponsor a RN to complete an approved NP program in return for service with the sponsoring organization. Since the program's inception, over 65 RNs have graduated, with the majority of positions filled in communities that include long-term care (Health Force Ontario, 2015).

To address ongoing barriers for APN role development and integration, DiCenso et al. (2010a) articulated, based on the Canadian Health Services Research Foundation (CHSRF) roundtable, the need for clearly defined APN roles and titling, role development based on identified client/community and stakeholder need, stable funding for and increased awareness of the role, and ongoing research that demonstrates the value the role brings. These are all factors that may be critical to the sustainability of APN roles.

Education of Advanced Practice Nurses

NP programs are offered at three educational levels: post-RN, graduate, and post-graduate. There are 28 NP university programs in Canada, with approximately 400 NPs graduating each year (CNA & CASN, 2013). In 2012, eight full-time faculty members were engaged in graduate-level NP education, and schools reported a 45.5% shortage of NP, graduate, and doctorally prepared nurses seeking academic positions to teach in APN programs (CNA & CASN, 2013).

At this time, and consistent with approved and adopted definitions of APN, the majority of Canadian programs are at the graduate level. What is lacking is a continued match between the education level and practice settings where APNs find themselves employed. Due to a number of issues, which include geographic boundaries, lack of available specialty programs, and funding, most NP programs in Canada are at a generalist rather than specialist level. The exceptions to this are neonatology education (see Chapter 16) and specialist education in Quebec (see Chapters 1, 3, 14, and 22). The result is that generalist-prepared NPs may work in specialized areas they were not educated for, but are expected to have the competencies to practice in (Martin-Misener et al., 2010).

There are few graduate programs in Canada that focus on CNS education. Hence, CNSs are prepared in generalist graduate programs. Given the lack of credentialing and title protection, any nurse can call themselves a CNS, whether baccalaureate or graduate-prepared. There is, therefore, a need for title protection and a credentialing mechanism (Martin-Misener et al., 2010).

Some stakeholders in Canada believe that national curriculum standards and a consistent core curriculum for NP programs are required, while others have voiced concern with the rigidity of such an approach (Martin-Misener et al., 2010). Although Canada is a vast country, there are only a relatively small number of APNs in relation to the large number and range of specialty areas, which is a barrier to how specialist education can be included in educational programs (DiCenso et al., 2010b).

There are, however, course commonalities across Canadian NP programs that include courses in advanced health assessment, pathophysiology, and pharmaco-therapeutic management. There is less consistency in the core graduate courses required in NP programs. In addition, there has been a lack of standardization in the number of clinical placement hours required and in the qualifications faculty and clinical preceptors should possess (CASN, 2012).

Doctoral Preparation of Advanced Practice Nurses and Faculty Development

In Canada, the only nursing doctoral degree that can be awarded is the Doctor of Philosophy (PhD) in nursing. The number of PhD-prepared nurses in Canada remained at 0.2% between 2007 and 2010 (CNA, 2012b). There are a relatively small number of schools (13.5%) that offer doctoral programs. Between the 2007/2008 and 2011/2012 academic years, admissions were between 80 and 84 students per year, but graduate levels decreased by 25.8% between 2011 and 2012 (CNA & CASN, 2013).

The Canadian Nurse Practitioner Initiative (CNPI) (2006) indicated that faculty who were actively engaged in clinical practice were best able to teach NPs, but were also expected to have a PhD. Currently, there has been, for some time, a shortage of nursing faculty who possess both current practice and a PhD (Martin-Misener et al., 2010). Additionally, PhD-prepared NP faculty are challenged in maintaining a practice while meeting the teaching, research, publication, and service criteria for tenure and promotion. These typically do not provide merit, in relation to tenure, to practice.

The introduction of the **Doctor of Nursing Practice (DNP)** degree in the US, a clinical doctorate, was originally discussed in 2004 as a mandate for entry to APN practice, commencing in 2015. While the number of DNP programs has been rapidly expanding across the US, there is currently no formal target date for changing entry to practice from a graduate to doctoral level. The primary difference between the PhD and DNP is in focus; the PhD primarily prepares nurse researchers, while the DNP prepares nursing leaders who are expert in knowledge translation in the practice setting (Acorn, Lamarche, & Edwards, 2009; Tung, 2010; Villeneuve & MacDonald, 2006).

The DNP has met with both resistance and support among various groups in Canada. CASN, in 2011, developed a position statement on doctoral nursing education in Canada, which did not support the concept of the DNP. This was primarily due to the low number of APNs, but also, as the 2013 CNA/CASN statistics show, because PhD programs are relatively small as well, therefore it would be potentially difficult for schools of nursing to sustain two doctoral programs. In addition, it has been suggested that another APN title may continue to cause role confusion (Brar, Boschma, & McCuaig, 2010). On the other hand, the 2013 CNA/CASN statistics also identified a shortage of faculty, including NPs, seeking academic positions that could teach in APN programs (CNA & CASN, 2013). Martin-Misener et al. (2010) identified, through focus group interviews, that there was importance placed on recruiting faculty who were academically and clinically qualified in order to meet the needs of APN programs.

Conversely, the CNA, in their 2020 vision of nursing (2006b), supported two streams of doctoral education and posited that the DNP provided an alternative for NPs who were exploring clinical roles in policy, administration, and clinical areas. A number of NPs who hold faculty positions across Canada have sought DNP education in the US, contributing in many areas of scholarship to APN knowledge and research. To inform a decision of the DNP, further research is required exploring this trend and the need for a practice doctorate so that consensus among policy-makers and provincial and national nursing organizations will be possible (Joachim, 2008). Otherwise, nurses will continue to seek DNP education elsewhere if it is not available in Canada, further demonstrating a desire to have an alternative level of doctoral education (Tung, 2010).

Preceptorship of APN Students

Graduate nursing education, specifically for NPs in Canada, relies heavily on **preceptorship** to prepare students for NP practice. Preceptors, acting as role models, provide clinical learning experiences for students that help them apply theory to real-life situations that support role socialization and develop APN competencies. The literature related to preceptorship is focused primarily on baccalaureate education. The CNA (2004), supporting the importance of preceptorship, developed a guide for preceptorship and mentorship. This document, and the literature relating to preceptorship, is relevant for APN education in relation to the roles of the student, faculty member, and preceptor.

The major problems associated with preceptorship are the recruitment, preparation, and remuneration of appropriate preceptors; competition with other students for clinical placements; the ability of the clinical setting to provide a supportive learning environment; and evaluation of the students (Ivey, 2006; Martin-Misener et al., 2010; Payne, Heye, & Farrel, 2014).

One of the biggest and most time-consuming challenges is the process of securing and maintaining a reliable cadre of experienced preceptors across programs that may be local, provincial, or distance. Some programs encourage students to find their own preceptors, but this too can be problematic if it creates added competition for limited placement sites. Problems encountered by preceptors include managing the dual duties of practice expectations and teaching the student, uncertainty about the expectations of the student and preceptor, and differences in learning styles and personality (Ivey, 2006; Payne, Heye, & Farrel, 2014).

In 2014, the Saskatchewan Academic Health Sciences Network (SAHSN) launched several initiatives to support preceptor education and recognition in any health science discipline, including a provincial website and online curriculum (www.saskpreceptors.ca), preceptor conferences, and a preceptor recognition fund. Although the focus is primarily on baccalaureate education, the Collaborative Nurse Practitioner Program (CNPP), a partnership between the Saskatchewan Polytechnic and the University of Regina schools of nursing, are utilizing this provincial resource.

With a focus on NP placements, the BC Preceptors Development and Support website (www.preceptordevelopment.org) supports collaborative placement efforts and provides a mechanism between the British Columbia Academic Health Council, the University of British Columbia, the University of Victoria, and the University of Northern British Columbia for managing the preceptor contact lists to facilitate successful placements.

The Ontario Primary Health Care Nurse Practitioner Program (PHCNP) consortium established in 2007, with provincial Ministry of Health funding, a Resource Centre for Preceptors and Employers via an online website, which continues today.

Subsequent to the publication of *Nurse Practitioner Education in Canada: National Framework of Guiding Principles & Essential Components* (CASN, 2012), CASN developed the NP Education Interest Group in 2013. From this group, a working preceptorship subgroup formed in 2014, which has developed a national survey to be administered to all NP programs in 2016 that seeks to understand how NP programs are supporting preceptorship, specifically in relation to recruitment and retention. The findings will be used to develop a draft document that furthers discussion of cooperative efforts for clinical placements in the future.

Remuneration and Trends in Employment

Between 2007 and 2011, the Canadian Institute for Health Information (CIHI) reported that the number of NPs had doubled from 1,344 to 2,777, and by 2015, the number further grew to 3,966 (CIHI, 2015). These increases are due to greater investments in NPs provincially, which has led to an increase in data submitted to the CIHI (Picard, 2012). Although this is a positive finding, a negative trend began to emerge in relation to where NPs were practicing. Over the five-year period, a 10% decrease was seen in NPs working in primary health care settings and a 10% increase was seen of NPs working in hospitals and long-term care (LTC) (The Canadian Nurse, 2012).

The reason for this trend is that **remuneration** and benefits in primary health care settings have not kept up with salaries in the tertiary care sector, where there is greater perceived job security, increased salary, and a pension plan. Since 2006 in Ontario, NPs in primary health care (i.e., Family Health Teams (FHTs), Community Health Centres (CHCs), Aboriginal Health Access Centres (AHAC), and NP-Led Clinics) have seen a wage freeze. With approximately 19% of unfilled NP positions being within the community, many of these NPs are choosing to leave for higher-paying jobs in hospitals or other health care settings. This is a concerning trend for the recruitment and retention of Ontario NPs (Association of Ontario Health Centres [AOHC], 2013).

Another reason for this trend is related to the age of NPs. Between 2007 and 2011, the highest proportion of NPs across Canadian jurisdictions was between 45 and 49 years of age. The CIHI (2015) found that 79.8% of NPs were employed full-time (39.6% in the tertiary care sector), and the proportion of NPs unemployed declined from 2.2% to 1.6%.

NPs who are leaving primary health care are practicing in emergency departments where they provide triage and care to patients experiencing episodic health-related illnesses/

conditions. Others are working in outpatient chronic care clinics related to diabetes, renal failure, and cardiac care. If primary health care NP positions cannot attract NPs or are left unfilled, problems related to accessibility and wait times will resurface, leading to an increase in emergency department visits. This will in turn result in increased health care expenditure and fragmented care delivery (The Canadian Nurse, 2012).

Regulation and Legislation for Practice

Recent Ontario legislation has expanded the scope of practice of NPs, allowing for fuller access without physician oversight to prescribing, diagnostic testing, admitting, treating, transferring, and discharging both in-patients and community outpatients to and from hospital. Unfortunately, existing **regulation** in many provinces does not allow NPs to work to the full scope of practice, including restrictions on what they can prescribe or diagnostic investigations they can order.

In support of a pan-Canadian approach for NP licensure and registration, the Canadian Council of Registered Nurse Regulators (CCRNR) launched, in 2014, a project to analyze NP practice across Canada. The purpose of the project is to provide a comprehensive description of the entry-level knowledge, skills, and abilities required in the three streams of NP practice: Family/All Ages, Adult, and Pediatric (CCRNR, 2015). The report is to be released in late 2015 and it is hoped that it will inform a national consensus on NP registration, licensure, examination requirements, and a description of the clinical services NPs provide to Canadians.

As stated previously, without regulation or a credentialing mechanism for CNSs in Canada, there is no title protection for the role and any nurse can identify themselves as a CNS in the absence of the requisite education and expertise for the role. CNSs are strongly advocating for title protection not only to strengthen the role, but also to ensure those in the role possess the requisite education and experience to enact it. This, in turn, would lead to accurate tracking of the number of CNSs and the roles they are performing across Canada (DiCenso et al., 2010b).

Conclusion

The roles of health care providers, including APNs, must be optimized to sustain the health system. Increases in chronic diseases related to an aging population will be a challenge for many Canadians, as well as for health care providers who will have to anticipate these demands within the health system. The continued shift away from illness to health has seen health care consumers become more educated and engaged in actively participating in maintaining their functional health status. A pan-Canadian approach will ensure continuity and consistency in education, legislative and regulatory mechanisms, and systematic planning to guide role development and practice across all three levels of government.

APNs are part of the solution to health system challenges and reforms that are anticipated in the future. New approaches to health care provision, based on interprofessional collaboration and practice, will improve access to timely health services and meet the health needs of individuals, groups, and communities in Canada.

Critical Thinking Questions

1. What are the opportunities for APNs to build on their role, both today and into the future?
2. Looking at the current practices for APNs, what do you think is the biggest challenge and what strategies will be needed to address it at local, provincial, and/or federal levels?
3. Where do you see the APN role in Canada in one year, five years, ten years, or even twenty years and why? Compare and contrast differences between where you live to other provinces or territories.

References

Acorn, S., Lamarche, K., & Edwards, M. (2009). Practice doctorates in nursing: Developing nursing leaders. *Nursing Leadership, 22*(2), 85–91.

Association of Ontario Health Centres (AOHC). (2013). *Toward a primary care recruitment and retention strategies for Ontario: Compensation structure.* Toronto, ON: AOHC. Retrieved from http://www.aohc.org/sites/default/files/documents/PC-Retention-and-Recruitment-Compensation-Structure-for-IPCOs-Report-to-MOHLTC-June-2013.pdf

Brar, K., Boschma, G., & McCuaig, F. (2010). The development of nurse practitioner preparation beyond the master's level: What is the debate about? *International Journal of Nursing Education Scholarship, 7*(Article 9). doi: 10.2202/1548-923X.1928

Bryant-Lukosius, D., & DiCenso, A. (2004). A framework for the introduction and evaluation of advanced practice nursing roles. *Journal of Advanced Nursing, 48*(5), 530–540.

Canadian Association of Schools of Nursing (CASN). (2011). *Position statement: Doctoral education in nursing in Canada.* Ottawa, ON: CASN. Retrieved from http://casn.ca/wp-content/uploads/2014/10/DoctoralEducation2011.pdf

CASN. (2012). *Nurse practitioner education in Canada: National framework of guiding principles & essential components.* Ottawa, ON: CASN. Retrieved from http://casn.ca/wp-content/uploads/2014/12/FINALNPFrameworkEN20130131.pdf

Canadian Council of Registered Nurse Regulators (CCRNR). (2015). *Nurse practitioner practice analysis project.* Beaverton, ON: CCRNR. Retrieved from http://www.ccrnr.ca/np-practice-analysis.html

Canadian Institute for Health Information (CIHI). (2015). *Regulated nurses, 2014.* Ottawa, ON: CIHI. Retrieved from https://secure.cihi.ca/free_products/RegulatedNurses2014_Report_EN.pdf

The Canadian Nurse. (2012). *Perspectives: NP numbers up, but employment trends concerning.* Ottawa, ON: CNA. Retrieved from http://www.canadian-nurse.com/en/articles/issues/2012/march-2012/np-numbers-up-but-employment-trends-concerning

Canadian Nurses Association (CNA). (2004). *Achieving excellence in professional practice: A guide to preceptorship and mentoring.* Ottawa, ON: CNA. Retrieved from https://www.cna-aiic.ca/~/media/cna/page-content/pdf-en/achieving_excellence_2004_e.pdf?la=en

CNA. (2006a). *Position statement: National planning for human resources in the health sector.* Ottawa, ON: CNA.

CNA. (2006b). *Toward 2020: Visions for nursing.* Ottawa, ON: CNA.

CNA. (2008). *Advanced nursing practice: A national framework.* Ottawa, ON: CNA. Retrieved from https://www.cna-aiic.ca/~/media/cna/page-content/pdf-en/anp_national_frame-work_e.pdf

CNA. (2012a). *Strengthening the role of the clinical nurse specialist in Canada.* Ottawa, ON: CNA. Retrieved from https://www.cna-aiic.ca/~/media/cna/page-content/pdf-fr/strengthening_the_cns_role_background_paper_e.pdf?la=en

CNA. (2012b). *2010 workforce profile of registered nurses in Canada.* Ottawa, ON: CNA. Retrieved from https://www.cna-aiic.ca/~/media/cna/page-content/pdf-en/2010_rn_snapshot_e.pdf

Canadian Nurses Association (CNA), & Canadian Association of Schools of Nursing (CASN). (2013). *Registered nurses education in Canada statistics 2011–2012: Registered nurse workforce, Canadian production: Potential new supply.* Ottawa, ON: CNA and CASN. Retrieved from https://www.cna-aiic.ca/~/media/cna/files/en/nsfs_report_2011-2012_e.pdf

Canadian Nurse Practitioner Initiative (CNPI). (2005). *Canadian nurse practitioner initiative technical report, education chapter.* Ottawa, ON: CNA. Retrieved from http://www.npnow.ca/docs/tech-report/section5/01_education.pdf

CNPI. (2006). *Nurse practitioners: The time is now: A solution to improving access and reducing wait times in Canada.* Ottawa, ON: CNA. Retrieved from http://www.npnow.ca/docs/tech-report/section1/01_Integrated_Report.pdf

DiCenso, A., Bryant-Lukosius, D., Martin-Misener, R., Donald, F., Abelson, J., Bourgeault, I., … Harbman, P. (2010a). *Clinical nurse specialists and nurse practitioners in Canada: A decision support synthesis.* Ottawa, ON: CHSRF. Retrieved from http://www.cfhi-fcass.ca/sf-docs/default-source/commissioned-research-reports/Dicenso_EN_Final.pdf?sfvrsn=0

DiCenso, A., Bryant-Lukosius, D., Martin-Misener, R., Donald, F., Abelson, J., Bourgeault, I., … Harbman, P. (2010b). Factors enabling advanced practice nursing role integration in Canada. *Nursing Leadership, 23*(Special Issue December), 211–238. doi:10.12927/cjnl.2010.22279

Donald, F., Martin-Misener, R., Bryant-Lukosius, D., Kilpatrick, K., Kaasalainen, S., Carter, N., … DiCenso, A. (2010). The primary healthcare nurse practitioner role in Canada. *Nursing Leadership, 23*(Special Issue December), 88–113.

Health Force Ontario. (2015). *Grow your own nurse practitioner.* Toronto, ON: MOHLTC. Retrieved from http://www.healthforceontario.ca/en/Home/Employers/Grow_Your_Own_Nurse_Practitioner_Program

Ivey, J.B. (2006). Fostering successful preceptorships for advanced practice nursing. *Topics in Advanced Practice Nursing eJournal, 6*(1), 1–4.

Joachim, G. (2008). The practice doctorate: Where do Canadian nursing leaders stand? *Nursing Leadership, 21*(4), 42–51. doi: 10.12927/cjnl.2008.20286

Kilpatrick, K., Harbman, P., Carter, N., Martin-Misener, R., Bryant-Lukosius, D., Donald, F., ... DiCenso, A. (2010). The acute care nurse practitioner role in Canada. *Nursing Leadership, 23*(Special Issue December), 114–39.

MacDonald-Rencz, S., & Bard, R. (2010). The role for advanced practice nursing in Canada. *Nursing Leadership, 23*(Special Issue December), 8–11. doi: 10.12927/cjnl.2010.22265

Martin-Misener, R., Bryant-Lukosius, D., Harbman, P., Donald, F., Kaasalainen, S., Carter, N., ... DiCenso, A. (2010). Education of advanced practice nurses in Canada. *Nursing Leadership, 23*(Special Issue December). 61–84.

Payne, C., Heye, M.L., & Farrell, K. (2014). Securing preceptors for advanced practice students. *Journal of Nursing Education and Practice, 4*(3), 167–179.

Picard, A. (2012, September 6). Nurse practitioners in Canada more than double in five years. *The Globe and Mail.* Retrieved from http://www.theglobeandmail.com/life/health-and-fitness/nurse-practitioners-in-canada-more-than-double-in-five-years/article1359892/

Statistics Canada. (2015). *Annual demographic estimates: Canada, provinces and territories. 2014.* Ottawa, ON: STATCAN. Retrieved from http://www.statcan.gc.ca/pub/91-215-x/2014000/part-partie2-eng.htm

Tung, T.K.C. (2010). In support of doctor of nursing practice education in Canada. *Topics in Advanced Practice Nursing eJournal, 11,* 1–4.

Villeneuve, M., & MacDonald, J. (2006). Toward 2020: Visions for nursing setting the stage for the future. *The Canadian Nurse, 102*(5), 22–23.

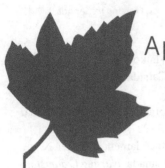

Appendix

Resources for Advanced Practice Nurses in Canada

National

Canadian Nurses Association/Association des infirmières et infirmiers du Canada (CNA/AIIC)

The CNA is the unified voice for RNs in Canada by advancing the practice and profession of nursing to improve health outcomes and strengthen Canada's publicly funded health system. CNA speaks for RNs and represents Canadian nursing to other organizations and governments nationally and internationally.
http://cna-aiic.ca/

Canadian Council of Registered Nurse Regulators (CCRNR)

The purpose of the CCRNR is to promote excellence and serve as a national forum and voice regarding provincial, national, and global regulatory matters for nursing regulation.
http://www.ccrnr.ca/

Canadian Nurses Protective Society (CNPS)

The CNPS offers legal advice, risk management services, and professional liability protection relating to nursing practice to eligible RNs and NPs.
http://www.cnps.ca/

Canadian Association of Advanced Practice Nurses (CAAPN)/Association canadienne des infirmières et infirmiers en pratique avancée (ACIIPA)

The mission of the CAAPN/ACIIPA is to improve the health of Canadians by promoting and influencing the development, growth, and integration of advanced practice nursing in health systems.
http://caapn-aciipa.org/

The Clinical Nurse Specialist Association of Canada (CNS-C)

The CNS-C recognizes that the CNS is an essential component of a sustainable health care system. It provides a leadership platform through which CNSs impact and influence cost-effective health care system change to support safe, quality care and superior outcomes.
http://cna-aiic.ca/

Provincial

British Columbia

College of Registered Nurses of British Columbia (CRNBC)
The CRNBC is the regulatory body that governs the regulation of RNs and NPs in BC.
https://www.crnbc.ca/

Association of Registered Nurses of British Columbia (ARNBC)
The ARNBC is the professional association representing RNs in British Columbia. It was launched and incorporated under the BC Society Act in 2010. Their strategic directions for 2014–2017 include engaging effectively with RNs and NPs in BC, advocating for evidence-informed policies to promote the health and health care of British Columbians, and developing and sustaining professional practice support structures and services for all RNs and NPs in BC.
http://www.arnbc.ca/

British Columbia Nurse Practitioner Association (BCNPA)
BCNPA is a non-profit, volunteer-based professional organization that supports and advances the professional interests of nurse practitioners, nurse practitioner students, and nurses who have an interest in NP practice. Its efforts support enabling NPs to provide accessible, efficient, and effective health care that meets the highest standards across NP practice.
https://bcnpa.org/

Clinical Nurse Specialist Association of BC (CNSABC)
The CNSABC supports the expert role of the CNS by promoting an environment in which members can network, contribute to knowledge, and access support that meets the highest professional standards of practice.
http://cnsabc.ca/

Alberta

College & Association of Registered Nurses of Alberta (CARNA)
The CRNA is professional organization and regulatory body for nurses in Alberta.
http://www.nurses.ab.ca/

Nurse Practitioner Association of Alberta (NPAA)
NPAA's mission is to advocate and advance NP practice to build a healthier Alberta.
https://albertanps.com/

Saskatchewan

Saskatchewan Registered Nurses' Association (SRNA)
The SRNA is the profession-led regulatory body for the province's RNs and RN(NP)s, and has professional practice groups for both NPs and CNSs working in Saskatchewan.
http://www.srna.org/

Nurse Practitioners of Saskatchewan (NPOS)
NPOS represents the professional interests of all RN(NP) in Saskatchewan and is a membership unit of the SRNA. NPOS advocates for accessible, high-quality health care by influencing the integration of RN(NP)s across the health care system.
http://www.npos.ca/

Saskatchewan Association of Nurse Practitioners (SANP)
SANP is a non-profit, volunteer-run, professional organization that supports and advances the professional interests of NPs, NP students, and nurses who have an interest in the NP practice.
http://www.sasknursepractitioner.org/

Manitoba

College of Registered Nurses of Manitoba (CRNM)
CRNM is the professional regulatory body for registered nurses in Manitoba. Their vision is to maximize health for all Manitobans through excellence in registered nursing practice.
https://www.crnm.mb.ca/

Association of Registered Nurses of Manitoba (ARNM)
The newly formed ARNM is the result of a transition in the CRNM membership position with CNA and is the professional voice of RNs in Manitoba.
http://arnm.ca/

Nurse Practitioner Association of Manitoba (NPAM)
NPAM is a non-profit, volunteer-run group that serves as a voice for NPs in Manitoba as a specialty practice group within the CRNM. It endeavours to support and advance the professional interests of NPs in order to provide accessible and effective health care to the public.
http://www.nursepractitioner.ca/

Clinical Nurse Specialists of Manitoba Interest Group (CNSMB)
The CNSMB serves as a provincial voice to enhance and promote the valuable contributions of the CNS to health and well-being of patient populations.
http://www.cnsmb.ca/

Ontario

College of Nurses of Ontario (CNO)
The CNO is the regulator for RNs, RPNs, and NPs in Ontario. Its role is to carry out entry to practice requirements, communicating and enforcing practice standards, overseeing its QA program, and acting in the public's interest by participating in legislative processes and sharing information about Ontario nurses.
http://www.cno.org/

Clinical Nurse Specialist Association of Ontario (CNS-ON)

The CNS-ON supports the role of APN in Ontario through the provision of professional networking opportunities and educational development activities for its members by clarifying and promoting the role of APN within the nursing profession and among other health care professionals, health care employers, consumers, and policy-makers. CNS-ON is an interest group of RNAO.

http://rnao.ca/connect/interest-groups/cns_association_of_ontario
http://cns-ontario.rnao.ca

London Region Advanced Practice Nurses (LRAPN)

The LRAPN is a professional group whose vision is to advance and promote innovative leadership initiatives in health care and nursing at the local, provincial, national, and international levels.
http://www.lrapn.org/

Nurse Practitioners' Association of Ontario (NPAO)

NPAO is the professional association for NPs in Ontario.
https://npao.org/

Registered Nurses' Association of Ontario (RNAO)

The RNAO is the professional association representing RNs, NPs, and nursing students in Ontario.
http://rnao.ca/

Quebec

Ordre des infirmières et infirmiers du Québec (OIIQ)

The OIIQ is the regulatory body for nursing in Quebec. It is mandated with protecting the public by administrating professional practice set out in the regulations of Quebec's Professional Code. Under the Nurses Act, there are regulations for classes of specialization for NPs and CNSs.
http://www.oiiq.org/

New Brunswick

The Nurses Association of New Brunswick/Association des infirmières et infirmiers du Nouveau-Brunswick (NANB/AIINB)

The NANB/AIINB is the professional regulatory organization in New Brunswick. It acts to protect the public and to support nurses by ensuring standards of practice for nursing education and practice are maintained, and through support of healthy public policy.
http://www.nanb.nb.ca/

Nurse Practitioners of New Brunswick (NPNB)
The NPNB are partners of the NANB and affiliated with CAAPN. Their goal is to promote sustainable, integrated, and comprehensive NP practice; enhance NP professional development; support ongoing development of APN; and to promote the health of New Brunswickers.
http://npnb.ca/

Nova Scotia

College of Registered Nurses of Nova Scotia (CRNNS)
The CRNNS is the professional body that regulates the practice of RNs and NPs to protect and serve the public interest in Nova Scotia.
http://crnns.ca/

Nurse Practitioners' Association of Nova Scotia (NPANS)
The NPANS' goal is to enhance the health of Nova Scotians through advocacy, support, and the development of the NP role.
http://www.npans.ca/

Prince Edward Island

The Association of Registered Nurses of Prince Edward Island (ARNPEI)
The ARNPEI is the professional organization and regulatory body for RNs in PEI.
http://www.arnpei.ca/

Prince Edward Island Nurse Practitioner Association (PEINPA)
The PEINPA's mission is to promote a social, economic, and political climate that supports NPs in the provision of accessible, patient-centred, and sustainable health care services.
http://www.peinpa.ca/

Newfoundland and Labrador

The Association of Registered Nurses of Newfoundland and Labrador (ARNNL)
The ARNNL is the regulatory body and professional association for all RNs and NPs, and advocates for healthy public policy in the public interest.
https://www.arnnl.ca/

Newfoundland & Labrador Nurse Practitioner Association (NLNPA)
The NLNPA represents the professional interests of NPs by advocating for accessible, high-quality health care for all citizens throughout NL.
http://www.nlnpa.ca/

Northwest Territories and Nunavut

Registered Nurses Association of Northwest Territories and Nunavut (RNANT/NU)

The RNANT/NU is the regulatory body and professional association for RNs and NPs in both NT and NU. Its functions serve to protect the public, and it strives to enhance the roles of RNs and NPs through professional advocacy and promotion.
http://www.rnantnu.ca/

Yukon

Yukon Registered Nurses Association (YRNA)

The YRNA is the regulatory body and professional association for RNs and NPs in the Yukon, and exists to ensure public protection with regard to nursing practice.
http://yrna.ca/

International

International Council of Nurses (ICN)

ICN is a federation of more than 130 national nurses associations (NNAs), representing more than 16 million nurses worldwide. ICN works to ensure quality nursing care, sound health policies globally, the advancement of nursing knowledge, the global presence of a respected nursing profession, and a competent and satisfied nursing workforce.
http://www.icn.ch/

ICN Nurse Practitioner/Advanced Practice Nursing Network

The Network is an international resource and forum for NPs and APNs, and others who are interested in these roles such as policy-makers, educators, regulators, and health planners.
http://international.aanp.org/

National Organization of Nurse Practitioner Faculties (NONPF)

NONPF is a US-based organization specifically devoted to promoting quality NP education at the national and international levels. NONPF has evolved as the leading organization for NP faculty sharing the commitment of excellence in NP education, and represents a global network of NP educators.
http://www.nonpf.org/

Copyright Acknowledgements

Index